CW00606876

KP

Korsgaard Publishing
www.korsgaardpublishing.com
© Vernon Coleman 2022
ISBN 978-87-93987-40-1

The Author

Dr Vernon Coleman MB ChB DSc FRSA was one of the first qualified medical practitioners to question the significance of the 'crisis' with which you may be familiar, telling readers of his website www.vernoncoleman.com at the end of February that he felt that the team advising the Government had been unduly pessimistic and had exaggerated the danger of the bug. At the beginning of March, he explained how and why the mortality figures had been distorted. And on March 14th he warned that the Government's policies would result in far more deaths than the disease itself. In a YouTube video recorded on 18th March, he explained his fear that the Government would use the 'crisis' to oppress the elderly and to introduce compulsory vaccination. And he revealed that the infection had been downgraded on March 19th when the public health bodies in the UK and the Advisory Committee on Dangerous Pathogens decided that the 'crisis' infection should no longer be classified as a 'high consequence infectious disease'. Just days after the significance of the infection had been officially downgraded, the Government published an Emergency Bill which gave the police extraordinary new powers and put millions of people under house arrest. Dr Coleman, a former GP principal, is a *Sunday Times* bestselling author. His books have sold over two million copies in the UK, been translated into 25 languages and sold all around the world. He has given evidence to the House of Commons and the House of Lords, and his campaigning has changed Government policy. There is a short biography at the back of this book.

COVID-19:
THE GREATEST
HOAX IN HISTORY

The startling truth behind the planned world takeover

Vernon Coleman

To Antoinette

Not many people have the joy of meeting and knowing the one person who means more to them than life itself. I thank God for bringing us together. You give happiness to people through your kindnesses but to me you give hope, joy and purpose. You are my delight and my salvation and the centre of my universe. You are everywhere I go because you live in my heart. You have all my love and all my caring. All I want in life is to be with you. You give me everything: love, friendship, understanding and kindness.

Table of Contents

Foreword

When I wrote my first book about the coronavirus (*Coming Apocalypse*) I was told that I was not allowed to mention the word 'coronavirus' anywhere in the title or the book itself. And so I went through the entire book and managed to write round the word 'coronavirus' around 250 times. Even so, I thought at the time that there was a real risk that all my other books (close to 100 of them in all) would be removed from sale because of the content of *Coming Apocalypse*.

I would like to thank my wife, Antoinette, for wholeheartedly supporting what was a hugely risky venture since our only earned income comes from writing books – we long ago agreed to refuse advertising income and together we chose to earn nothing from the videos or the website – if the books had been removed from sale we would have been left with a diet of dandelion leaves and tree roots. Antoinette has worked tirelessly despite being in almost constant pain as a result of the closure of the hospital physiotherapy department which should have been helping her deal with the pains which are an unwelcome souvenir of the surgery and radiotherapy which she undertook last year for breast cancer. Without her unceasing work and enthusiasm and support, none of these videos would have been made. She has been ahead of this story from the very beginning. The videos and website articles have been a joint effort though I take full responsibility for everything that has been written and recorded.

When I first started making videos I was aware that the use of the words 'vaccine' and 'vaccination' were considered illegal by some if used in association with criticism of any kind. Experience has, however, told me that these words are (surprisingly) now slightly less of a problem than they were when I published *Coming Apocalypse*. Also, it now appears that it may be possible to use the words 'coronavirus' and 'covid-19' in some circumstances. The attention of the self-appointed authorities has been directed to words such as 'masks' and 'social distancing'. These are now 'dirty' words and using them will attract a long period in detention, 500 lines and a meeting with the headmaster in his study.

It is difficult to know precisely when the coronavirus hoax really started – or who was responsible for initiating what has, without question, turned out to be the greatest fraud in human history. This book explains just how a bunch of crooks are using the fear which has been deliberately created out of a fairly ordinary flu bug to take over the world. Making huge profits has been effectively disguised as philanthropy.

The usual suspects are, of course, the Rothschilds, the Rockefellers, the Bliderbergers and the Jesuits. But a variety of modern billionaires and self-styled philanthropists (such as Gates and Soros) have been added to the mix.

It is vital to remember that behind the whole fraud lies the global warming scam.

This fraud, which first surfaced back in the 19th century, was resurrected in the 1990s and deliberately chosen by the Club of Rome as a means to an end: the excuse to create a New World Order.

The hysterical simpletons who are now scaring themselves silly over global warming don't realise that the only thing which is man-made about the scare is the scare itself.

But in fact the climate change hoax came relatively late onto the scene and was introduced merely to tighten the screw on the global population. The current global crisis, which is rapidly removing all our freedoms, started much earlier and can be traced back for decades. However, the plan really accelerated into action after the Second World War.

You don't have to look too hard to find the evidence.

The World Health Organisation was founded in 1947, and its first director general was a fellow called George Brock Chisholm who is largely forgotten now except for his enthusiasm for world government. Chisholm is famous (or infamous) for having said: 'To achieve world government it is necessary to remove from the minds of men their individualism, loyalty to family tradition, national patriotism and religious dogmas.'

That should have rung alarm bells. But at the time no one much noticed.

At this time, of course, senior Nazis who had made their fortunes out of concentration camps and who had, with the help of the Americans, successfully avoided much in the way of punishment were busy creating the foundations of the European Union out of what was left of Europe. (I have dealt with the way the Nazis achieved this apparent impossibility in my books *The Shocking History of the EU* and *OFPIS.*)

The usual suspects, the world's bankers, were also planning a world government. In February 1950, when he appeared before the US Senate Committee on Foreign Relations, banker James Paul Warburg said: 'We shall have world government, whether or not we like it. The only question is whether world government will be achieved by conquest or consent.'

To those early events we must add the more recent influences of the United Nations and the World Economic Forum. The United Nations is, of course, the mother organisation of the World Health Organisation, and its original charter bears close kinship to the communist manifesto. It is the United Nations which created Agenda 21 – the programme for a 'new world order'. The contribution of the World Economic Forum has been the proposed 'global reset'.

Using covid-19 as a flimsy excuse, these organisations have proposed changing every aspect of our lives. There are now strong moves to get rid of cash and to replace it with digital currency (on the curious grounds that cash is reckoned to be more likely to transmit the covid-19 virus than any other), to close down traditional farming (and replace natural produce with factory produced artificial replacements), to move whole populations into high rise apartments in smart cities (leaving rural areas uninhabited), to confiscate private property and to move shopping, health care and education online (with high street shops, doctors' surgeries and schools largely closed). There are also plans to introduce a modest national wage for all, to replace many jobs with robots and to use implanted chips to control human beings from afar. The whole evil scenario has been produced and promoted by a small bunch of unelected billionaires who clearly believe they have the right to impose their bizarre and dangerous personal views on the rest of us. Just because many people have, over the years, forecast the end of civilisation (usually at the hands of a bunch of scheming madmen) it doesn't mean it can't happen and it certainly doesn't mean it isn't happening this time.

And, today, with software billionaire Bill Gates and a small army of well-paid shills pushing DNA/RNA based vaccines, the use of which will result in the genetic modification of the human race (and spending hundreds of millions of dollars on ensuring that he has a good press) it is not difficult to feel that we are being assailed from all sides.

All these proposed changes have become public only since the appearance of the coronavirus, and are being promoted as an answer to the health problems of dealing with what is widely being 'sold' as a pandemic. It is clear, however, that all have been planned for many years.

The origins of the virus which devastated the world in 2020 are shrouded in mystery, disguised by deceit, confused by lies and deliberately clouded by misinformation. The very existence of the virus, or indeed of viruses at all, is questioned by many but this seems to me to be irrelevant. It really doesn't matter whether there is or is a not a virus. What matters is the way the authorities are using the current hoax to remove all our freedoms. Those of us who care about freedom (including freedom of speech, which I believe to be fundamental) are too busy trying to fight the vaccine proposals, the cashless society and other scary proposals.

It has, for some months, been widely acknowledged by medical experts that the risks associated with covid-19 are no greater than the risks associated with an ordinary winter flu. This was the claim I first made in February and March of 2020, and which immediately led to my demonization. It has now been acknowledged that death totals associated with covid-19 have been deliberately and massively exaggerated and the original predictions (which led to the lockdowns) have been shown to be absurdly over-pessimistic. There is now widespread agreement that the lockdowns which were unnecessarily introduced in an attempt to stop the spread of the coronavirus will result in far more deaths than the infection itself. The health care problems and economic problems produced by the hoax will result in the worst social and economic crisis in global history.

My first book about the coronavirus and covid-19 (entitled, *Coming Apocalypse*) dealt with the early stages of the manufactured crisis, the hysteria and the immediately apparent consequences.

This book is a collection of the articles published on my website and the transcripts of my videos broadcast on YouTube (including the transcripts of the videos which YouTube took down and banned). Some of the essays appeared on the YouTube channel and some appeared only on my website but most appeared on both. (This explains the occasional duplication of dates which usually relate to the date when a video was put online but in some cases relate to the date of writing.) The narrative develops as I acquired more and more information and as the evidence showed just how deep the conspiracy really is. There is no little irony in the fact that the conspiracy theorists like to demonise those of us telling the truth and exposing the real conspiracy as – conspiracy theorists! It's an old psychological trick.

These articles and transcripts date from the end of April 2020, immediately after the publication of my book, *Coming Apocalypse*, and continue up until the end of August.

I have excluded the material which was written before the publication of *Coming Apocalypse* to avoid repeating material already available in that book. The excluded material includes my first video script which was entitled 'Coronavirus scare: The hoax of the century' since that was dealt with in *Coming Apocalypse*.

This collection has brought together a collection of most of the material I wrote and recorded about the coronavirus and covid-19 during those four months. The only changes I have made have been to edit (very lightly) the transcripts to remove some of the references which were appropriate on the videos and which now seem redundant. I have, however, left some references to the videos where these seemed significant and where removing those references would have led to serious changes in tone or emphasis. Occasionally, you will see that facts have been repeated – this is simply because when videos were removed I re-used a vital fact that had been censored into oblivion. I make no apologies for this.

I realise that all this material is available without charge as recordings and on my website (and I have no doubt that some kind souls will draw attention to this when giving this book a one star review) but some people prefer to read material in book form. Besides, I am primarily a book writer. And it will be nice to earn a little money from a new book for the first time in 2020. The book will be made available at the lowest price allowed. Believe me, if I had wanted to make money I would have either written something else quite different or I would have monetised (what a horrible word) the YouTube channel and taken money from advertisers.

The essays show how the hoax has unfolded, and as things have become clearer it has become increasingly apparent that we are dealing with the greatest fraud in our history. Never before in history have so many people been deliberately deceived for the profit of a few. It became clear during the period that governments had hired military specialists and psychologists to induce a sense of fear in the population. Governments had become the enemy of the people. Adapting the essays for book form has not been particularly difficult since although I worked as a television presenter for a while in the 1970s and 1980s, I am first and foremost a writer and the scripts for the videos were written as essays rather than as scripts.

I had originally intended to put the dates on each essay. But then I hit a problem. Should I put on the date when the essay was written, when it was recorded as a video, when it was placed on YouTube or when it first appeared on my website? In the end I confused myself so much that I decided to settle for putting the essays in roughly the order in which they were written. Most of the essays are just between 10 and 25 minutes long when read but some of the essays took at least a week to write – and much longer to research. Antoinette and I have worked on researching and writing these essays for almost every hour of every day since the onset of the hoax. This is her book just as much as it is mine.

Originally the recordings appeared once a week or so, then for a while we put up a recording every evening and then when we were too exhausted to continue with that, we put up recordings twice a week – on Sundays and Wednesdays at 7 p.m.

I had also intended to put on the dates when YouTube had banned/censored/removed some of the videos. But I had to abandon this idea for the simple fact that I couldn't keep up – and I certainly could not keep the list up to date. Towards the end of August, YouTube was taking down videos almost every day.

If you really want to know which recordings were censored (or, in YouTube language removed for violating something or other) then all you have to do is compare the contents of this book to the videos available. The transcripts of the banned videos are shown separately on my website www.vernoncoleman.com under the 'Health' button. Of course, by the time you read this there is a very good chance that the entire channel will have been removed. And that is another reason for reproducing these essays in book form. I think the whole drama needs to be recorded for posterity.

Throughout the months to which these essays relate, the laws being brought in around the world were changing almost daily, and the only consistent factors were the ever-growing power of the World Health Organisation (whose primary financial supporter are the fanatically pro-vaxx Bill and Melinda Gates of the Bill and Melinda Gates Foundation) and a complete disinterest in any of the available science. How many coincidences make a conspiracy?

Finally, please remember my specially written triptych – designed according to the psy-op principles used on the British people.

Distrust the Government

Avoid Mass Media

Fight the Lies

And remember too: you may feel like you are alone, but more and more people are waking up. You are not alone. And we will win this war.

Vernon Coleman, September 2020

Hidden Agendas

I would not be so committed to the notion that the coronavirus is being used to control us, if it were not for the fact that our freedom and our freedom of speech have been thoroughly torn apart. And, of course, no government anywhere could possibly be as inept as governments now appear to be – unless there was an ulterior motive.

One clear result of the lockdown and the extraordinarily misleading propaganda about the coronavirus has been to turn people against one another. The police have actually been asking people to ring them with information about neighbours who may have broken the (vague) laws about exercise or shopping. Worse still, the police have asked citizens (a nice old-fashioned word because although they want us to be prisoner-slaves we are still citizens) to report material on social media which may 'radicalise' members of the public. I actually read the other day about an unfortunate woman who was named and shamed by her community because she had failed to go out onto the street and clap health workers at the designated time. I accidentally missed a one way route in a supermarket and was subjected to abuse. This now appears to be commonplace. Orwell saw it all coming. When we all distrust one another there is little risk of real rebellion from those who wish to share truths but the fearful will turn on one another like cornered rats.

The house arrest of millions has turned many into long-time recluses. People who have been forced into isolation for a long period often find it difficult to adapt to a 'normal' society. The advantage for the authorities is that recluses are fearful and obedient. I have seen people (and particularly teenagers) displaying the sort of repetitive behaviour exhibited by bored animals in zoos.

People have been deprived of their spiritual comfort. One of the most shameful things to happen has been the closure of the churches. The leaders of the Church of England and the Catholic Church should be thoroughly ashamed of themselves. If supermarkets can open why the devil can't the churches? Most churches are fairly empty and could easily allow worshippers to keep well apart. Spiritual comfort is, for many, as essential as bread and beans. Depriving people of spiritual comfort at their greatest time of need helps to break down their morale. Am I the only one to have noticed that, purely by accident of course, we are becoming a curiously Muslim looking society? Our churches are shut, we are told we must cover our faces, our pubs are shut, parties are banned, an attempt was made to stop the sale of Easter eggs and make-up is considered a 'non-essential'. This comment is not in any way intended as a criticism of the Muslim religion but merely a suggestion that maybe our society is being redirected towards something called Chrislam. (Chrislam is dealt with later in this book.) Small businesses are being destroyed. The Corporate Finance Network, which represents 12,000 accountants, has estimated that 800,000 small businesses do not have enough cash to survive longer than a month. Governments have long been opposed to small businesses – which they regard as a nuisance and an unwanted complication.

The elderly are being targeted (as I predicted they would be). In the UK, the old are being denied health care. They are being urged to sign Do Not Resuscitate forms. My fear is that not allowing relatives or friends to visit means that the elderly can be denied health care without objection. It is likely that State pension rises will in future be cut. Many old people will die of hunger and the cold before they even fall ill. Older patients with cancer, heart disease and whatever else have been sent home from hospital to die, untreated, in care homes (where, inevitably, the deaths are counted as coronavirus deaths).

Companies are being told to stop paying dividends. Interest rates are lower than they have ever been before. This will impoverish millions of old people who rely on their pensions and it will also impoverish those who hoped to achieve financial independence. I suspect that negative interest rates will soon be the 'norm'.

We are being nicely set up for mass vaccinations. All the talk is about how we cannot be safe until a vaccine is made. The Government in the UK is planning to make criticism of vaccines and vaccination illegal – even when the criticism is factually based.

As predicted, cash is now being outlawed. The banks have long wanted to get rid of cash. And governments don't like it either. Cash gives people freedom of movement and behaviour. The banks were in serious trouble before the coronavirus panic began. But they will now be rescued with loans. The loans will be paid for by taxpayers. Bank bosses will, of course, continue to enjoy their obscene salaries and huge bonuses.

The truth is being manipulated and distorted in many ways. Around the world, one billion people rely on the $715 billion sent back to poor countries from workers in rich countries. The media doesn't seem to have given much space to this. Nor have journalists asked why, in the UK, there are four times as many empty beds in UK hospitals than there usually are at this time of year and so why, as a result, cancer patients needing surgery or radiotherapy or drug treatment are going completely untreated.

Governments have given themselves massive new powers. In the UK, the Emergency Bill has given the Government complete power. MPs of all parties are apparently happy to allow the UK to be run by a dictator. The police now have total power to do virtually whatever they like. The police can send you home if you venture out of your home – even if you are going shopping or taking your allowed exercise. The range of activities now banned is extraordinary. In the UK it is now illegal to wash a motor car.

The cost of the 'crisis' will be met by massive rises in taxation – which will lead to the further impoverishment of the hard-working middle classes.

We now have no freedom and we have no freedom of speech. That is the ultimate hidden agenda. My new, just completed book *How to Survive the Post Coronavirus Apocalypse* has been banned. The book contains nothing illegal or dangerous or misleading or unsafe. It merely contains facts, and my assessment of how things will work out over the coming months and years. But I cannot publish it. There isn't even a single copy available for the authorities to burn. I have had books banned in China but never before in the West. My website has frequently been pushed into a dark corner. (If you would like to help please put a link to www.vernoncoleman.com on your website!) I have been banned from social media such as Facebook – even though all I want to share are facts and some professional judgements. No newspaper or magazine will even mention my name, let alone print an article or review a book. The Wikipedia page in my name has been distorted and unbalanced in a clear attempt to damage my reputation and destroy my credibility. Anyone can edit a Wikipedia page but, bizarrely, the subject of a page is not allowed to correct errors. If you want to help then there is a list of useful references on my Biography page on www.vernoncoleman.com – look at the entry marked Biographical Detail. And an analysis of how the Advertising Standards Authority (a private body in the UK) refused to look at scientific evidence before reaching a bizarre conclusion is published on my website. (Note: only after I removed the word 'coronavirus' from *Coming Apocalypse* was I allowed to publish it.)

April 28th 2020

The Hidden Agendas behind Government Lies and Deceits

In Britain they started off by telling us that eight million would need to go to hospital and that 500,000 would die. There was much talk of fighting and war and the Spanish Flu in the early 20th century and the black death plague which killed around half of the people in Europe. The coronavirus was made a notifiable disease and put into a special category along with rabies and Ebola. The doom mongers had a field day.

Much the same happened everywhere else around the world. Panic was suddenly in fashion. But right from the start it all seemed wrong. The figures weren't right. Back in February, on my website, I suggested that there were hidden agendas. Since then everything I have said and written has been proved absolutely accurate.

Everyone seemed to forget that the ordinary old-fashioned flu can kill 650,000 a year. In the UK alone it regularly kills tens of thousands.

Why was this coronavirus so very dangerous?

Well, it quickly turned out that it wasn't.

On March 19th the UK Government's advisory committee of experts decided that the coronavirus didn't deserve to be classified as a 'high consequence infectious disease'. It was put back into the flu category where it belonged.

You'd have thought that governments would have back pedalled a little.

But no. Not a bit of it. A few days later the UK was put into lockdown. Many other countries had done the same thing.

Even though the bug had been downgraded the government didn't say whoa, sorry folks, we got a bit overexcited.

Instead they took a 358-page Emergency Bill out of a drawer and put most of the country under house arrest. They call it lockdown but it's house arrest.

Handy that they just happened to have a 358-page document ready. The experts had just downgraded the bug.

The Government was relying on a bloke called Neil Ferguson who does forecasts based on mathematical models. He is professor of mathematical biology at Imperial College in London and on the basis of his advice, the politicians decided we should be locked in and subjected to social distancing rules.

Has this bloke got a great track record?

Well not exactly.

This is what the Government knew about Ferguson when they decided to put all their trust in him and his team:

In 2001, the Imperial team did the modelling on foot and mouth disease which led to a cull of six million sheep, pigs and cattle. The cost to the UK was around £10 billion. But the Imperial's work has been described as 'severely flawed'.

In 2002, Ferguson predicted that up to 50,000 people would die from mad cow disease. He said that could rise to 150,000 if sheep were involved. In the UK, the death total was 177.

In 2005, Ferguson said that up to 200 million people could be killed by bird flu. The total number of deaths was 282 worldwide.

In 2009, Ferguson and his chums at Imperial advised the Government which, relying on that advice, said that swine flu would kill 65,000 people in the UK. In the end swine flu killed 457 people in the UK.

Finally, Ferguson has admitted that his model of the covid-19 is based on undocumented 13-year-old computer code that was intended for use with an influenza epidemic.

No one seems to have questioned Ferguson's work on covid-19 – despite the fact that if he is wrong again (which I believe he is) the nation will be pushed back into the Dark Ages as a result of his work. As far as I know his work has never been peer reviewed.

When I started to criticise the Government's stance, I was vilified and lied about with great enthusiasm. I don't allow adverts on my videos but someone has put a plug for the Government's website on them. There used to be a time when questioning the Government was considered to be a good thing. No more. Telling the truth is apparently unacceptable. The British government has announced that it intends to treat anyone who tells the truth about vaccination as a terrorist. So much for free speech. In future, people won't dare speak out and free speech will be nothing more than a memory. A few years ago I was banned in China. I never thought it would happen here but I can feel it coming and it's scary. I tried to open an account on Facebook for the first time. I was told that I couldn't in order to protect the Facebook community. If the Facebook community needs protecting from me then they've got big problems.

My critics (and there are a great many of them – including, it seems, the UK Government) might like to look at the list of accurate warnings and predictions I have made in the years gone by. I was the first author to write about the excessive power of the drug companies – in my book

The Medicine Men in 1975. I was the first doctor to warn about the danger of benzodiazepines, in a series of articles and TV programmes in the 1970s. I warned about badly organised medical research in a book called *Paper Doctors* in 1977. I was the first doctor to warn that stress could cause massive harm to the human body, in my book *Stress Control* in 1977. I was the only doctor to rightly judge that the Government's warnings on AIDS were wild exaggerations. In 1988, I was the first doctor to warn about the demographic problems caused by an ageing and sick population. In the 1990s, I wrote about the link between meat and cancer. I have also written and broadcast against animal experiments and vaccination, and I'm no longer allowed to broadcast about those issues not because I was wrong but because I won every public debate I ever took part in on radio and television. The opposition was happy to debate with me until they started losing the arguments.

Excuse me for suggesting that my track record is a bit better than Ferguson's.

Sorry about the slight diversion but I think it's relevant.

The result of the Ferguson inspired lockdown is that tens of thousands of patients with cancer are not being treated. And even the Government has admitted that more people will die because of the lockdown than will die of the coronavirus. The Government's own guess is that 150,000 people will die in Britain as a result of the lockdown. The coronavirus isn't going to kill anywhere near that many – even with fiddled figures.

I know how painful this is for those involved. My wife had treatment for breast cancer last year, and the surgery and radiotherapy have left her with a very painful shoulder. She desperately needs physiotherapy. She had one session. And that's it.

And millions of people are terrified out of their wits. I have massive respect for the shop assistants and delivery drivers and others who are working on. Some of them are scared. In one shop I saw an assistant dressed as for an operation. She wore a gown, an apron, a hat, a mask and surgical gloves. Power-crazed police have made things worse. A supermarket delivery driver told me that he was stopped while driving his delivery truck and asked to explain the purpose of his journey.

And the Government continues with the lies and deceit. They can't stop – perhaps because they realise that if they admit they screwed up then they will all be looking for jobs.

Every day they produce new figures showing that the coronavirus has killed many people. Not as many as the ordinary flu it is true. But many people. And those figures aren't true. Many people who die of cancer or heart disease are being put down as covid-19 deaths to boost the figures.

We are being told that people are dying in care homes. Well, I'm afraid that people in care homes are often near the end of their lives. That's why they are there. Every year around 600,000 Britons die. That's over 11,000 a week.

The key is to look at the overall number of deaths. And when you do that it's clear that the total death rate is much the same as it always is. The only difference is that everyone is now officially dying of coronavirus.

Meanwhile we have more empty ITU beds than there were before the scare started. And nearly half of hospital beds are empty.

And here's something else.

Back in March, Professor Ferguson, the Government's advisor, admitted to the House of Commons Science and Technology Committee that up to two thirds of the people who would die from the coronavirus in the next 9 months were likely to have died from some other cause anyway. So the official figure for coronavirus deaths can sensibly be cut to a third.

There are only two conclusions

Britain and the rest of the world are being run by incompetent buffoons who have managed to hoodwink unquestioning journalists.

That's very possible.

The BBC for example, has been a propaganda machine ever since the organisation started taking millions of euros from the EU. You knew about that, of course.

If the press reported every time someone died of ordinary flu we would all live in constant terror – or simply ignore their reports.

But can politicians really be as stupid as they seem?

Or are there hidden agendas?

I've compiled a list of a dozen ways in which governments will benefit from all this nonsense –a dozen hidden agendas

The first of my 12 hidden agendas is that people have been turned against one another. One police force has even asked citizens to report material on the internet which might radicalise members of the public – in other words material which might encourage them to reject the status quo and to question the validity of our having been turned into a police state.

It seems that it is now considered illegal to tell the truth if by so doing you embarrass the Government. If you believe in free speech then you might find that worrying.

I seem to remember the Chinese, the Soviet Union and the Nazis had rather similar policies.

Other hidden agendas? We've been turned into recluses who are fearful and obedient – perfect for a police state. The elderly have been marginalised. We've been prepared for regular, compulsory vaccination, we are all going to be impoverished and less independent than before, cash is going to be outlawed, freedom of speech will soon be a memory, churches have been shut and people deprived of spiritual comfort, small businesses are being destroyed, taxes will rise massively and so on.

My list of 12 hidden agendas appears in more detail on my website www.vernoncoleman.com

There have been serious attempts to hide the site but it's still there at the moment.

There is one easy way for the politicians to prove that there aren't any hidden agendas.

Sack Ferguson, forget the social distancing rules and abandon the lockdown.

Now.

And then there may be a hope that we can salvage something from the mess they've made of the world.

It is governments not the coronavirus which threaten our lives

When will the morons in charge stop lying to us about this damned mangy virus?

At the beginning of this fiasco I couldn't quite make up my mind whether the whole coronavirus panic was the result of a cockup or a conspiracy.

Politicians and their advisers can and do make many stupid decisions. But this has gone way beyond cockup. It is inconceivable that so many leaders could get so much so wrong unless there was a reason for their apparent stupidity.

And so we're left with the conspiracy theory.

Since they have taken over the world and now rule our lives without mercy, there can no longer be any doubt about what is happening. As I pointed out half a lifetime ago, if the politicians really felt this was an important disease they'd have done extensive testing and put the sick into lockdown – not the healthy. They didn't do mass testing though did they? If they had done they would know that people have had the bug without being very ill. And that wouldn't be convenient.

Most sensible, intelligent people now realise that the whole coronavirus crisis is a hoax, a piece of outrageous flummery. Only the terrified and the gullible can possible still accept the nonsense about this being the new plague. Our local council wrote to me yesterday to remind me that sunbathing in parks isn't allowed because it puts everyone's health at risk. How, in the name of everything, does sunbathing put everyone's health at risk?

The politicians are still lying through their teeth.

Here are the biggest lies they are telling:

The first lie is that the coronavirus is a big killer.

The numbers are wrong. Completely wrong. They have worked desperately hard to push up the numbers by listing every death as a coronavirus death. No one dies of flu or cancer or heart disease these days. If there was an aeroplane crash the people on board would all be put down as dying from the coronavirus. The politicians shed crocodile tears over all the deaths but they are using those individual tragedies for their own purposes. They've managed to get the global number of deaths up to 250,000, and although that's a fake figure they seem excited by it. But, as I pointed out in the middle of March, the ordinary flu can kill 650,000 people in a season. The coronavirus is not a big killer. It can kill, and that is always a tragedy, but for most people it is nothing more than a nuisance. And remember the ordinary flu can kill babies, children and healthy adults. Even governments now admit that far more people are going to be killed by the lockdowns than will ever be killed by the coronavirus. Most of those who catch it have no symptoms at all. Most of the rest get the symptoms of a cold or the flu. Around 99.9% of those who catch it will recover. Around 90% of the people who die have pre-existing health problems and are even older than I am. Those are the facts. The coronavirus is no bigger a killer than the flu can be.

The second lie is that lockdowns are essential.

Keeping people under house arrest is not going to help anything – but the lockdowns are doing massive damage and they are killing far more people than the coronavirus. When the lockdown was introduced in the UK, the hypocritical Neil Ferguson (the one who broke the lockdown rules to see his mistress) had originally forecast that 500,000 Britons would die. There was talk of 8 million people being hospitalised (in a country with 140,000 hospital beds). That was all absolute garbage. Ferguson has an appalling track record. The so-called scientific modelling may have been modelling but it was not scientific.

Only a complete moron would persist with keeping a country in lockdown – unless there was an ulterior motive. The lockdown will not protect us against anything but it weakens individuals and it weakens nations in every conceivable way. It helps to ensure that there will be another outbreak in the autumn. Today, in the UK, the hospitals are still largely shut for non-coronavirus patients. Patients with cancer are being untreated. Even dentists are shut. Businesses are dying. This is blatant lunacy. Is it the plan to go on with lockdown forever? The only conceivable explanation is that there are ulterior motives. The politicians want to weaken us, frighten us and control us. Read the facts about the hidden agenda on my website.

The third lie was that the health service needed protecting because it wouldn't be able to cope.

Heavens knows who thought up this piece of garbage. It was never true. But as a result of the lie, doctors were told to stop treating cancer patients. There was never any justification for that. Never. And the doctors who obeyed these inhumane instructions – and who are still obeying those wicked instructions should damned well be ashamed of themselves. They don't deserve clapping – they should be clapped in irons. Hospitals and ITUs are emptier than they have ever been. The lawyers are going to have a field day when this is all over.

Finally, if you still doubt that there is a hidden agenda here let me remind you of two things:

On March 19th the UK's public health bodies and the Advisory Committee on Dangerous Pathogens decided that the new coronavirus infection should no longer be classified as a 'high consequence infectious disease'. The coronavirus was downgraded to common or garden status. Like the flu.

On March 26th (after the bug had been downgraded), the UK Government published a 358-page Emergency Bill giving itself massive powers. That Bill took away our freedom and turned Britain into a police state. And we were shut in our homes under house arrest. Elections everywhere were postponed for no good reason.

You cannot possible reconcile the second event with the first event unless you believe that we have lost our freedom for a purpose.

Oh and there's that other odd thing that people who have had the disease won't get immunity and will still need to have a jab. (I'm just a doctor so I'm not allowed to use the other word in public or my government will want to have me arrested.) This claim seems to me to have originated in Grimm's Fairy Tales. Why would you not get immunity from the real disease but then get immunity from an expensive jab that gives you a mild dose of the same disease? What a puzzle that is. A real mystery. I've been studying jabs for 50 years and probably know more about them than most people but I can't even begin to explain it. It sounds to me like something doctors like to refer to as total bollocks.

If we want to get our democracy back we have to demand that politicians explain exactly why they are persisting with stupid lockdown policies. Why all the secrecy? It's our world and we are not at war. Well, most of our governments are at war somewhere in the world but none of them has anything to do with the coronavirus.

We are entitled to know what evidence they are using. They're being secretive because there isn't any damned evidence to show it makes sense.

You probably try to avoid conspiracy theories. I certainly do.

But when you eradicate all the other possibilities, what is left?

And what is behind it all? Look for who benefits. Follow the money. And read the section on hidden agendas which is on my website.

You'll also find all the facts about this damned fiasco. And don't believe anything the politicians or the mass media tell you. Paranoia is now the only sensible, healthy, sane condition.

And please try to educate everyone you know. Tell them to watch the videos and visit the website before I'm banned completely for the terrible crime of telling the truth.

They'll arrest us all if we go out onto the streets or into the parks to protest. So use the internet to spread the truth to as many people as you can.

Ask the frightened, who still believe the official garbage, to read the facts and then they'll perhaps understand what is happening to us all. The threat doesn't come from the coronavirus – it comes from our governments.

We need to let the politicians know that we don't trust them, we don't believe them and that the ones who still persist in unscientific, dangerous lockdown policies will be voted out of power at the first opportunity – and never voted in again.

That is, of course, if they ever let us vote again.
These are scary times.

May 2ⁿᵈ 2020

How Many Million Will the Global Lockdown Kill?

Around the world, millions of people are going to die because of absurd lockdown policies. Serious illness has been ignored. Patients with cancer, heart disease and other threatening diseases have been pushed aside as many hospitals have closed their doors to the patients who really needed help. The coming global recession will result in massive, long-term unemployment and mass starvation.

All those responsible for this stupidity should be fired and banished from positions of responsibility.

Despite the fact that more and more doctors around the world now agree with me that the coronavirus scare was viciously oversold and that the lockdowns, mass hysteria and panic have done far more damage than the damned disease, there is no sign of governments abandoning the lunacy.

Experts also now agree (belatedly) with my suggestion (made weeks ago) that governments should have tested everyone and shut in the people who were infected so that the disease couldn't spread. Simple but very effective.

Huge publicity was recently given to the tragic fact that around the world, 250,000 people are alleged to have died with the coronavirus. But many (possibly most) of those patients did not die because of the coronavirus, they died with it. The two things are very different.

Why are the UK figures the worst in the world?

Well, massive immigration means that England is the most overcrowded nation in Europe but that isn't the only cause.

I believe the enthusiasm for blaming the coronavirus for just about all deaths was originally inspired by the need to justify the wicked Emergency Bill which gave the police unprecedented powers.

But everyone got too enthusiastic and the trick backfired – leaving the UK with the world's worst figures and causing the Government massive embarrassment. I doubt if half of the 30,000 alleged to have died of the coronavirus were actually killed by it.

I believe the UK has had the worst people imaginable dealing with the coronavirus.

The important thing that no one ever mentions is that even if 250,000 people had died globally (and they clearly have not) then the coronavirus would still not be as deadly as the flu – which can kill 650,000 worldwide in a single season.

No one gets hysterical about the flu, do they?

Around 600,000 people a year die in the UK, and I expect the number of deaths from flu and pneumonia will fall as the number linked to the coronavirus has risen. (I'd bet that the mortality figures for flu are going to be very low this year. The drug companies will claim the credit for that. You can guess why.) Later in the year (and next year) the number of deaths from cancer and other abandoned diseases will rocket – as, I fear, will the number of suicides and murders.

Governments and media everywhere (and particularly in the UK) have deliberately built up the terror.

I know that the coronavirus is a very nasty disease. (We both believe we had it back at the start of the year and Antoinette was horribly ill.) But so is the flu. I've had bouts of the flu that I thought would kill me. And flu can kill people of all ages – young and old, fit and unfit.

But the coronavirus terror has been built up out of all proportion.

I went into a shop two days ago and the assistant was dressed in a surgical gown, plastic apron, mask, surgical cap covering her hair and rubber gloves. She stood behind a plastic screen and looked terrified. I cannot imagine why she felt she needed to cover her hair. She was holding her hands in the air as though ready to start diving into the chest, abdomen or skull of some invisible patient. The poor woman looked as if she were about to set off to a fancy dress party or to take on a role in a gory horror movie. What is she going to do when the nonsense stops? Will she suddenly leave off all her protective equipment or will she do some grotesque, slow strip tease and lose one item a day?

The UK Government's pathetic attempt to end the crisis they created will be a failure. Allowing people to have picnics on the beach will make the problems worse. People have been off work too long. Many don't want to go back to work. Government paycheques have made life comfortable in a rather couch potato sort of way. There are no holidays or big events to look forward to. Everything is grey. And the fear will still be there. So, even if the jobs are there, why go back to work?

The only solution is to act fast and definitively. End the lockdown immediately. Abandon all the Ferguson inspired nonsenses.

My book, *Coming Apocalypse*, explains how we got into this mess and what is going to happen now. Having analysed the past, I did my best to assess the future that Ferguson, Johnson et al have created.

Everything I put on my website has been proved accurate. Now we are facing more serious threats to our health and freedom.

Ferguson and Johnson et al thought that we were heading for an apocalypse. They were right. But the apocalypse will not be caused by the coronavirus but by their so-called 'cure'. It no longer matters how much of it was due to a cock-up and how much was due to a conspiracy.

Antoinette and I worked hard to put *Coming Apocalypse* together as quickly as possible, and then fought to get it published, in the hope that if enough people read it (and understand the future we face) then we might be able to put pressure on the politicians to act decisively. There is far too much text to put onto the website (the book is 133 pages long) but the prices of the eBook and the paperback are, as always with my books, the cheapest possible. I'll spend the royalties on adverts for the book (if anyone will sell me advertising space!) so that more people know the truth.

Whatever happens, we have to prepare ourselves for a very different world.

The Bank of England says that although a recession is coming, it may all be fine by next year. So, given the Bank's track record, I think that is as good a guarantee as you are likely to see that we are well and truly stuffed for eternity and a half. (I wish I could get hold of a crate of whatever it is that the highly paid BoE staffers are quaffing. It must be pretty potent stuff.)

May 7th 2020

Is Boris Taking Advantage of the False Coronavirus Crisis to Steal Our Democracy?

We no longer live in a democracy. We live in a police state.
Here's the evidence from my new book, *Coming Apocalypse*:
On March 19th the UK's public health bodies and the Advisory Committee on Dangerous Pathogens decided that the new coronavirus infection should no longer be classified as a 'high consequence infectious disease'. The coronavirus was downgraded to common or garden status.
On March 26th (after the bug had been downgraded) the UK Government published a 358-page Emergency Bill giving itself massive powers. That Bill took away our freedom and turned Britain into a police state. And we were shut in our homes under house arrest. Will we ever get our democracy back?
We have to demand that Boris Johnson explains exactly why he is keeping us in lockdown. What evidence does he have proving that the lockdown will help? It's our country and we are not at war. There is no need for secrecy. We are entitled to know what evidence Boris is using. Is he still relying on Ferguson?
The lockdown has reduced the incidence of the infection in the country. But that just makes us all more vulnerable. Having little herd immunity means that there will almost certainly be a second wave epidemic in the autumn. Flu bugs always kill more when the weather gets bad. And so there will be more panic and even stricter lockdowns. Is that what Boris wants?
In situations like this it is vital to see who benefits.
We have to follow the money.
And you already know where that trail leads.

May 8th 2020

How Medical Truths Are Suppressed

I have been writing about the way the drug industry controls the medical profession since the 1970s. In my first book, *The Medicine Men*, I pointed out that doctors had become nothing more than a branch of the pharmaceutical industry.

The book was well received at the time. There are reviews for *The Medicine Men* under the Biography and Contact Details section of www.vernoncoleman.com

But things have got much worse since then. These days my books are hammered or ignored because the drug industry controls just about everything.

Indeed, these days, doctors only get to read and hear what the drug industry wants them to read and hear. I can prove this.

A few years ago I was invited to speak at a conference in London. The conference was, I was told, intended to tackle the subject of medication errors and adverse reactions to prescribed drugs. The company organising the conference was called PasTest. 'For over thirty years, PasTest has been providing medical education to professionals within the NHS,' they told me. 'Building on our commitment to quality in medical and healthcare education, PasTest is creating a range of healthcare events which focus on the professional development of clinicians and managers who are working together to deliver healthcare services for the UK. Our aim is to provide a means for those who are in a position to improve services on both national and regional levels. The topics covered by our conferences are embraced within policy, best practice, case study, clinical management and evidence based practice. PasTest endeavours to source the best speakers who will engage audiences with balanced, relevant and thought-provoking programmes.'

Goody, I thought.

Iatrogenesis (doctor-induced disease) is something of a speciality of mine. I have written numerous books and articles on the subject. My campaigns have resulted in more drugs being banned or controlled than anyone else's.

In addition to my speaking at the conference, the organisers wanted me to help them decide on the final programme. I thought the conference was an important one and would give me a good opportunity to tell NHS staff the truth. I signed a contract.

PasTest wrote to confirm my appointment as a consultant and speaker for the PasTest Conference Division.

And then there was silence. My office repeatedly asked for details of when and where the conference was being held.

Silence.

Eventually a programme for the event appeared on the Internet. Curiously, my name was not on the list of speakers.

Here is part of the blurb promoting the conference:

'Against a background of increasing media coverage into the number of UK patients who are either becoming ill or dying due to adverse reactions to medication, our conference aims to explain the current strategies to avoid Adverse Drug reactions and what can be done to educate patients.'

Putting the blame on patients for problems caused by prescription drugs is brilliant. Most drug related problems are caused by the stupidity of doctors not the ignorance of patients. If the aim is to educate patients on how best to avoid prescription drug problems, the advice would be simple: 'Don't trust doctors.'

The promotion for the conference claims that, 'It is estimated errors in medication...account for 4% of hospital bed capacity.' And that prescription drug problems 'reportedly kill up to 10,000 people a year in the UK'.

As I would have shown (had I not been banned from the conference) these figures are absurdly low.

The list of speakers included a variety of people I had never heard of including one speaker representing The Association of the British Pharmaceutical Industry and another representing the Medicines and Healthcare Products Regulatory Agency.

Delegates representing the NHS were expected to pay £250 plus VAT (£293.75) to attend the event. Delegates whose Trust would be funding the cost were asked to apply for a Health Authority Approval form.

So why was I apparently banned from this conference?

This is what PasTest said when we asked them: 'certain parties felt that he (Vernon Coleman) was too controversial to speak and as a result would not attend.'

Could that, I wonder, be the drug industry?

Is the drug industry now deciding whom they will allow to speak to doctors and other NHS staff on the problems caused by prescription drugs? If I was banned at the behest of the drug industry, do NHS bosses know that people attending such conferences will only hear speakers approved by the drug industry and that speakers telling the truth will be banned? (I think it is safe to assume that I won't be invited to speak at any more conferences for NHS staff.)

Why are people who had me banned so frightened of what I would say? It can surely only be because they know that I would have caused embarrassment by telling the truth.

The scary bottom line is that the NHS paid a lot of money to send delegates to a conference where someone representing the drug industry spoke to them on drug safety. But I was banned.

Because I had a contract, PasTest paid me *not* to turn up. I used the money to buy advertisements for my book *How to Stop Your Doctor Killing You.*

May 9th 2020

Another Disgraceful Incident Involving Vernon Coleman

Wikipedia editors have been scouring the internet for exciting incidents from my long forgotten past which they can use in their attempt to discredit me.

Here is one they seem to have missed.

In the distant days when I was a GP, family doctors did a lot of home visits. And inevitably the calls occasionally came at inconvenient moments. Quite a few came through while I was conducting a morning or evening surgery.

Sometimes patients were happy to wait until the surgery had finished. But on other occasions they needed a visit immediately. I always used to ask: 'Do you want me to visit now or can you wait until the surgery has finished?' Simple.

On one occasion, I remember receiving a call from a woman who thought her husband was having a heart attack. She wanted me to go immediately. I told the receptionists that I would have to leave the surgery, left apologies for the patients in the waiting room and hurried off to the patient's home.

It was about 5.30 p.m. and naturally the roads were busy with people going home from work. I turned on my hazard flashers so that people could see me coming and drove as fast as I could. I was, I remember, driving a bright orange Saab 99 at the time. It had, I seem to remember, a turbo model with a fine turn of speed.

The patient wasn't having a heart attack. I stayed a few minutes, soothed him and his wife, prescribed whatever was appropriate (I can't remember what it was) and drove back to the consulting rooms to finish the evening surgery.

I didn't think any more of it until a day or so later when I received a telephone call from the secretary to a local Chief Superintendent who was something significant in the local police station. His secretary wanted me to go along to the local police station. Apparently, the policeman had been one of the cars I had passed while driving to my patient. Maybe he had tried to catch me but had failed. He had taken my car number and traced me to the surgery.

I didn't see why I should go along to the police station, so I didn't go. And a few days later, I received a summons for driving with my hazard flashers on.

I had to go to court, and the Medical Defence Union sent a high powered lawyer up from London to defend me.

In the end, I was fined £5 for driving with my hazard flashers switched on. That was it. My driving licence remained unblemished. It was, apparently, illegal to drive a moving motor car with the flashers flashing. I was told that only bus drivers can drive with their flashers going and only then when they have been hijacked and need to attract the attention of the constabulary.

The story hit most of the national newspapers, and one reporter asked me why I thought the policeman wanted me to go along to the police station.

I said I assumed that he wanted to tell me off.

And at this point things got very silly.

One of the papers reported that I had said that the policeman had wanted to browbeat me into making an apology.

I had never said any such thing but that, apparently, was no defence when the Chief Superintendent sued me for libel.

At that point the whole story got very silly.

A very eminent barrister in London said he would have loved to have the policeman in the witness box but sensibly suggested that the case really wasn't worth the effort. I ended up paying £200 in damages for the comment I hadn't made, and agreeing to the printing of a small apology in the local newspaper. Heaven knows what the legal costs came to. Mine were paid by the Medical Defence Union and the policeman's were, I think, paid by some sort of police body.

So, there is another story about me that Wikipedia could use. I'm sure they could get a few juicy paragraphs out of it.

It happened in the late 1970s or the early 1980s, so a couple of weeks digging through newspaper and court reports would doubtless prove immensely fruitful.

May 10th 2020

Why Did YouTube Ban My Video?

I was shocked but not surprised when YouTube took down one of my videos recently.

I was shocked because everything I said in the video was absolutely accurate and honest. The only conceivable problem was that the video didn't follow the authorised line being heavily promoted by governments all over the world.

A huge number of doctors now agree with me that governments have made huge mistakes in the way they have dealt with this virus. I've been saying this since February. Their propaganda has created much fear and I don't think anyone in government now denies that the number of people dying because of the lockdowns – the so-called 'cure' for the coronavirus – will be far, far greater than the number who will die from the virus itself. Governments everywhere have distorted truths and misled their populations.

My only aim has always been to provide some truths and, hopefully, some reassurance. I never allowed advertising or sponsorship on my videos or my website. Both exist as what used to be called a public service. I don't make TV or radio programmes and I don't write articles or columns any more. Everything I've written or recorded about the coronavirus has resulted in my reputation being trashed so much that I would have been far better off if I'd kept my thoughts to myself.

I've never been able to do the sensible thing. My life has been one of fighting for lost and difficult causes and truths. I've spent most of my many years battling for people and animals without enough care for the consequences. And I'm pretty used to being banned and lied about, sneered at and patronised.

I said I was shocked but not surprised by YouTube's decision.

I wasn't surprised because YouTube has got itself an unfortunate reputation for censoring people who put up videos on its channel.

Well, it's their channel. They are the publishers. So they can, if they like, allow only State approved lobbyists to put up videos. (The odd thing is that publishers usually have legal liability for whatever they publish. I suspect that YouTube would deny that they were publishers if they were asked to take any sort of responsibility.)

But if anyone from YouTube ever bothers to watch this before deciding to ban it, because it doesn't follow the official party line, I've got a thought for you...

Some years ago I resigned from a well-paid column on a British Sunday newspaper because the editor refused to print a column questioning the validity of the Iraq War. I didn't believe in the weapons of mass destruction claims and I thought we were being lied to. I didn't see the point in writing a column if I wasn't allowed to express my honestly felt views. Resigning from that column on a matter of principle meant that I didn't get any more newspaper work. Editors don't much like columnists who have principles – and it cost me dearly in financial terms.

But that newspaper has been slowly dying since then.

The circulation fell by around 90% in the years which followed. Now, you could argue that the circulation fell that much because I left and I wouldn't stop you if you did but I wouldn't really believe it. And you could argue that the circulation fell because all newspapers are losing circulation and that's true. But this particular newspaper has lost a devil of a lot more circulation than it should have done.

And I know why.

It is slowly dying because it lost its integrity. It doesn't stand for anything. It didn't respect its readers. And the readers saw or sensed that lack of respect.

In a way it's tricky being a publisher.

If you're going to retain your integrity and ensure that your readers or viewers know that you respect their intelligence then you have to put up with people wanting to write or say things you don't agree with. When the men and women in suits tell you to ban this or censor that, you have to have the guts to say 'No' or someone else will come along and put you out of business.

You obviously have to censor people who tell blatant lies or want to publish dangerous or illegal material. But you can't suppress the truth and expect to retain respect and goodwill. Leaving people alone to tell the truth or share their opinions needs courage and basic integrity. You have to recognise that you cannot have freedom without a free press. Remember those newspaper editors in old cowboy movies? They always had the courage to print the truth.

It was, remember, HL Mencken who wrote that the relationship of a journalist to a politician should be that of a dog to a lamppost. And it was Theodore Roosevelt who, to paraphrase slightly, wrote that thinking there must be no criticism of the establishment is not only unpatriotic and servile but morally treasonable.

It seems to me that the people at YouTube don't have either integrity or courage. More importantly, they don't realise that the heart and soul of any publishing company belongs to the readers.

The video of mine which YouTube took down contained nothing but the truth. I've been researching and writing about medical matters for a long time. I'm not stupid. I'm not going to write or say something I think is wrong.

Why did they try to censor me?

They could, I suppose, be like those terrible students who want to ban anyone who says something they don't like. But I don't think that's it. That wouldn't make commercial sense.

Maybe they just prefer to follow the safe route and specialise in publishing videos of ducks on roller skates.

But I don't think that's it. That wouldn't make commercial sense either.

Or, maybe they just disapprove of original thinking that doesn't fit neatly into government approved propaganda.

I was banned in China years ago so I know how that works. Statist, fascist, establishment organisations have been doing it for a long time. Look at what happened to Dr John Snow, Dr Ignaz Semmelweiss and many, many more.

I think YouTube has been got at. I don't think it's YouTube any more. I think it's ThemTube.

I think they're suppressing material which the authorities don't want publishing. I think that the men and women in suits have convinced them that anyone who questions authority is a mad, dangerous conspiracy theorist. Well look at my track record – it's all listed on my website. I'm not mad and I'm not a conspiracy theorist – though I suppose that if you're a fascist dictator I might be considered dangerous.

This time it's a lot easier for me than when I resigned as a columnist. I don't get paid to put videos on YouTube. Working out what to say and recording videos takes time and energy and there are lots of other things I'd rather be doing with the time and energy I've got left.

If I pack up making these little videos I'll just put the same stuff on my website. It means I won't have to comb what's left of my hair and I won't have to struggle with YouTube, which I don't find as user friendly as it could be. I don't want to be a guest on someone's channel if they don't want me there.

I did consider taking down all my videos but decided not to for now – though if they remove this one I won't put up any more. I don't want to be associated with a channel which serves only as a mouthpiece for fascist, statist, oppressive propaganda.

So, I don't really care what YouTube decides to do.

If they want to restore a little of that lost integrity they could put back the video they banned – it was called 'Why You Are Now in Great Danger' and the script, in its entirety is on my website so that anyone who is interested can read it and wonder why the devil they censored it.

Let's see if YouTube has the bottle to leave this video in place.

Or if the channel run by wee cowering timorous beasties is so desperate to suck up to the establishment that they ban this one as well.

And if the sycophants at YouTube ban me completely I really don't give a fig.

I was banned and suppressed long before YouTube appeared – long before the internet appeared.

Once before when I was banned I wrote that I would, if necessary, write out my articles and hand them out on street corners. Or sell my books from a wheelbarrow. And I still mean that.

If they do remove this or any of my other videos then everyone who cares about freedom and free speech will know that YouTube is no more than a worthless propaganda vessel – specialising in indoctrination.

The script of this video is going onto my website and I hope everyone who can do so will put the tape in places where YouTube can't remove it. I'm banned from Facebook and so on because I'm considered a threat. It's the modern day version of book burning.

So put this tape on your Facebook page or Twitter or whatever.

Or put a link to my website so that people can read the truth directly.

Tell everyone to watch or listen or to read my website. It's all free. No ads. No sponsors. No one ever tells me what to write.

Stand up for the truth. It's really quite important.

From the old bloke in the chair, thank you for watching and thank you for all your support.

May 13th 2020

Seventeen Things You Should Know About Face Masks

The world is now awash with conflicting reports on how or when or whether to wear a mask to protect you against the flu, the lurgy or the embarrassment of having egg on your chin. Some people, such as the Mayor of London, want masks to be compulsory though no one has provided evidence for the compulsion. The Mayor has allegedly threatened to order people to wear masks in London if the Government does not do so.

There are videos and books explaining how to make your own mask out of unwanted bits and pieces found lying around the home. It is possible to make two excellent face masks out of the cups of an old brassiere, using the straps to fashion loops to go around the ears or the back of the head. Naturally, the size of the bra has a big influence on its suitability for turning into a face mask, and a bra measuring 44JJ is probably going to be a little on the loose side for most people. And if you need fresh masks every day you will need a large supply of bras.

Here are the 17 things everyone should know about masks:

The World Health Organisation recommends that disposable masks should be discarded after one use.

The WHO doesn't seem to have any guidelines for masks made out of washable material but it's a fair guess that it would recommend washing thoroughly at a high temperature after every use.

The WHO says that if you are healthy you only need to wear a mask if you are taking care of someone who is suspected of having covid-19 infection aka 2019-nCoV.

Masks are effective only when used in combination with frequent hand washing with soap and water or an alcohol based hand rub.

Fabric masks may allow viruses to enter and are not considered to be anywhere near as protective as surgical masks.

A study called 'Optical miscroscopic study of surface morphology and filtering efficiency of face masks' concluded that face masks made of cloth are not very good at filtering out viruses because the pores are much bigger than the particulate matter that needs to be kept out.

One study showed that facemasks may have pores five thousand times larger than virus particles. If this is accurate it means that the virus will wander through the face mask much like a mouse wandering through Marble Arch.

Washing cloth face masks makes them even less effective. The more you wash the mask the less effective it becomes.

Masks are only really effective if they fit perfectly and if the wearer does not move their head.

Surgical masks are worn to stop bits of saliva, food or hair falling from the surgeon or nurse into a wound. They will stop some bacteria but will not usually stop viruses.

Much of the air we breathe in and out goes around the side of the mask unless it is very tight fitting.

The Centers for Disease Control and Prevention in the US recommends that everyone wear masks in public places where it is difficult to stay six feet from other people.

Touching a mask appears to stop the mask providing protection. It has been suggested that you should put on a new mask if you have touched the one you are wearing.

People with breathing difficulties (such as asthma or bronchitis) may find that wearing a mask makes breathing even more difficult.

Does wearing a face mask reduce your immunity levels? No one seems to know the answer for sure but it seems possible that if people wear face masks for long periods (months or years) then the absence of contact with the real world might well have a harmful effect on immunity – if the face mask works.

Do face masks prevent us developing immunity to particular diseases? This depends on many factors – mainly the effectiveness of the face mask.

Everyone seems to have a view on whether or not wearing face masks is a good thing. But no one seems to have any evidence to prove their viewpoint. And the effectiveness of a mask depends massively on the nature of the mask, how it is worn and how often it is changed. I have studied yards of scientific studies on the subject and as a result of much dull reading, I am totally confused. The only certainty seems to me to be that no one is certain. Wearing a mask may or may not do any harm but it may give the wearer a false sense of confidence.

Please note the date at the bottom of this article. Things are forever changing.

May 16th 2020

A Population Control Plan?

I work hard at avoiding conspiracy theories. I have always believed that cock-ups are more common than conspiracies.

But I have long given up thinking that the global response to the coronavirus is a series of cock-ups (though there have, along the way, been many incidental cock-ups). The evidence makes it clear to me that we are being manipulated.

Here is a summary of some of the reasons why I am convinced…

First, in the UK, the Government's advisers ruled in March that the coronavirus was not a high consequence infectious disease. As far as I know, only my website reported this momentous piece of front page news.

Second, within days of this reassuring news, the UK Government had published its 358-page Emergency Bill and put the country into lockdown.

Third, the total number of alleged coronavirus deaths around the world is 300,000 (though this figure has been manipulated and is, in reality, widely believed to be much lower). This is a tragedy. But we have to remember that up to 650,000 people die in a bad flu season. And I don't remember countries being put into lockdown or social distancing being introduced for the flu.

Fourth, all opposition to the establishment's view point is being silenced. (For example, YouTube is closing down platforms belonging to broadcasters who produce 'unacceptable' information which questions government views. After YouTube banned two of my videos for absolutely no good reason that I could see, I decided to beat them to it by banning YouTube before they could ban me. However, three of my original videos and my two videos questioning the YouTube policy are, surprisingly, still available for the time being.)

Fifth, governments everywhere are promoting fear. I will come back to the mass hypnosis techniques they are using to control whole populations.

In a previous article on www.vernoncoleman.com, I have discussed the various hidden agendas behind the grab for power and control.

But there is one more hidden agenda which I forgot to include on that list: population control.

Look at the evidence.

The world is overpopulated.

The coronavirus is not going to kill enough people to affect the overpopulation problem.

But the twin evils of social distancing and lockdowns will have a massive effect on the population in many ways.

Obviously, we are all being made afraid and prevented by law from meeting new people or forming groups which might question what is happening.

But look at what is happening to young, single people.

They are being told to wear masks. So they cannot see what anyone looks like. No smiles can be exchanged.

They are being told that they must keep six feet apart from people who aren't in their own household.

They cannot go to nightclubs or pubs to meet people.

They cannot go to the cinema together unless they are already in the same household.

So, there isn't much (or any) chance of new relationships developing.

Forget the jokes about the lockdown causing a population boom in December.

The medium and long-term result is going to be a massive drop in young people meeting partners.

And an inevitable, massive fall in the population.

Another big win for those who want to control the planet.

May 16th 2020

Why the Economy Won't Bounce Back

Central banks and economists are predicting that economies damaged by the coronavirus 'crisis' will bounce back quickly.

I don't think they will.

The bankers and the economists are not thinking straight because they see everything in hard, fiscal terms. They think that if governments throw huge amounts of money at the problem they have manufactured, then large businesses will recover and soon begin operating as they did before. (They don't give a damn about small businesses. Indeed, part of the plan is to destroy small businesses which are difficult to regulate and inefficient in taxation terms.)

This confidence is embarrassingly naïve.

Even if governments cancelled lockdowns and social distancing straight away, the damage done by a series of deliberately terrifying and oppressive regulations will last for decades and probably for generations.

And that, of course, is the aim.

The politicians and Bilderbergers know what is going on.

But most economists and many bankers are not at the top of the food chain.

The fact is that the fear and anxiety which has been created is not going to disappear overnight.

There is much anger among those of us who see exactly what governments are doing: the thinkers, the sceptics and so on.

But a large part of the population is too overwhelmed by fear to see the truth.

Millennials and children, in particular, have been devastated by the way their lives have been disrupted. They see very little future.

Those in their late teens and early twenties who are usually the backbone of any protest movement, are now too terrified to do or say anything. They want to be told what to do and when to do it. They have lost their drive, their ambition and their sense of identity.

Younger children, equally terrified, have seen their world turned upside down and inside out. They no longer have any certainties other than fear and foreboding. Education skills, now fractured, will probably never develop. Ambitions have been smashed. Many will see no further than a government paycheque and a life lived in quiet obedience.

It has been noticeable that most of the protests about lockdowns and social distancing have come from the over 40s. It is older folk who see what is happening and who are feisty enough to stand up for themselves and their country. And it is mainly those in the older age groups who find it difficult to understand why nations have been shut down for a virus which has so far killed less than half the number of people likely to be killed by a nasty winter flu. (As I write, the coronavirus is alleged to be responsible for 300,000 deaths worldwide. The flu can kill 650,000 people in a season.) And it is those people who realise that without people and businesses back at work and paying taxes there won't be any money for health care, education, roads or unemployment benefits.

The economists and the central bankers don't realise that most people's habits will now be changed permanently.

People have become distrusting and suspicious. They don't trust anyone or anything outside their immediate circle. Many relationships have been fractured permanently. The effect of the stress they have been under will produce permanent damage. When (or if) GPs surgeries eventually reopen there will be queues and long waiting lists as people report their depressions and anxieties and ask for help. With no suitable training, and no time, GPs will hand out vast quantities of anxiolytics and anti-depressants – most of which are addictive. Tens of millions will be turned into prescription drug zombies.

In the future, shopping is going to be largely done online. People will want to hoard essentials because they know that there are likely to be more lockdowns ahead. Vast numbers of small businesses will move online since their bricks and mortar businesses are no longer viable. People won't travel as much as they used to do. If holidays are taken, they will be relatively low key and most people will probably not travel outside their home country. Millions are going to lose their jobs and become reliant on government paycheques. Millions more will work at home. Most people will get their entertainment entirely from the television set.

The consequence will be that many large businesses will fail as it becomes clear that their business models are no longer valid.

In my view, the economists and the bankers have got it all wrong. There is not going to be a rapid recovery from the coming recession. But, then, I don't think that the politicians and global leaders ever expected that there would be. They arrested the wonderful bloke who used to wander up and down carrying a sign saying 'The End is Nigh'.

I fear his time has come.

We are heading for a global depression like nothing there has ever been before. We are being manipulated and we're going back to the days before the Industrial Revolution days.

And I'm afraid I don't think it's happening by accident.

May 17ᵗʰ 2020

Protecting the Oil Supplies

As I have said many times before, I no longer believe the current fake crisis is the result of a cock-up. (Though there have certainly been many mistakes made – particularly in Britain where the Government has proved itself astonishingly inept.)

I think the crisis is the result of a power grab – which has worked very effectively.

And it is a power grab which has many facets.

I explained on www.vernoncoleman.com how the 'crisis' is being used as a tool to control the size of the global population.

But there are other things happening.

The oil, for example. I have, for many years, argued that the oil is running out and that the nature of our world will, therefore, have to change.

Governments have welcomed and encouraged climate change protestors in order to find an excuse for oil preserving policies which have nothing to do with the fake global warming arguments and everything to do with the knowledge that if we don't reduce our use of oil there soon won't be enough of the stuff left to fill a lawnmower – let alone the tank of a presidential limousine.

The coronavirus hoax has, within weeks, enabled governments to do what they could have never hoped to do otherwise for decades.

Millions of people are now going to work at home.

Energy sapping small businesses are being replaced by internet based companies which are far more efficient.

Public transport is being cut back and will be side-lined.

Air travel (for business or pleasure) will soon be so unpleasant and expensive that the only people boarding aeroplanes will be the 20,000 climate change protestors regularly jetting off to their conferences.

Spectator sports are going to become television events and millions of sports fans will stay at home to watch their favourite teams. And so the depleted oil supplies will last longer.

If you want to know more about the oil shortage – and how it is going to affect our lives – you will find everything I know on the subject in my book *A Bigger Problem than Climate Change* – it's available on Amazon as a paperback and an eBook.

May 19th

We Are Breeding a Race of Psychos: Act Now to Stop the Politicians' Damaging, Deadly Lies

My wife, Antoinette, is the only person in our home who understands things which require electricity and therefore the only one capable of finding stuff on the internet.

This morning, Antoinette showed me several images which will haunt us both for years.

One photo showed schoolchildren in a playground, each child confined within a chalk square drawn on the ground. The children were not allowed to play with one another. They were not allowed to touch one another. They had to play games by themselves.

Solo marbles.

Try playing tag by yourself.

The quickest game in the history of playground sport.

No football. No cricket. No rounders. No racing around screeching for no apparent reason other than the fact that you have joy in your heart and energy to waste.

Another photo showed children in a classroom sitting yards apart from one another – each one wearing a mask and a plastic visor.

This is utter, utter madness. It is also wicked cruelty.

In the UK, it is alleged that if a child falls or has any sort of accident then they must not be helped by other children or by teachers.

The child who falls and grazes a knee will have to attend to it themselves.

The child who is so terrified that he or she has a leakage of some kind must deal with it alone.

No caring. No hugs.

Enough. The lunacy has gone far enough. Who in the name of all things holy thinks up these barbaric madnesses?

Has anyone in authority any idea of the permanent damage this will do to those poor children?

Children will be scarred for life by what has already happened to them. We are breeding a new race of weirdo, loner psychopaths.

Do teachers want to create a generation of uncaring psychos or are they doing it because they are ill informed and too lazy to look at the facts?

Teachers are educated people. They should care about the science.

A study by paediatricians could not find one case of a child passing on the coronavirus.

Not one.

One boy who did have the disease failed to give it to 170 people who were classified as contacts.

If teachers want to protect children from danger they would do better to insist that all children wear crash helmets in case meteors fall on their heads.

And then there are the adults.

I saw a picture of diners in a restaurant sitting in what looked like a small greenhouse. The waiter was passing them their food on a plank of some kind.

Professional footballers (whose risk of suffering any serious illness as a result of the coronavirus is minute) were delighted to be practising alone. Each one had half a pitch on which to practice. But they weren't allowed to pass the ball to anyone else.

And, if and when they play a match, they will be encouraged to look away when tackling.

The churches are still shut. That was the biggest abrogation of responsibility in history. I hope no one ever enters a church again. Put the well-paid bishops out on the street. Formal religion failed people when they needed it.

The dentists in the UK are still shut. Thousands of people with toothache are becoming addicted to opiates. That's great for the drug companies. Why the hell are the dentists shut? They wear masks, gloves and work in sterile conditions. My wife, who is bravely trying to retain a sense of humour said that if all her teeth fall out she can at least wear a mask to cover her mouth.

Councils are defying the Government and still keeping parks, public toilets and car parks shut so that people can't sunbathe or take exercise. Hasn't anyone told them about the need for vitamin D? That'll be another few hundred thousand sick people. Councillors work for us. It's not their country. It's our country. The councils will be broke next year and they'll put up taxes and blame the virus. But it's their fault. Not the virus.

There were tears in Antoinette's eyes as she told me about the agonies she'd read about: the children who don't understand and the patients in pain.

Our society is falling apart.

Antoinette and I went shopping.

There were only three shops open.

And it was a miserable, soul searing experience.

At one shop I was ordered to stay outside until another shopper had left. Not asked. Ordered. (You may be surprised to hear that I'm not good with being given orders.)

At the next I was shouted at for paying with cash.

And in the third I was screamed at by a youth with powerful jackboot tendencies, for failing to follow a one way system that would have foxed a maze designer. There was, incidentally, no one else except the two of us in the shop at the time.

All this is allegedly being done to 'save lives'.

Anyone who still believes this is all necessary is ill-informed or stark raving mad. Or both.

I can laugh at the pathetic diners and the even more pathetic footballers.

And we will do our shopping online.

But what the hell are we doing to our children?

How can we allow teachers to do this?

The wicked teachers who agree to draw chalk lines and putting down tape and inventing rules that would have embarrassed the Nazis, should all be sacked and permanently banned from any employment that involves people.

The madness has gone too far.

It has to stop.

Why do so many apparently intelligent people put up with all this garbage? What next? Will we be ordered to kill all the Jews, gays or just the people over 70? Why do so many people believe the lies they are told about the coronavirus? The worst and most dangerous lies aren't coming from conspiracy theorists – they are coming from governments.

Remember the evidence proves that in terms of mortality levels, the bloody coronavirus is less dangerous than a bad flu. Back in mid-March, in my first video, I described the coronavirus scare as the biggest hoax in history. I was right. Governments, for their own reasons, chose instead to treat mathematical modellers as though they were scientists instead of putting them where they belong – along with fortune tellers and economists.

I know YouTube wouldn't like me saying that because it's an inconvenient fact.

Remember: so far, in a season the coronavirus has killed less than half of the number the flu can kill in a season. If you don't believe me just look at the figures.

Check out the number of people alleged to have died worldwide from the coronavirus. At the moment that's about 300,000 alleged deaths. And then check out the number of people who can die worldwide from a bad flu. That's around 650,000.

You can suppress that truth but you can't ignore it.

If YouTube cared about their viewers they would suppress the politicians and the media and the mathematicians producing a constant stream of unjustifiable scare stories.

The problem, of course, is that governments want to keep us terrified and compliant and obedient. They don't want things to change. They are enjoying the power and are persisting with the biggest confidence trick in world history.

And as a direct result, people are dying in their tens of thousands – because they are being denied treatment.

So when will they re-open the hospitals and the dentists and the GP surgeries?

If they don't then everyone will have died of something else.

People are already pulling their own rotten teeth with the old string and doorknob trick.

I would not be surprised to hear that someone had removed their own appendix with a grapefruit spoon and a bread knife.

And prospective patients are now as nervous of hospitals as Parisian citizens were of the Hotel Dieu half a millennium ago.

The problem is that politicians want to keep social distancing and they will keep the lockdowns as a threat. It's working brilliantly for them. If we get too complacent they warn us of a second wave of the virus.

They warn the virus will last forever. They tell us we won't be safe until we have a damned vaccine and then admit that there may not be a vaccine for years.

Remember the only figure that really matters: the flu can kill 650,000 in a single season. And even governments now admit that their 'cure' is going to kill more people than the coronavirus.

There is only one solution.

Professionals everywhere have got to find the guts to stand up to the politicians and their crazy policies.

Doctors and nurses have got to find the balls to stand up, tell everyone the coronavirus crisis has been wildly oversold and announce that it is safe to open hospitals and surgeries and start to deal with the backlog of patients who will otherwise be dead by Christmas. Any health professional who doesn't do this will have blood on their hands and some difficult questions to answer in a year or two's time.

I believe responsible doctors and nurses will do that now if they care about their patients and their responsibilities.

Dentists should open their surgeries.

Teachers should insist on opening up schools that children can be taught again. No daft rules. No stupid chalk squares. No plastic visors.

Bishops and clergymen of every hue, collectively responsible for the greatest act of corporate cowardice in history, should open up all places of worship. Though to be honest they do not deserve to have any congregations after such a wanton act of abandonment.

Everyone has more power than they think. If doctors, nurses, teachers, dentists and so on threatened to resign then the politicians would have to back-peddle.

(I know that isn't easy but sometimes it's something that has to be done. For the record, I resigned from a job as a GP as a matter of principle. And I resigned as a columnist on principle.)

Dealing with this flu-like virus has distorted our priorities.

We have to stop this distortion before things become impossible to repair.

Those who disagree will doubtless say, 'Oh, but lives are at stake and breaking the lockdown and social distancing is too risky'.

But anyone who says this doesn't understand the facts and is missing the point. Not breaking the lockdown and not smashing the social distancing nonsense is far riskier, and will definitely result in far more deaths than the coronavirus will ever kill.

I absolutely agree that health takes priority.

But why are people who are dying of cancer or heart disease less important than people who might die of the coronavirus?

Thank you for reading. And my thanks to those who have given my wife and me your kind support.

And maybe the unkind individuals who prefer abuse and threats to rational, constructive thought and campaigning will one day realise just how much they have been manipulated by people who don't give a damn about anything other than power and control.

You can help by sharing the articles on www.vernoncoleman.com with as many people as you can. That's how we can stop this wicked, dangerous nonsense.

May 19th 2020

Mental Health Problems Will Now Soar

It's been pretty obvious for over two months that the mental health issues arising from the absurd and unnecessary global lockdown and social distancing policies will be unprecedented. There will be twin, genuine pandemics of anxiety and depression. Mental health problems will rise massively because of deliberate government policies.

It has also been clear from the start that the medical profession will be quite incapable of dealing with the massive demand for help.

The response of doctors will inevitably be to prescribe drugs such as tranquillisers, sedatives, hypnotics and anti-depressants which will do little or nothing to help the patients for whom they are prescribed but which will produce a mass of dangerous side effects including addiction and an increased risk of suicide.

So far so bad, but it gets worse.

I have been studying the effects of stress on human beings for nearly 50 years. My book *Stress Control* was published in 1978 and was the first mass market book to introduce the concept of stress as a factor in mental and physical health. At the time it was considered heretical and controversial to regard stress as having any influence whatsoever and one Professor of Medicine called for me to be struck off the medical register for daring to suggest that stress might have an effect on blood pressure.

As the days and weeks of this manufactured fake crisis have passed by, I have become increasingly convinced that what is happening is not a result of a combination of misjudgement, misfortune and incompetence but a result of manipulation and oppression.

I didn't come to this conclusion lightly. Whenever things go badly wrong it is always more likely to be a result of incompetence than of conspiracy in high places.

But the evidence in favour of a conspiracy is now irresistible.

Right from the start it has been clear that the coronavirus was not a new plague. Back in March, the UK's public health bodies concluded that the virus was not 'a high consequence infectious disease'.

And yet, just days after this, the UK Government introduced the most tyrannical bill ever passed by a British parliament – the 358-page Emergency Bill which took us back to pre Magna Carta days. King John himself would have been proud of Johnson's ruthless and unnecessary power grab. Unfortunately, we don't have a King Richard to ride to our rescue. Not even during the Black Death plague was so much power taken from the people. Our civil rights have disappeared and there is no sign of them returning. It is no exaggeration to say that many people in the world now live in police states.

Everything I have written to date has been proved right. Experts now agree that we should have done far more testing in March and that Ferguson (the mathematical modeller whose theories decided Government policy) had mistakenly exaggerated the risks. I am by no means the only person to realise that Ferguson's track record is appalling. His predictions seem to me as reliable as those of a fortune teller using an upturned goldfish bowl to guide her.

Ferguson's initial claim that 500,000 Britons would die of the coronavirus is still being quoted, even though the estimate has been discredited and the modelling questioned, to put it politely.

Much fuss is made of the fact that 300,000 people are now alleged to have died around the world. I doubt if many doctors still believe this figure for there is little doubt that it is a wildly exaggerated number. And though every one of those deaths is a tragedy the figure has to be put against the figure of 650,000 which is the number who can die of flu in a single season. Malaria can kill over 600,000 in a year without rolling up its sleeves and without anyone turning a hair. And tuberculosis recently killed 1,500,000 million people in a single year. I don't remember councils taping up park benches to protect us from that danger.

The UK Government's appalling record on testing puts it in 41st place in the world, far below Lithuania, Luxembourg and Cyprus. Several studies have suggested that a huge percentage of the population has already had the virus and that those people are, therefore, now immune. The Minister responsible for this failure should be looking for employment elsewhere.

There is also now widespread medical support for my contention that the lockdown was not only unnecessary and counter-productive in controlling the infection but also guaranteed to cause far more deaths and mayhem than the virus itself. In my book *Coming Apocalypse*, I have described the future we face and every day that passes produces yet more evidence that every forecast I made is going to come true.

Sadly, and rather worryingly, such views are however frequently suppressed or mocked in the mainstream media. YouTube banned three videos of mine which as far as I can see broke none of its guidelines.

I can only see two possible conclusions from all this.

The first is that the politicians and the Government's scientific and medical advisors are all stupid and I am brilliant.

The second is that there has been a conspiracy to exaggerate the danger of the coronavirus in order to grab power and damage our rights and freedoms.

I cannot see any other explanation.

Now, as much as I would like to accept the first conclusion, I am old enough and realistic enough to know it is not very likely.

The second conclusion is far more likely.

And once we accept that there is a conspiracy then all bets are off and we must re-examine everything that is happening.

And this takes us back to mental health and the coming twin pandemics of anxiety and depression which are going to do infinitely more harm than a pesky virus which has clearly done far less damage than some flu bugs.

And it quickly becomes apparent that governments have done everything possible to create more anxiety and exacerbate the incidence of depression.

Everything the Government in the UK has done has been designed to create loneliness and a sense of fear. The lockdowns and absurd social distancing policies were never necessary but are now destined to be part of our lives indefinitely. The threat that lockdowns will be reintroduced will be kept hovering over heads like the sword of Damocles. And we are told that social distancing policies must be maintained indefinitely in case this well-marketed virus reappears. When the lockdown rules were slightly relaxed in England on 20th May, a Government minister told the world that a son could meet his elderly parents if he met his father in the morning and his mother in the afternoon, but not together. And the meeting should take place out of doors and the participants should keep six feet apart. What the devil would they advise if the plague came back big-time?

Incidentally, why must people keep six feet apart? In some countries the required distance is three feet. And if social distancing were based on science then people would have to keep at least 24 feet apart because that is the distance that a cough or a sneeze might send an infection.

And so the fear will be maintained. The screw will be kept tightly turned.

Millions are already so terrified that they hardly dare leave their homes. It is a bizarre new variation of cabin fever.

Closing hospitals, GPs surgeries, dental surgeries and so on has added a new fear. Those who are already ill are suffering agonies as they wait for treatment. Those who are not ill are terrified that help will not be available if they need it. Around the world, 28 million surgical operations have already been cancelled or postponed, and every week that the disruption lasts will result in another 2.4 million cancellations. The UK has built ten brand new, huge and expensive hospitals for dealing with the coronavirus but only two have ever been used. The NHS has 100,000 acute medical beds. Around 40,000 of those lie empty. The number of people visiting A&E departments has fallen by more than half because people are terrified to leave their homes even when they need medical attention.

You can see the effect of the social distancing policies if you walk down the street or enter one of the few shops allowed to open. Many people step aside with terror in their eyes. They cover their mouths and turn away. We are being taught to regard our neighbours as angels of death. We are creating a world in which enjoyment will be just a memory.

I read somewhere that the coronavirus 'crisis' will result in people being kinder to one another.

I have rarely read such nonsense.

This fake 'crisis' will lead to ever more suspicions, fears, distrust, resentment and clinical anxiety.

I have previously pointed out that school-children, teenagers and people in their 20s will suffer most.

Cruel school and college distancing policies will inevitably lead to generations of young people suffering serious psychological problems. We are breeding lonely, frightened people. Many will become very seriously mentally ill; dangerously withdrawn and unhinged.

And all the time, politicians and advisors around the world are creating ever more fear by exaggerating the risks, by withdrawing promise and regularly contradicting one another so that confusion is created. In the UK, we had the absurd sight of a senior minister suggesting that a son who wishes to meet his parents should meet his father in the morning and his mother in the afternoon. Moreover the meeting should take place out of doors and the participants should remain a six foot distance apart.

We are told that there will be no summer holidays (though if we behave ourselves we may have an extra bank holiday in the autumn) and no sporting events except on television.

And so we are denied the chance of brightening our lives with events to which we can look forward. No dinners, no celebrations, no big matches and no trips. In the unlikely event that hotels, restaurants and pubs survive the social distancing rules, visiting them will be about as much fun as root canal surgery.

And just in case we allow ourselves a glimmer of hope for the future, we are warned of massive tax rises, shattered pensions, penury and joblessness lasting for decades. We are told that even if the virus goes away it might return or mutate. There is much threatening, scary talk of the 'second wave'. We are warned, quite bizarrely in my view, that we may be able to catch the disease more than once and so no one will ever be safe. (Curiously, however, it is said that magic vaccines will be prepared which will provide protection. Indeed, we have been told that a vaccine will be available within months though it usually takes years to create a vaccine.)

So, why have they done all this?

They couldn't possibly have been as incompetent as they appear to be so there has to be a reason.

It's power. We live in a police state. We have no control over our lives. And power brings money.

And a menu of hidden agendas – population control, preserving the oil supplies, replacing cash with plastic cards which can be regulated, and, of course, as I predicted in my very first video back in the middle of March, demonising and marginalising the elderly.

May 21st 2020

The Only Shops Which Will Survive…

Antoinette and I went shopping the other day.

When I say that we went shopping that is something of an exaggeration.

We visited a garden centre, a supermarket, a newsagent, a pharmacy and a greengrocer.

Nothing else was open.

It wasn't a great deal of fun.

We were shouted at by several shop assistants (in some cases more than once).

'Don't go that way!'

'You can't come in here until someone leaves.'

'Move back!

'You have to follow the arrows.'

'We don't take cash.'

It was a miserable experience.

In future we will do as much shopping as we can online.

It's quicker and less painful. And often cheaper too.

I realise that shop assistants have been scared witless by the Government's constant threats. I understand that.

But you can't shout at customers, or treat them like prisoners, and expect them to return.

I fear that in the short-term, the only shops which will survive the manufactured coronavirus 'crisis' will be the shops which make shopping a special, pleasant experience.

And for the medium and long-term, shops and shoppers need to campaign to push governments to abandon social distancing laws which will destroy our society if they are maintained. We don't have social distancing to protect us from the flu, which can kill more people than the coronavirus. And we don't have social distancing to protect us from other killer diseases such as tuberculosis – which kills far more people than the coronavirus.

The way things are going at the moment, Mr Bezos is going to own the world within a few months.

May 23rd 2020

Passing Observations (May 23rd 2020)

For some years I included on my website a series of pieces called Passing Observations in which I detailed items which seemed worth a short mention – but not a longer article.

I saw a photo the other day of a barman wearing a mask over his mouth. The mask did not, however, cover his nose. Wearing a mask that covers one aperture but not the other is utterly pointless – and does more harm than good in that it probably gives the wearer a completely false sense of security. Incidentally, I wonder if people in nudist camps and on nude beaches will wear masks and gloves.

Governments have been so effective at terrifying populations that it will take a good deal of work to persuade people to leave their homes and start returning to a new variety of normal life. But do governments actually want people to leave their homes? Moot point.

England has the highest population density of any country in Europe. Mass immigration, constantly under-estimated by the Home Office, and resulting from absurd and onerous EU laws, has caused massive overcrowding in towns and cities. Overcrowding is a well-known factor in the spread of many types of physical and mental disorders including, of course, infectious diseases.

By insisting on ignoring the UK Government's laws about lockdown, the leaders of the toy parliaments in Scotland and Wales may have pleased the bureaucrats in Brussels but they have caused confusion and bewilderment. In refusing to allow English citizens to cross their borders they are guilty of blatant racism – which will be remembered long after the coronavirus 'crisis' is over.

Regular readers will know that I believe that the BBC is a treacherous organisation. Despite the grave situation in Britain, the BBC is still sending out threatening letters to those who haven't paid its wretched annual licence fee. The default position of the BBC seems to me to be that anyone who hasn't paid the licence must be guilty of a criminal offence – even if they don't need or want a licence. Even if a citizen tells the BBC they don't need a licence, the organisation's 'gestapo' will still threaten to come round to check that they aren't watching television. I ignore the BBC's letters since I do not have to reply, and if their goons turn up on our doorstep I do not have to let them in. The BBC gets enough money from the EU – it's not getting any of ours.

After YouTube had taken down my video entitled 'Why did YouTube Ban my Video?' I protested that the video did not infringe any of their guidelines. YouTube then restored the video. However, YouTube has still banned two more of my videos – even though these did not appear to break any of their published regulations.

The National Education Union (a misnamed organisation if ever I found one) is opposing the reopening of schools and is also opposing remote learning for primary school pupils over the internet. The organisation is offering advice to teachers on how to sue schools that are 'too keen' to reopen the doors. My contempt for this organisation and its officers and members is almost tangible.

People who live in rural and seaside areas are complaining about town-dwellers being allowed to visit for the day. They want car parks kept locked and public loos kept closed so that no one can walk along their lanes or sit on their beaches. The police are busy slapping penalty notices on cars which are parked near to pleasant places. 'Having no visitors and holidaymakers here has been wonderful for six weeks,' said one aggrieved local. But Antoinette and I are well aware that allowing visitors to share the landscape is a price that those who live in pleasant parts of the country have to pay for being lucky enough to live in beautiful places. Heavy traffic and badly parked cars can be annoying but it's the cost of living. The resentment of would-be visitors will be massive and when holiday areas are reopened many will remember how they were treated. Many rural and seaside towns rely on visitors. In future they will, I fear, have to find some other way to make a living. Good luck to them.

The Times newspaper estimates that denying people access to healthcare has already killed a similar number of people to the number killed from Covid-19. The death rate from the latter will almost certainly fall. The death rate from the former will certainly rise.

Just two of us research, write and produce the articles and videos which carry my name. Half of the work is done by my wife, Antoinette, who in addition to researching and editing material is also entirely responsible for doing everything which requires electricity. I write out much of the material in longhand on large writing pads. And from then on it's Antoinette who is responsible for fighting the hardware and software in order to publish the material. I would also like to point out that taking on the establishment isn't an easy or risk-free business – it can be worrying to wonder if the men in boots are going to come and kick down the door or pop a summons in the post.

And Antoinette shares those worries too. Ginger Rogers once said that she had to do all the dance steps with which Fred Astaire dazzled us all but that she had to do them all backwards in high heels. Antoinette has to do all this in constant pain because her cancer treatment has left her with pain which cannot be treated because the hospitals in England are cruelly closed to everyone who isn't a coronavirus sufferer. I am not a great lover of the NHS at the moment and I have not been clapping on Thursdays.

May 23rd 2020

There Is No Science Behind Social Distancing

The theory behind social distancing is that it will protect people from other folk who sneeze or cough. The lunatics who are currently running the asylum say that we will have to maintain social distancing forever.

Forever.

Really. That's what they've been saying.

But there isn't any science to it.

In some countries people have to keep three feet apart. In others they must keep four and a half feet apart. In Britain adults and children are told they must keep six feet apart. The latest rule in Britain is that two people can meet one person but one person cannot meet two people. I've thought about that a lot and I don't think I'm completely potty just yet but I can't get my head round it.

Two people can meet one person but one person cannot meet two people.

That's the law. And it is, quite possibly, the most completely stupid piece of advice ever given to anyone anywhere. But if you break the law you can be fined. I've no idea how much. I'm still too busy trying to work out how the law works to care what the fine is.

There is no uniformity to the rules between countries because they are just made up by people who think they are a good idea.

Our lives are being regulated and destroyed by rules which somebody somewhere thought were a good idea.

Forcing us to stay in our homes is also something that was just made up.

And it's pretty clear that the authorities – the people who dreamt up the rules and who insist that we follow them – don't bother to take much notice of them.

I've lost count of the number of senior public figures who have been caught flouting the rules. They always have a good excuse, of course. But then we all have good excuses for flouting the rules.

Am I the only one to have noticed that the police don't seem to take much notice of the social distancing rules when they are out hunting for people who are sunbathing or sitting on park benches?

And when the police attend demonstrations against the lockdown, they completely ignore the social distancing rules – standing close to one another and then getting very hands on with demonstrators.

The police are certainly breaking the social distancing laws when they arrest people.

So why should the police not arrest themselves?

Or maybe the demonstrators could arrest the police for breaking the social distancing laws.

Apart from the massive social and economic implications, there is of course one big problem with the social distancing rules.

A sneeze doesn't stop at three feet or four and a half feet or six feet. And nor does a cough.

A cough can spread droplets for 18 feet. And a sneeze can travel 24 feet.

So these social distancing rules are arbitrary and utterly pointless.

If we were going to have effective social distancing then we would all have to keep at least 24 feet apart – preferably 30 feet apart.

But that would bring the world to a complete standstill, everyone would go bankrupt, no one would ever be able to buy any food and we would all starve to death.

How many people can you get in a bus or a railway carriage if everyone has to be 30 feet from everyone else? If there's a driver on a bus the passenger will have to run behind.

So they made up these lower figures.

And even these figures are destroying lives and will destroy businesses and everything which makes our world good.

Social distancing forces friends to shout to one another and prevents grannies hugging their grandkids. Social distancing makes people fearful. It breeds distrust, suspicion and even hatred. Passers-by step to one side and walk on the road if they see someone coming towards them. Social distancing will prevent meetings and demonstrations.

It is difficult to think of a business which won't be adversely affected by social distancing. Restaurants are told they will have to throw out three quarters of their tables and then try to make a profit. How many waiters can serve food from six feet away? A bowl of tomato soup will cost £200. Airlines have been told that they have to throw out a third of their seats, and airline bosses have pointed out that if they do that then they will never be able to fly again. Hairdressers will need to use scissors that are two yards long. Sports arenas can only seat people if they have six feet of space all around them. Cinemas and theatres will have to close off most of their seating. Most commercial kitchens will only be able to accommodate only one chef. Who is going to tell the bloke in the big white hat that he has to do all the washing up?

Hotels are doomed by social distancing.

Can you imagine trying to get back to your room after breakfast?

'I'm afraid there is a one hour queue for the lift, sir. We're only allowed to put two people into one lift. And when sharing a lift you must both face the walls.'

I sense that the people who made up the social distancing rules are beginning to weaken.

The sensible solution is to push our so-called leaders into forgetting about social distancing laws.

When they know that we don't believe their lies and that we do know what is going on – and how they are trying to take over our lives with their power grabbing emergency legislation – then they will back off. They want to stay in power and if we shout long enough, loud enough and hard enough then they will listen.

And to encourage old-fashioned good manners; to encourage everyone to cover their mouths and noses if they sneeze or cough. That'll protect us all against all the diseases which can be transmitted this way.

If we do these simple things we can go back to living ordinary lives. We can eat out, watch live sports and talk to people we meet without having to shout at them.

If we must have laws to control our behaviour then introduce a law which says that if you don't cover your mouth and nose when you sneeze then you will be punished.

And we must have a punishment for breaking the law, bring back the stocks that were popular in England a few hundred years ago. People who don't cover their mouths and noses will be sentenced to 24 hours in the stocks where the rest of us can stand and throw rotten fruit and vegetables at them.

Oh, and tell local authorities to install more public loos with decent hand washing facilities. One of the most insane things done during the last few weeks has been to close public loos. The people who decided to do that should be put in the stocks too.

May 24th 2020

You've Been Brainwashed (Here's How They Did It)

Governments have been using a range of Orwellian mind control tricks during the coronavirus 'crisis'. The slogans, the clapping and the symbols have all been carefully used to enable the authorities to take control of our thinking.

I am grateful to Dr Colin Barron, a former NHS doctor and eminent hypnotherapist who is the author of the book *Practical Hypnotherapy*, for pointing out to me just how our minds have been taken over and how we have been very successfully and skilfully manipulated into believing the lies we have been fed.

Elected governments, aided by specialist behavioural scientists, have been brainwashing millions into accepting the coronavirus propaganda. The mind is a wonderful thing. It responds in sometimes unpredictable ways. So, for example, if you see a headline which says: 'Boris Johnson is an alien' then most people will probably dismiss it quite readily. But if the headline says 'Is Boris Johnson an alien?' readers will be more likely to suspect that the British Prime Minister might indeed be from another planet. And research shows that if people see a headline which says, 'Boris Johnson is NOT an alien' then their suspicions will be raised still higher.

Manipulating and tricking the mind is a professional business.

You've been brainwashed and the brainwashing has been very subtle. We've all been quietly hypnotised and indoctrinated to accept the new mass hysteria generated by governments everywhere. Many people now enjoy the lockdown and don't want it to end. It enables them to avoid responsibility for their own lives.

Do you remember who said: 'Through clever and constant application of propaganda people can be made to see paradise as hell and also the other way round, to consider the most wretched life as paradise.'?

It was Adolf Hitler, who was a master at mass manipulation and the use of subliminal techniques. And it was Hitler who also commented that it was good fortune for governments that the mass of people did not think.

The Nazis were very good at controlling people's minds.

Goebbels, who was Hitler's propaganda chief, once said that if you repeat a lie often enough then people will believe it. He also pointed out that if you want to control a population and you have to deal with opposition then you should accuse the other side of the sin or the trickery which you yourself are using.

So, governments everywhere have been accusing those who are telling the truth of spreading fake news. Anyone who doesn't toe the party line is dismissed as a dangerous conspiracy theorist – though the big conspiracies have all been coming from governments.

Countries around the world have been promoting slogans to persuade their citizens to behave as required. In China there was a slogan which said 'If you love your parents, lock them up'. In Taiwan people were told: 'To visit each other is to kill each other'.

At first glance the slogans which are heavily advertised in the UK seem harmless enough. We all recognise them.

Some such as 'We're all in this together' seem fairly innocuous, though we might all be forgiven for adding the rider that we are all in this together unless we work as advisors to the Prime Minister.

The first trio of phrases which were promoted everywhere were:

Keep your distance

Wash your hands

And

Think of others

More recently new phrases have been added to the repertoire:

Stay home

Save lives

Protect the NHS

The rhythm and pattern used in these phrases is not a coincidence. There are usually three words in each phrase and the phrases run in threes. This isn't a coincidence; it isn't happenchance.

Using phrases of three words, presented in groups of three, is a technique known as the rule of three in psychological conditioning. And that's the reason for the three phrases with which we are all being bombarded. We've being trained and taught at the same time. It's behavioural psychology.

Other hypnotherapists have pointed out that if we repeat phrases often enough then the words and thoughts become implanted in our subconscious minds and then become a belief which motivates our behaviour. And so governments repeat slogans which become beliefs. It's called auto suggestion – along the lines of 'every day in every way I am getting better and better'.

Hitler was also a believer that if a lie was repeated often enough it would eventually be confused with the truth by the greater part of the population.

'People more readily fall victim to the big lie than the small lie,' said Hitler, 'since it would never come into their heads to fabricate colossal untruths, and they would not believe that others could have the impudence to distort the truth so infamously.'

Hitler used these techniques to control and manipulate the German people and to persuade them to accept the evil things he wanted them to do.

George Orwell who invented Newspeak, also understand the importance of the triple three word phrase. In 1984, his futuristic novel which was written in 1948, Orwell invented the slogan: 'War is peace, freedom is slavery, ignorance is strength'.

If you want a picture of the future, wrote Orwell, imagine a boot stamping on a human face – forever. Power, he reminded us, is not a means, it is an end.

Everything else that has been happening since February 2020 is part of the brainwashing process.

It has been noticeable that the instructions we have been given have been more like orders. The signs that have popped up like dandelions say Stand here, not Please stand here. And why not? You don't say 'Please' to prisoners do you?

And then there are the weeks of clapping for carers and medical staff. Clapping, which probably started innocently and with good intentions, covers up the paradox – the quiet insistent terror that comes from knowing that for all practical purposes there is no health care and we have all been betrayed by politicians and bureaucrats who decided to devote entire health care programmes to caring for a relatively small number of patients who have, or might be thought to have or be susceptible to a flu like virus.

Dr Milton Erickson, an eminent hypnotist, used to give his patients simple tasks to do. He would send them home to clean the attic or count the books they owned. All this was done as part of the process of mind control. Telling people to stand on their doorsteps at 8 p.m. on Thursdays and to clap is a simple, repetitive task which is part of the mass hypnosis. The clapping may have started out innocently but it was quickly and enthusiastically promoted by the people influencing our lives.

Persuading people to do what you want them to do is part of the hypnotherapy process. Getting people to clap was also important in that it made people believe in the danger of the coronavirus and the bravery of those working in health care. It helped people accept the fact that there were no beds available for patients with cancer or any other disorder.

The rainbow which has suddenly started to appear everywhere is another part of the brainwashing process. Thousands have been so successfully brainwashed that they willingly take part in promoting the symbols and the slogans.

Even the confusing rules about who we can and cannot see were part of the programme. A minister recently told Britons that two people could meet one person but that one person could not meet two people. An obvious contradictory nonsense.

If you confuse and bewilder at the same time that you are frightening people then you unsettle them and create an anxious and obedient population.

And that is what has been going on for weeks.

Bearing all this in mind I have prepared my own triple phrased slogan. Three words and three phrases:

Distrust the government

Avoid mass media

Fight the lies

My slogans fit the brainwashing requirement perfectly. Simple, effective, honest.

So try to remember them: Distrust the government. Avoid mass media. Fight the lies

May 26th 2020

Patients Who Have Been Betrayed

I have absolutely no doubt that all around the world people have been betrayed by their politicians. Whether you think they have done it deliberately or through incompetence there can be no doubt that they have turned a health threat that has so far killed far fewer people than a bad flu into the biggest health, economic and social crisis that the modern world has ever seen.

But that's no great surprise. We expect politicians to let us down. They are selfish and they always betray the electors. It's the only thing they're any good at. No group of people in the world are quite as corrupt or as mendacious as politicians.

I am, however, surprised and massively saddened by the way we have been betrayed by people we might have expected to protect us – the leaders of three professions: the medical profession, the nursing profession and the dental profession. And it is the leaders I blame – the medical establishment.

These professions seem to have abandoned anyone not suffering from the coronavirus.

Around the world there is no consistency. In some areas hospitals are shut entirely. In other areas hospitals are open and even functioning fairly normally. In some countries patients who don't have the coronavirus, or might not have the coronavirus, are completely ignored and rejected as irrelevant and unsuitable for treatment. There is no science or logic behind the closures and the refusal of hospitals and medical centres to treat patients.

Lockdowns and social distancing rules have been imposed without much sense. It is now fairly widely known that most of the people who have died from the virus, or have been ill with it, were obese or diabetic or both, and many had more than three chronic diseases. The UK's Prime Minister probably suffered badly from the coronavirus because of his weight.

So why haven't governments selectively protected the individuals most likely to be at risk? As I said back in early March it was nonsense to pick on perfectly fit over 70-year-olds to be the first to be put under house arrest.

The current treatment of patients with cancer, heart disease and other dangerous but treatable diseases is a grotesque scandal which has taken health care back to the Middle Ages. Patients, doctors and nurses have all been betrayed by the profession's leaders and by their governments and governmental advisors. Mental health problems are growing too. In California, a hospital has reported that it has seen a year's worth of suicide attempts in just four weeks.

It's the same with dentistry.

In some countries, people with dental problems are being treated normally. I gather that in Ireland and Germany, for example, at least some dentists are providing treatment. In America there seems to be some confusion about what is and is not allowed. In Britain, there is virtually no dental care available – even though most dentists say they are well-equipped with the necessary masks and gloves. Many dentists, particularly those in private practice are desperate to get back to work. Dentists working for the Government may still get paid but private dentists are receiving nothing, and their insurance policies are probably not any good. Many dentists warn they will go bankrupt and are desperate to get back to seeing patients.

Strangely, in the UK, it seems that no one within the dental profession itself has the authority to force dentists not to work. The General Dental Council says it cannot force dentists to close, and the Care Quality Commission also says it cannot force dentists to refuse to see patients. But dentists are closed because they are worried about the Government's general lockdown and social distancing rules – and there will inevitably be legal worries too.

There is, it is said, some sporadic emergency dental treatment available in some areas but I have seen reports suggesting that the only service available is the removal of teeth – rather than attempts being made to keep teeth in place.

All this could go on indefinitely.

How the devil do you ever fill a bad tooth from six feet away? And although dentists and dental nurses can all wear masks it's a little difficult for a dental patient to keep a mask on while having treatment. Meanwhile, millions of patients are missing essential dental work. Many are in agony and are desperate for relief. Hundreds of cases of mouth cancer will be missed. Patients with gum disease who need regular work to keep their mouths healthy will lose teeth that they didn't need to lose.

All of this is a tragedy and a scandal unlike any other.

The leaders of the medical profession and the dental profession aren't doing anywhere near enough to end this appalling state of affairs.

At least I don't feel quite so lonely these days.

Five hundred brave doctors in the United States agree with me and have told Donald Trump to end the coronavirus shutdown for the reasons I have explained.

The bottom line is that patients who think they might have cancer aren't being treated, even though everyone with a basic diploma in emptying bed pans knows that speed is of the essence when treating cancer. That's why doctors arrange screening programmes, for heaven's sake. Patients who had the first signs of cancer three months ago will, whatever happens, have to wait another three, four, five or six months for treatment – while the system catches up with the backlog. My wife has breast cancer. Last year she had surgery and radiotherapy and now she has constant pain in her shoulder. It is a common consequence of the treatment and it can be treated with physiotherapy. But the hospital physiotherapy departments are shut so she struggles to do exercises which don't make much difference. She is also due to have another mammogram. But she hasn't heard a word from the hospital about that. And we cannot get the physiotherapy or the mammogram done privately because the Government has commandeered all the private hospitals just in case it needs them for coronavirus patients. It hasn't needed the hospitals because the predictions made by the mathematical modellers were absurdly pessimistic, and so the hospitals are empty and the staff don't have anything to do except on Thursday evenings when they lighten their week with a little brisk clapping to congratulate their colleagues in the health service – who also have relatively little to do because the Government admits that most of the hospitals in Britain are half empty. If you detect a slightly bitter note in all this then give yourself full marks. I am angrier than I have ever been. And I am incredibly disappointed with the way patients have been betrayed.

A friend of ours who was diagnosed with cancer a few months ago is still waiting for her treatment to start. Meanwhile her cancer, unhindered, is undoubtedly doing what cancer does best. It's growing unhindered.

My wife found this on the internet:

'My cancer treatment has been cancelled and interrupted throughout this pandemic. I have found it hard as the nurses allocated to advise and offer support have been redeployed onto empty covid wards and so are unavailable to cancer patients. I have felt quite alone and unimportant compared to virus sufferers.'

How can anyone not be angry?

What the hell is going on?

Are governments trying to kill people? Is this some crude population control plan?

It's not as if the problem is unrecognised.

Governments have admitted that thousands and thousands of patients will die because they are being denied treatment. In the UK it has been admitted that the closure of health services could lead to 150,000 deaths – far, far more than will ever die from the coronavirus. I think that figure is a massive underestimate. The figures show that so far 60,000 people have died unnecessarily in the UK because they have been denied treatment. That's in the UK alone and it is a far, far higher figure than the number of coronavirus deaths. Why, in the name of everything holy, do those deaths matter less than coronavirus deaths? The majority of people who died from the coronavirus are over 80-years-old and seriously ill with other diseases. They would, it is admitted, have died within a few months anyway. This is exactly the same sort of way that flu usually kills so many people. But the patients with cancer being denied treatment are often otherwise healthy and frequently quite young.

Around the world tens of millions of operations have already been cancelled and millions more get cancelled every week. All operations are essential, some more so than others. With the possible exception of some cosmetic surgery, no one has an operation they don't really need. Screening tests and investigations have also been abandoned and delayed. Patients with symptoms and signs of serious disease have been told they will have to wait months to find out if their problems are likely to kill them or are benign. In such situations the waiting is almost unbearable. Only those who know the awful pain of waiting for test results will understand just how terrible the situation is at the moment.

Moreover, doctors now report that vast numbers of patients have been so terrified by their government's hysterical over-reaction to the risk that they won't go near a hospital in case they catch the coronavirus bug and die of that. Even when medical care is available patients prefer to do nothing. And that problem is likely to persist unless the hysteria is reversed.

At the end of World War II, the concentration camp guards who had done appalling things in places like Dachau and Auschwitz. People who had closed their eyes to what was happening were also arrested. They were all taken to the War Crimes Tribunal and almost to a man and woman their defence was that they were just doing what they were told to do. The excuse didn't get them anywhere, of course.

The medical administrators and the leaders of the professions may think they are immune from criticism because they are obeying orders from their governments.

But I'm afraid they are not.

And they aren't innocent in moral or ethical terms either.

The senior bureaucrats who have ordered that hospitals and GPs and dentists close down are all guilty of a crime against humanity.

Indeed, the irony is that not even the bureaucrats, the politicians and the civil servants appear to believe that the coronavirus is any more dangerous than a bad flu.

Time and time again, in recent weeks we have seen people who've been telling us that we must stay in our homes ignoring their own advice. Ferguson, whose now widely disputed advice led to the lockdown, allowed his mistress to visit him at home. The Prime Minister's closest advisor, Dominic Cummings, travelled more than two hundred miles, and back again, at the beginning of the lockdown. When there were calls for him to resign or be fired, the Prime Minister defended him – appearing to many to make a mockery of the law and of the sacrifices made by millions of people who all had their own very good reasons to break the lockdown but didn't dare do so. The Irish prime minister – having a picnic with friends in a public park.

Thinking folk will inevitably suspect that if these people broke the rules in such a cavalier way then they probably didn't think we are dealing with the plague.

Doctors do have one weapon that they could use.

They could certify their own leaders and the bureaucrats and the politicians insane and incapable. Those individuals could then be removed from their positions and we could get back to a more caring world. It's a rather off the wall solution. But then we're hardly living in normal times, are we?

May 26th 2020

Passing Observations (May 26th 2020)

I can pretty well guarantee that the 'temporary' powers the Government has given itself (and the police) will turn out to be permanent. When Governments grab power they tend to hang onto them. As Milton Friedman once observed 'nothing is as permanent as a temporary Government programme'. In the UK, one former Supreme Court Judge, is reported to have talked about 'collective hysteria' and to have used the phrase 'police state'.

The Government knows where all pensioners live but, despite having forbidden relatives or friends to visit them, has made no effort to ensure that the elderly are receiving food supplies. How many old people will starve to death? How many dead bodies will be found behind locked doors?

Some pathologists have decreed that dead patients who have the coronavirus must now be cremated without examination. I've seen a briefing which states: 'If a death is believed to be due to confirmed covid-19 infection there is unlikely to be any need for a post-mortem examination to be conducted and the Medical Certificate of Cause of Death should be issued'. The key word here is surely 'believed'.

In the UK, shops are due to open in June. There is talk that people will be reluctant to go back to the High Street because they are too frightened of the coronavirus. This is partly true. But it is part of the propaganda. (Encouraging us to remain fearful.) The truth is that shopping is going to be a miserable experience. And the closure of many public loos will make shopping impossible and impractical for many people – especially the elderly and those with children. (Remember that back at the beginning of March I predicted that part of the plan was to marginalise the elderly? Well closing public loos is part of that.)

The BBC Director General, speaking on a BBC programme which was reported on the BBC website, claims that 94% of the population accessed a bit of the BBC in the 3rd week of March. We can assume that this was their best week and, of course, I am sceptical of anything the BBC says about anything, but it is worrying that anyone still uses the BBC. I hope no one relies on the BBC for news. The woman along the way with the curlers and the pinafore provides a much more reliable source of news than the BBC.

The United Nations estimates that worldwide 25 million jobs will be lost as a result of the coronavirus. Some claim the figure could be as high as 190 million. Actually, virtually no jobs will be lost because of the virus. It's the lockdowns and social distancing which will cause the job losses.

Every fact I have provided has been absolutely accurate. Every prediction I've made has been proven accurate. So why don't the authorities admit that they got it wrong? Even if they wanted to do so the scientists, the politicians and the media are now wedded to this deceit. Even if they wanted to, how could they possibly admit that they got it all so very, very wrong?

By exaggerating the number of deaths, the authorities are endangering us all. You cannot investigate a disease when you don't keep proper records. As the weeks pass by we should be able to learn a good deal about this coronavirus. But we won't be able to do any useful research because we don't know who really died from it and who died from something else. We can't work out whether the disease mostly affects people who are meat eaters, or who have been vaccinated against the flu or who have red hair because the information we have is inaccurate and useless.

The UK Government has admitted that the NHS has 2,295 empty intensive care beds. The average number of empty intensive care beds before the coronavirus 'crisis' was 800. So, the NHS has 1,495 more empty intensive care beds during the coronavirus 'crisis' than it had before the so-called 'crisis' began. And it has been reported that almost half the beds in some English hospitals are lying empty.

It is difficult to take the lockdown laws seriously when so many senior figures seem to take little or no notice of them – or bend them to suit their 'special' circumstances. Could it possibly be because those senior figures know the truth about the danger of the coronavirus?

The Government in the UK admits that 60,000 people have now died unnecessarily because health care has been devoted to the coronavirus. That figure will soar. As I predicted many weeks ago, it will continue to rise. It is crucial that hospitals are opened up to everyone who needs help.

May 26th 2020

The End for NHS Dentistry?

I don't usually bother with rumours but this one could be important.
I've heard that in the UK, the Government is going to force dentists to
see no more than one patient an hour. There is no logical reason for
this but logic plays no part in anything these days (and 'science' is just
an old-fashioned word which is now entirely irrelevant as far as our
'leaders' are concerned).
If this rumour is true (and I think it could be) then it will destroy NHS
dentistry.
Dentists working in the NHS don't get paid much per patient and so
rely on numbers. They need a lot of patients to make a living.
If a dentist is only allowed to see one patient an hour then private
dentists will probably cope (though I suspect many will have to put up
their prices).
But there will be no more dentistry within the NHS.
The Government will say it was simply saving lives.
And it will blame dentists for quitting the NHS.
But the end result will be no more NHS dentistry.
And those who cannot afford private dentistry will be left with no
dental care at all.
Was this all part of the mad, indefensible lockdown and social
distancing strategies?

May 27th 2020

Passing Observations (May 27th 2020)

Opticians are closed, of course. So millions of people will be suffering enormously. And what about motorists who need eye tests in order to retain their licences? No one in government cares. What about patients with developing eye problems? No one in government cares about them, either. Cataracts, glaucoma and macular degeneration will all go undiagnosed. Will this lunacy ever end?

Dominic Cummings was supposed to be the brains of the Conservative Party. He is, it was said, the man who understands what the public wants. I read that he was able to manage public opinion. Really? If he is the best brain the Conservatives have then heaven help us all. His absurdly arrogant behaviour has destroyed the British Government's lockdown policies (not a bad thing, so thanks to him for that), split the Conservative party (serves them right for employing him), wrecked the Prime Minister's credibility and lost any reputation he had himself. Brilliant. Not bad for a highly paid advisor who was supposed to work behind the scenes and help the Prime Minister run things. If the fellow had integrity, self-respect or respect for his employer he would have resigned ages ago. If he was employed in the private sector I suspect he would have been fired for arrogance, incompetence and simple, old-fashioned stupidity. But he's a sort of uncivil servant so what can we expect?

Attempts are constantly being made to 'monster' Sweden and to fake the Swedish mortality figures. The problem for the UK and other countries is that Sweden hasn't really had a lockdown. The Government there trusted the people to behave sensibly. And the death rate has been a fraction of the death rate in the UK. Britain's aggressive lockdown and social distancing policies have been an utter disaster. And the utterly pathetic Boris Johnson will be remembered for having got just about everything wrong. If he hadn't contracted the bug himself and then had a child with his mistress he would by now be as popular as Corbyn used to be. The Buffoon Boris is surviving only on public sympathy.

Big energy companies are now banning customers from joining their cheapest deals unless they have smart meters fitted. That suggests to me that smart meters are 'good' for big energy companies. And we already know they are good for the Government – because smart meters enable the authorities to turn your supply on and off when they feel like it. Smart meters certainly aren't much good for customers! The inconvenience and disruption simply isn't worthwhile. As we all lose all trust in the Government, it is important to stay alert. We won't be letting the energy company install a smart meter.

We acquire our immunity to a whole range of minor infections through being in daily contact with other people. Being in contact with many infections keeps our immune systems in tip top condition. When groups of people are isolated they become dangerously vulnerable to infections. And so forcing millions of people to stay under house arrest for considerable periods of time will make them very vulnerable to infections of many kinds when (or perhaps that should be 'if') their isolation ends. This is well known to everyone except governments around the world and their highly paid scientific and medical advisors who seem to have a combined IQ of 11.7 when the wind is blowing in the right direction, and who either don't know this simple truth – or don't care.

Much is being made of the claim that 100,000 people are alleged to have died of the coronavirus in America. Might I suggest that those who find this figure (which is generally agreed by doctors to be a wild exaggeration) a good reason for the lockdowns and social distancing, take a look at the number of people who died in America last year of the flu (the figure for which is generally agreed to be accurate).

It seems that in the UK, the Government is planning to allow hairdressers to open before dentists. Both lots of workers get up close and personal with their patients. But dentists work in sterile surroundings and are well accustomed to wearing masks, gloves and so on. So, what is going on? I believe this is all a deliberate attempt to destroy NHS dentistry – and save huge amounts of money. (See the piece about NHS dentistry on this website.)

In order to satisfy social distancing requirements there are plans to widen pavements everywhere. The cost of this will, of course, be phenomenal. But the side effect will be to make roads narrower and, inevitably, to make all sorts of motorised travel (cars, lorries, etc.) even more difficult. And so less oil will be used. There is no doubt that all this is part of the plan to save our rapidly diminishing stocks of oil. (If you want to know more about what is happening I suggest you read my book, *A Bigger Problem than Climate Change* which is available on Amazon.)

On 27th May the EU announced that they would be putting together a recovery fund of 750 billion euros. This was widely reported by newspapers and TV. In my book, *Coming Apocalypse* (published in April) I suggested, in the March 14th entry, that the EU would need to raise £700 billion. (The truth, I am afraid, is that my keyboard doesn't have the sign for a euro and so I put my estimate down in sterling. Still, pretty close.)

I now think it was a pity Jeremy Corbyn didn't win the last election in the UK. We would have had a communist government but I don't think it would have been quite so communist as the government we've been given by Comrade Boris.

I'm not surprised to see China getting heavy with Hong Kong. Nor, indeed, will the readers of my book, *Coming Apocalypse* be surprised. Here is what I wrote in that book (my entry for April 14th): 'It's illuminating to think back to the days before the panic began. In France, the yellow vest riots were still in full flow. President Macron had pretty much lost control of his country. In Hong Kong, the demonstrators were causing mayhem and the Chinese Government was facing serious problems. All over the world, protestors were causing chaos with demonstrations inspired by climate change campaigners. In Europe there were increasing tensions as countries such as Italy and Greece struggled with a currency that was too strong for them. The German people were becoming very tetchy about the future cost of supporting the European Union. And the issues over Brexit were still causing serious concern among hard-line Remainers – who were still hoping to overturn the democratic will of the British people. In the United States, the ideological battles were heightened as the Presidential election got underway. The world was, in short, in rare turmoil. Today, the world is pretty much one big police state. Demonstrations of any kind are outlawed. Public meetings are outlawed. Elections have been cancelled. And there is now talk that social distancing will have to be indefinite. Researchers talk of a need for more surveillance. Convenient, eh?

May 27th 2020

These Tests for New Drugs Will be Dangerously Misleading

There's a lot of talk at the moment about the need for a new wonder drug to tackle the coronavirus. The media are desperate for it to all happen very quickly. A new drug by next Thursday would be nice. Wednesday would be better.

But when it comes how will we know that a new drug is safe?

Well, although there will be some trials on human patients, though they won't tell you what the long-term dangers might be, the basic safety tests will involve animals.

And I fear you may now be in for something of a shock.

I have spent a good portion of my life fighting animal experiments – vivisection. Sadly, the fight has proved ineffective. It's been an unequal battle. On the one side there have been a few people like me who know that animal experiments are not only inhuman but are also entirely worthless. Actually – worse than useless. On the other hand there are the huge international drug companies who pay for most animal experiments and who do so because animal experiments enable them to pretend that the drugs they sell are safe for human beings.

I've debated with vivisectors many times in public but for a long time now they've refused to debate with me – for the very simple reason that they always lost. Not because I'm particularly good at debating but because the facts are so much on my side. My last debate was due to take place many years go at the Union at Oxford University but they couldn't find any vivisector to debate with me so they cancelled me. I thought that was rather cowardly of them. They should have threatened the vivisectors that if they didn't turn up they'd let me debate with a chair.

Animal experimentation is a big and dirty business. Every thirty seconds vivisectors around the world kill another thousand animals. They use kittens, cats, dogs, puppies, horses, sheep, rats, mice, guinea pigs, rabbits, monkeys, baboons and any other creature you can think of. While waiting to be used in laboratory experiments, animals are kept in solitary confinement in small cages. Alone and frightened they can hear the screams of the other animals being used.

Oh, and some of the animals used in laboratory experiments are pets which have been kidnapped, taken off the streets and sold to the vivisectors.

The animals used in experiments are blinded, burned, shot, injected and dissected. They have their eyes sewn up or their limbs broken. Chemicals are injected into their brains and their screams of anguish are coldly recorded. Three quarters of the experiments performed by vivisectors are done without any anaesthetic, and most vivisectors have no medical or veterinary training.

Vivisectors claim that animals are not sentient creatures and are incapable of suffering mental or physical pain but I suspect that most people watching this will know that's not true. It's just one of the many lies told by animal experimenters.

There are many problems with animal experimentation. For example, all animals respond differently to threats of any kind depending on their circumstances (diet, cage size, etc.). None of these factors is allowed for by vivisectors. By locking an animal up in a cage, experimenters have already invalidated their experiment because by altering the animal's surroundings the experimenter alters the animal's susceptibility, its habits, its instincts and its capacity to heal itself. Since these variations are not controlled (cages and surroundings differ) experiments performed on animals kept in cages are of no scientific value.

Even animal experimenters don't deny that drug tests done on animals can produce dangerously unreliable and misleading information. Thalidomide safely passed tests on animals. Penicillin and aspirin both kill cats. When Alexander Fleming discovered penicillin growing on a culture dish in 1928, he tested the drug on rabbits and discarded it when it seemed useless. Later the drug was tested on a cat and a human patient at the same time. The cat died and the human being lived. If doctors had relied upon animal experiments to decide whether or not penicillin was of any value the drug would have been discarded long ago. Penicillin even kills guinea pigs – the classic test animal for many drugs. Aspirin can be toxic to rats, mice, dogs, monkeys and guinea pigs as well as cats. Morphine sedates human beings but excites cats, goats and horses. Digitalis, one of the best established and most effective drugs for the treatment of heart disease, is so toxic to animals that if we had relied on animal tests it would have never been cleared for use by humans.

Here are the two main reasons why animal experiments are worse than useless.

First, vivisectors admit that most animal experiments are unreliable and produce results which are not relevant to human patients. But they will also admit that they don't know which experiments are unreliable and which might be reliable. Logically, that means that all animal experiments are useless. If you don't know which experiments you can rely on, you can't rely on any of them.

It is, however, my second argument which is the real clincher.

Drug companies test on animals so that they can say that they have tested their drugs before marketing them. If the tests show that the drugs do not cause serious disorders when given to animals the companies say: 'There you are! We have tested our drug – and have proved it to be safe!' If, on the other hand, tests show that a drug does cause serious problems when given to animals the companies say: 'The animal experiments are, of course, unreliable and cannot be used to predict what will happen when the drug is given to humans. We have, however, tested our drug.'

You may find this difficult to believe but it's true: tests which show that a drug causes cancer or some other serious disease, or which even kills, when given to animals are ignored on the grounds that animals are different to people. And tests which show that a new drug doesn't kill animals are used as evidence that the drug is safe for human consumption.

The drug companies cannot possible lose. Scores of drugs which cause cancer or other serious health problems in animals are widely prescribed for human patients. There is a list of some of the drugs which are widely prescribed but which cause cancer and other serious problems on my website – www.vernoncoleman.com

As a result, it isn't surprising that four out of ten patients who take a prescribed drug which has been tested for safety on animals can expect to suffer severe or noticeable side effects and doctor induced disease is, along with cancer and circulatory disease, now one of the big three killers of human beings.

If you don't believe me go to the animal issues button and then scroll right to the bottom – there is a list of 50 drugs which cause cancer and other serious disorders in animals but which were passed fit for use by human patients.

Animal experiments are fraudulent and they are a major cause of illness and death.

And now you know just one of the many reasons why the drug companies don't like me. If this truth gets out then they'll have to start testing new drugs properly. It will cost them many billions – and a lot of dangerous but enormously profitable drugs will never get to market.

And it's one of the reasons why the internet is stuffed to the corners with lies about me.

May 28th 2020

Will Social Distancing be Permanent?

'Human lives are worth more than anything else. We must never put anything about the saving of one human life.'

It's a commonly expressed feeling.

And I absolutely agree with the principle.

Who could not agree with it?

If someone you love needs a treatment which will cost a trillion dollars a day you would rightly demand that the treatment be provided – and damn the cost.

I would.

But if you spend a trillion dollars a day saving Mr X's wife or Mrs Y's husband or their two-year-old child Z, there will be nothing left to pay for any other health services. Hospitals will have to shut. Operations will cease. There will be no medicines available. Millions of people will die unnecessarily.

And that is the dilemma.

Health care resources are finite.

And doctors always have to make decisions about how best to allocate those limited resources.

That's what triage is all about.

In an army surgical unit doctors assess the incoming wounded and decide who needs to be seen first. (These days triage is usually practised by nurses and receptionists though how well this works is open to question.)

When the coronavirus first appeared, mathematical modellers looked at the small amounts of evidence available, multiplied a bag of carrots by a golf ball, divided by a hamster, added a packet of peanuts and concluded that millions of people were going to die.

In Britain, the mathematical modellers led by Ferguson concluded that eight million people would be hospitalised and that 500,000 would die. Showing all the skills of life insurance salesmen, they sold this theory to the politicians – and convinced them that their projections were accurate. (Curiously, the normally sceptical politicians needed very little persuading.)

The mathematical modellers were wrong, of course.

They should have left out the peanuts and the hamster and divided by a rhinoceros.

But the politicians accepted what they were told. And life changed.

How the devil could they have all got everything so wrong?

I knew back in February that the coronavirus wasn't going to kill us all. In mid March I was vilified for recording a YouTube video in which I called the whole coronavirus 'crisis' the hoax of the century. I thought it pretty obvious that the mathematicians were wrong.

The wise will at this point wonder whether politicians leapt on the nonsense because they saw an opportunity or whether the politicians were looking for an opportunity and waiting for the nonsense to be served up to them.

The suspicions of the wise will be strengthened by the fact that this bizarre error was repeated all over the world and duly endorsed and encouraged by eager politicians.

And so the hysteria and the panic become global – even though the bug was downgraded to flu level back in March.

Politicians and compliant journalists ignored this inconvenient truth because they didn't want their plans damaged.

The next stage in this lunacy was for politicians, advisors and health care chiefs to decide that the threat from the virus was so great that the health services should be devoted in their entirety to the care of patients with this one disease. They decided to clear the wards, cancel operations and build new hospitals.

Patients with cancer, heart disease and other serious illnesses were shunted aside so that doctors and nurses could be ready to deal with the eight million patients Ferguson had told them to expect.

Suddenly, the coronavirus was the only thing that mattered.

In the UK, the Prime Minister conveniently fell ill with the disease and was taken to hospital. Every minor celebrity who had a sniffle became front page news.

Doctors and nurses obediently cleared their wards and prepared themselves. The nation came to a halt. Schools were closed. Factories and shops were shut. Even dentists and opticians were told to lock their doors to keep the virus at bay.

The panic was institutionalised.

And, as a result there will be eight million Britons on waiting lists for surgery by the autumn. Many of them will die waiting for treatment.

This abrogation of duty by health care bosses appals and enrages me.

The death rate has already started to rise – not because of the coronavirus but because people are being denied medical care.

Britons were told to 'save the NHS'.

But why? What for? For most of us there is no NHS. Hundreds of thousands are going to die because the NHS has for weeks been closed for business.

As it became clear that this massive overreaction was unjustified, strenuous attempts were made to maintain the myth and to justify the measures which had been taken.

Patients who died with the coronavirus were added to the list of patients who had died of the virus. A House of Commons committee was told that up to two thirds of the people said to have died of the virus would have been dead anyway within months.

And so, even though it was clear that the policy was killing far more people than the disease, the panic was kept at fever pitch.

It is now clear that if more people die this year than last year it will be entirely because patients have been denied lifesaving medical care.

And so the 'cure' will be far deadlier than the disease.

Nevertheless, there are already suggestions around that social distancing will be permanent.

In the UK, the Government and the supine media (none more supine than the treacherous BBC, of course) have raised the fear to terror and when Johnson's Government elected to slightly soften the lockdown in England (the leaders of the quasi governments in Scotland and Wales chose to take the United out of United Kingdom in a move that must have thrilled Remainers and the fascist bureaucrats in Brussels) the majority of the population reacted in horror and insisted on checking the door locks, drawing the curtains and crawling under their beds. (Some were undoubtedly inspired by the fact that after several weeks at home, being paid by the Government to do nothing, they found the prospect of going back to work rather unattractive.)

Governments everywhere have boosted the fear by talking of a second wave of infection and, having promoted the idea of a vaccine as the only saviour, confessing that there may never be one available.

Politicians want to control us. And they are doing very well.

It is difficult to see how we are all going to escape from this fake crisis. Of course, if this wasn't a conspiracy to turn us all into subdued, apprehensive and obedient zombies they could announce that they had made a bit of mistake and that the coronavirus is no worse than the flu. Whoops. Sorry. Pardon. Ferguson meant well but got his sums upside down.

They are not going to say that. Ever.

They could say that the coronavirus has become less dangerous.

Or they could say their brilliant lockdown and social distancing policies have worked brilliantly and have saved us all so that it now safe to come out from under the bed.

But they don't want to do that because they want to keep the threat of a second wave available to scare us with if we start getting cocky and comfortable.

And they don't want to get rid of social distancing because it is social distancing which gives the politicians a massive amount of power; it is social distancing which is running our lives and which will weaken us as individuals. It is social distancing which will result in millions of job losses. It is social distancing which will wreck education for millions. And, most important of all, it is social distancing which is wrecking health care and which result in huge numbers of people dying unnecessarily.

Governments will enthusiastically promote social distancing as the only way to keep us safe.

I believe that's why my honest and seemingly innocuous video on social distancing was removed from YouTube.

Unless we stand up and fight, social distancing will be with us for years – possibly forever. And, as a result, our lives will be ruined in any conceivable way.

Share this article with everyone you know.

May 30th 2020

How They Deliberately Terrified Us

This is the true story of how a government threatened, manipulated and deliberately terrified its citizens for a bug they knew was no worse than the flu. The Government I've described is the British Government but I have no doubt that the facts I'm outlining here would fit a good number of other countries too.

When the coronavirus was first identified, the British Government's advisors decided that it was a dangerous infection and they put it into the same category as rabies, Ebola fever and a few other deadly diseases.

But then on March 19th the public health bodies in the UK, together with the Government's Advisory Committee on Dangerous Pathogens, decided that the coronavirus should no longer be classified as a 'high consequence infectious disease'.

So they downgraded it – and effectively put it back into the same category as the flu.

That was on March 19th.

This decision was rather tucked away on the Government's website and although I put the decision on my website, the mass media ignored it. I'll show in a minute why they did so.

It was also announced that in future it would not be necessary to manage patients with the infection in special treatment centres only. It was effectively decided that the infection did not need to be regarded as anything more hazardous than the flu and that it could be dealt with in the same way that the flu is managed.

I confess I was rather excited by this decision which totally vindicated my original view, based on a mixture of information and experience, that the bug was nowhere near as dangerous as had been advertised. I naively assumed that the Government would back off, stop pretending that we were threatened by the plague and let the country get back to normal.

I now feel rather foolish for making that assumption. I should have realised that something bigger was under way from the fact that the Government did not publish this decision for two days.

A bigger game was already in play and the Government was already planning to put huge chunks of the nation under house arrest.

And then the Emergency Bill was passed by a compliant House of Commons which gave Comrade Boris and his bunch of ministers and advisors more power than any government has ever had in Britain. The House of Commons handed total control of the country to Boris Johnson, Neil Ferguson and Dominic Cummings. What a trio.

When the coronavirus bug was downgraded, the Government had already decided to take full advantage of the situation.

And the flu-type bug was used as a weapon to trigger a coup that would give the Government total control over the people.

I have already described many of the astonishing things that have happened but yesterday I was shown a document which made my blood run cold.

The document is entitled 'Options for increasing adherence to social distancing measures' and it is dated 22nd March 2020 – three days after the bug was downgraded and it was clear that it was no longer going to put eight million in hospital and kill 500,000 people as had been predicted by Ferguson and his chums at Imperial College.

The committee responsible for the document was named the scientific pandemic influenza group on behaviour so they presumably knew that we were dealing with a type of flu.

The document I'm going to quote from was prepared by a bunch of behavioural scientists working for SAGE – a surely appropriate James Bond like acronym for an organisation which deserves about as much respect as SMERSH or SPECTRE. The full title of SAGE is the Scientific Advisory Group for Emergencies and the first thing we need to do when we get our country back is to disband it.

I feel qualified to say this since, with all due modesty, the evidence shows that right from the start I've been rather more accurate than SAGE. And if an old man in a chair can produce better advice than a government committee then it's probably a good idea to get rid of the government committee.

Anyway, that's all for the future.

What concerns me at the moment is the document prepared by the behavioural science subgroup – a document which shows how the Government was advised to control the way we think and to manipulate the way we behave.

In the end, I think, our politicians and their advisors, deliberately set out to create mass hysteria. I think the advisors were perhaps remembering the way teenagers became hysterical when they had watched the film, The Exorcist.

The document was designed to offer advice to SAGE itself and here are some quotes which I assure you are not taken out of context:

First, under the heading 'Perceived threat' the Government's advisors wrote: 'A substantial number of people still do not feel sufficiently personally threatened.' And they suggested that the media be used to increase a sense of personal threat.

So now you know who was pulling the strings which kept the TV and newspapers building up the scare story. In the old days this was called propaganda. Actually, we should still call it propaganda. And so we now know that those inflammatory, scary headlines were written under orders from the Government. To sweeten the deal, the Government agreed to purchase massive newspaper advertising for three months. The Government's advertising, paid for with our money, replaced the advertising which was lost because of the lockdown and social distancing. Financially, the newspapers have come out of this very well.

I suspect the BBC will be rewarded for its propaganda by having the threats to remove the licence fee removed.

It's fair to suppose that a few editors will also be expecting knighthoods in the next honours list.

And the advisors went on to say: 'The perceived level of personal threat needs to be increased among those who are complacent, using hard-hitting emotional messaging.'

In other words the behavioural scientists advised the Government to make people more frightened of a bug which they knew had just been downgraded to flu level.

Second, under the heading 'incentivisation' the Government's advisors wrote: 'Communication strategies should provide social approval for desired behaviours and promote social approval within the community.'

The other side of that coin as the advisors doubtless knew, is that people who behaved inappropriately, and who preferred to be guided by the facts, would be demonised and shunned. No one seemed worried about that. And in due course the Government deliberately split communities into two – those who believed all the lies they were told by the Government and those who sought out the truth.

Third, under the heading 'coercion' the advisors we paid for said: 'Consideration should be given to use of social disapproval but with a strong caveat around unwanted negative consequences.'

Well, they managed the social approval but they didn't do much about avoiding the unwanted negative consequences. And they damned well knew that people would be abused. Let's hope that some of the unfortunate souls who suffered because they forgot to go out and clap on Thursday evenings will eventually get over the harassment and the abuse they received from their neighbours. I know a little about abuse. The minute I started exposing the truth about the coronavirus I was viciously attacked and unscrupulous attempts were made to destroy my reputation. I have dealt with some of these attacks on my website and I'll deal with more in a special video I'm preparing about precisely how individuals are being monstered.

Fourth, under the heading 'Enablement' the behavioural scientists pointed out that the public were being asked to give up valued activities and access to resources for an extended period and suggested that as compensation we should be given access to opportunities for social contact and rewarding activities that could be undertaken in the home, and to resources such as food.

I like that last bit.

I don't know what the rewarding activities were, I don't think the Government ever got round to that – other than the stupid clapping and the drawing of rainbows, but I am grateful to the scientists' suggestion that we be allowed access to resources such as food. Very generous of them.

And so in response to this advice, Boris Johnson's Government deliberately terrified the voters because of a flu bug and allowed them access to food.

It's no exaggeration to say that Comrade Boris's behaviour has been downright criminal. Here's why.

First, hundreds of thousands of citizens have been terrified out of their wits by the propaganda. Since the word pandemic is now fashionable, there will be a pandemic of mental illness and suicide.

Second, the level of terror is so great that many people are unwilling to go to hospital when they are ill. Parents won't let their children go to school. And teachers won't teach them. The absurd restrictions which will create mental havoc among children are a direct result of all this dangerous gibberish. Millions won't want to go back to work. The economic and social consequences will push Britain back centuries. Civilisation has been wrecked for a bug that was downgraded on March 19th and is no more dangerous than the flu.

And third, the people in charge of our hospitals are still following the social distancing rules that seem to have been created because no one listened to the expert advice lowering the risk level of the coronavirus. They still seem to believe that the coronavirus is as deadly as Ebola or the plague. Have they too been manipulated into a state of terror? Doctors and nurses must by now know the truth and yet operations are still being cancelled and cancer patients are still abandoned and left in limbo by a health system which seems irrationally obsessed by the coronavirus.

It's no wonder that the media are busy demonising Sweden, where the Government had no formal lockdown and have suffered far fewer deaths. It's no wonder that the British government has exaggerated the number of deaths from the coronavirus. They must now be desperate that the truth never comes out.

The bottom line is simple.

To make sure that you aren't unduly terrified by your government, and to protect yourself against manipulation, remember the slogan I introduced for my piece about brainwashing:

Distrust the government

Avoid mass media

Fight the lies

May 31st 2020

Snitches, Sneaks and Quislings Are Killing Families, Communities and Society

The Government in Italy is reported to be hiring 60,000 professional snitches to monitor their friends and neighbours and to sneak on anyone they see who is not wearing a face mask and obeying social distancing rules.

We really are moving well into the uncomfortable landscape of George Orwell country.

The professional snitches will not wear uniforms or badges so that they can merge into society unnoticed – and so they can spread their odious tittle tattle without being identified.

It's happening everywhere.

Several police forces in the UK have asked citizens to report anyone who mentions or discusses conspiracy theories on the internet – though to be honest no one is promoting conspiracy theories in the UK more than Comrade Boris, the man who was voted in as a Tory but who has, I suggest, rapidly turned into Britain's first communist Prime Minister. A conspiracy theorist is sometimes defined as someone who represents a point of view not generally accepted by the majority. Well, I think that makes Comrade Boris, Comrade Dominic, Comrade Neil and the rest of them fully fledged conspiracy theorists because I doubt if Comrade Boris would win a majority if we had a vote about his policies.

As in Italy, the police around the world have urged citizens to snitch on neighbours who might have broken lockdown or social distancing rules – though to be honest if anyone can work out precisely what the rules are I congratulate them. The rules seem to vary according to who is speaking and what day of the week it is. The confusion is, of course, all part of the plan to unsettle us and to make us uncomfortable – though some of the police forces who are encouraging people to tell tales on their friends and neighbours seem to be enjoying their new powers rather too vividly and I suspect that one or two police officers might have been watching too many movies about totalitarian societies. In the UK, at least four police forces have set up dedicated hot lines to make it easier for people to snitch on folk whom they think might have broken a law or two.

The bottom line is that snitches are bad for any society for exactly the same reason that they are good for governments.

The forces of law and order will always want to ensure that its laws are upheld (unless they are inconvenient for senior government figures). They will want to catch offenders, punish them as severely as they can get away with and make sure they don't do it again – and that others don't do it either.

Snitches and quislings are good for governments because they operate as additional members of the occupying force.

When you don't know who the quislings are you become paranoid and worry about everyone. In such a world everyone is a potential snitch and everyone is a threat. That's a miserable way to live but it is, it seems, the way we are now expected to live.

I mentioned 'occupying forces' and I was serious; that's how I, and many others, now see our governments – as occupying forces. That's why I use the word quisling to describe the snitches who making life easier for the oppressors.

Some governments around the world, including the UK Government, have used the coronavirus as an excuse to bring in whole rafts of oppressive legislation, turning democracies into police states and removing freedom and privacy as if they simply did not matter.

In the UK the Government's new Big Brother spyware track and trace system seems to me to have been designed to remove the last vestiges of privacy and independence. Anyone who tests positive for the coronavirus will be contacted by the NHS Test and Trace staff and will have to give the names and contact details of everyone with whom they have 'recently interacted' (that's the Big Brother jargon). It's all rather reminiscent of the McCarthy era inquisitions in the United States.

Those individuals who have been named must then isolate for 14 days. It is quite possible that within three months entire cities will be permanently in lockdown. I suspect that only Comrade Boris's closest advisors will be exempt from the new laws.

(Incidentally, Comrade Boris and company are calling them rules and not laws but in my world if I can be arrested, fined and imprisoned for not obeying an order then it's a law so let's forget the Newspeak and call things by the proper names, please.)

The system also seems designed to limit the number of people we meet. Anyone who has an active social life and meets lot of people will be forever being put into unnecessary periods of lockdowns. Meetings of all kinds, including protests and demonstrations, will be things of the past. Now, there is a surprise: no demonstrations against the Government.

And how safe will all this very private and personal information be? Well, the woman that Comrade Boris has put in charge of the scheme is Baroness Harding, the wife of a Conservative MP and the former head of a British phone company called Talk Talk. While she was the boss there the company lost the personal and banking details of 157,000 customers to hackers. Her company was fined £400,000 for security failings which allowed the data to be taken with ease and the company shareholders are said to have lost £60 million as a result. Boris hired Ferguson, the mathematical modeller who gave us lockdown and Cummings, the advisor who ignored the lockdown. And now he has hired a woman most famous for losing personal information to be in charge of collecting personal information. There is at least a pattern there.

Experts are lining up to applaud the new system and to warn that reducing lockdown is dangerous. I think they're looking at the wrong part of the problem. They are looking to see how many people are likely to catch the bug. And that is the wrong question. They should be concentrating on how dangerous the bug is. And the answer to the question they aren't asking is: no worse than a bad flu. That was obvious back in March, when I recorded my first YouTube video. Everyone who disputes that should remember that the total number of worldwide deaths so far from the coronavirus is around half the total number of flu deaths in a bad year. Some experts are also ignoring the number of deaths caused by the lockdown – and that is already higher than the disease itself.

The Government's scientists seem to me to be over-complicating things. It is a perfect example of groupthink where a group of people meet, talk and then think alike.

This is, perhaps, a good moment to point out that the death rates seem to show that Britain's policies have been among the worst in the world. The Norwegian public health authority concluded the other day that the virus was never spreading as fast as had been feared and was already on its way out when their lockdown was ordered. Countries where the people have been trusted to behave sensibly (covering your mouth when you cough or sneeze for example) have done much better than Britain – with its onerous lockdown policies. And it is worth pointing out that Vietnam, which is rather close to China, has had 327 cases but no deaths. Africa hasn't had many lockdowns or many deaths. Of course, the way Britain has been counting the deaths probably has something to do with Britain's very high death rate. Boris has a dilemma – if he keeps the total low then the house arrests look like overkill. If he lets the total rise too much then his policies look as stupid as they are.

There is no doubt that the police state will be strengthened by Comrade Boris's absurd, impractical and entirely unnecessary laws – which will incidentally, destroy a number of industries. For example, no one will ever dare risk money making a movie or even a television programme in Britain if they know that the whole multi million pound enterprise could be brought to a screeching and very expensive standstill if one extra or assistant wardrobe mistress develops a sniffle.

The UK seems to have more vicious new laws than any other major country. It's a safe bet that the UK is going to come out worst when this farce eventually struggles to a conclusion. British companies are doomed and that won't do much good for the unemployment figures which are going to reach new records. The only people looking forward to the future are the police – it must be fun being a policeman in a police state.

As an aside I should mention that the police seem to be enjoying themselves everywhere. In the United States a woman was wrestled to the ground by police officers for not wearing her mask properly and a woman was arrested for taking her children to a park so that they could play and get a little fresh air. All over America clergymen have been arrested for trying to hold church services.

And inevitably, there have been some Americans eager to do their very best to support the police. Yesterday I saw a video of a woman being chased out of a store for not wearing a mask. The people doing the chasing were, of course, all dutifully wearing masks.

Heaven knows how people would behave if they were at risk of catching a serious disease. I wonder how many of these folk know that the coronavirus of which they are all so terrified has killed around half the number of people killed by a bad flu bug. I wonder how many wore masks last winter to try to protect themselves against the flu.

Finally, I wonder if snitches and sneaks know how much damage they are doing. The police are doing enough harm without members of the public joining in.

Snitches and quislings damage our trust in one another – they create fear, uncertainty, anxiety and distrust and attempt to force us to suppress our individuality and our sense of freedom and personal dignity.

That's the real danger.

The snitches and quislings probably don't realise it but they are doing permanent, fatal damage to our sense of society and our sense of community.

May 31st 2020

How and Why Thousands of Old People Have Been Murdered

I won't see 30 again, unless it has a one in front of it, and, as a result, I am, I have to say, definitely feeling unwanted, superfluous and generally surplus to requirements.

My government and the health service clearly regard me as a nuisance, though the former is happy to send me income tax demands and to accept my cheques and the latter is doubtless ever ready to blush daintily if I should be overcome with the desire to enliven my Thursday evenings with a little light clapping or saucepan banging – though to be honest even if I had been inclined to follow this most curious custom, I would have felt a little foolish since we have no neighbours and I fear the rabbits in our garden would have been a trifle startled if I had lost my mind, stood on the doorstep and tapped a wooden spoon on the bottom of an ancient saucepan.

Some of the young do not seem too concerned about the way their elders have been treated in recent months. A few, indeed, have actually cheered as folk in their 70s, 80s, 90s and more have been ignored, pushed aside and subjected to the biggest mass murder in the so-called civilised world since the Second World War.

The elderly are the new Jews and if you think the word 'murder' is pushing it a bit just stay tuned to this channel as they used to say and I will explain why it isn't.

The young who have ignored what has happened to the elderly should not feel so comfortable or be so sanguine because what has happened to their grandparents will happen to them with the sole difference that it will happen sooner – a lot sooner. Sixty will soon be the new seventy.

When I recorded my first YouTube video back in mid-March of 2020, I explained why the coronavirus scare was a hoax. The title was 'Coronavirus scare: the hoax of the century'. I suggested that it was either a hysterical over-reaction to a disease no more deadly than a common or garden flu, or a devious ploy to terrify the world in order to create a fearful, obedient population which would accept a scary array of new laws in the belief that by doing so they might just survive a form of the flu which was being promoted as a disease slightly deadlier than the plague.

I said back then that I suspected that one of the underlying aims of the politicians who were over-selling the coronavirus bug was probably the demonization and marginalisation of the elderly.

Oh, how they laughed and sneered.

I was, of course, widely demonised and lied about on the internet – largely by ignorant and anonymous bullies who wouldn't recognise a fact if it came in a box with the word FACT stamped on the side in big black letters.

But I fear I was right and I have no doubt that even as I speak a thousand red-faced trolls will be penning their grovelling apologies and begging forgiveness for their arrogance and stupidity.

Right from the start of the absurd and entirely unnecessary process of putting people under house arrest, it was the elderly who were the first to be locked up, or locked in if you prefer.

For absolutely no good reason the elderly were told that they had to stay in their own homes to protect themselves, hospitals and the world. There was never one shred of real evidence for this. On the contrary, it was clear from the start that this cruelty was based on political expediency rather than scientific necessity. Men and women over 70 were told that they couldn't see their loved ones and many were told they would be refused medical treatment – whatever might be wrong with them. People who died, for whatever reason, died alone – abandoned by a system they had helped create and pay for.

It was all total bollocks, of course.

The elderly aren't likely to die from the coronavirus just because they are old.

The people most likely to die from the coronavirus are the people who are most likely to die from the flu – people who are frail, unfit, overweight or suffering from serious, long-term health problems.

As a doctor I can tell you there seem to be just two big differences between the coronavirus and the ordinary flu virus.

First, the flu virus can kill more people.

Second, no flu virus has ever got this much attention or put an entire civilisation back several centuries.

The fact is that the risk of dying from this coronavirus is, for healthy adults, minute.

However, there have been more deaths than there should have been because of the government policies. It isn't just the lockdowns and the terror that have killed people unnecessarily but the way the coronavirus has been mismanaged – either deliberately or through gross incompetence.

If the mathematical modellers, the medical and scientific advisors, the so-called experts and the politicians had all gone on holiday last January, at least 100,000 people around the world would still be alive. The whole damned fuss has been unnecessary and many of the deaths were unnecessary too.

I haven't forgotten about my charge or murder. I'll come to that soon. But before I do, I just want to say a few more things about the way the elderly have been abused during all this unscientific bullying and blatant discrimination. And it was and is discrimination. Just imagine the fuss there would have been in the posh papers if it had been announced that all homosexuals or women or Methodists were being put under house arrest. Imagine the fuss if the governments had, more sensibly announced that everyone overweight had to stay indoors to protect the health services. That would, at least have had the merit of being logical.

The elderly were, in parts of the world at least, denied all medical care. Many were manipulated into signing 'Do Not Resuscitate' forms – effectively signing their own suicide notes. By being locked away for longer than anyone else, their immune systems were weakened. Many, without internet access, had real difficulty in obtaining food supplies because, despite its promises, their government made virtually no effort to ensure that the elderly received food. The elderly were told that they couldn't see their families. The big lie was that this was to protect the hospitals though no one ever even tried to explain why this should be, and the nonsense was highlighted by the fact that in some areas the elderly were told that they wouldn't be treated in hospital whatever was wrong with them.

None of this was a real surprise, of course. The elderly have been demonised by the media for a long time. They have been blamed for the poverty, the weather and anything else you can think of – despite having worked and paid taxes all their lives. Governments see the elderly as worthless and an expensive drain on society. If you doubt that just look at the sentences given to thugs who attack the elderly. Mug a 40-year-old and you will be punished severely. Mug an 80-year-old and you'll get a light slap on the wrist at worst.

And, of course, the elderly are sneered at and laughed at. When a movie based on my novel, *Mrs Caldicot's Cabbage War* was released, the reviewer for the London *Sunday Times* dismissively and patronisingly described that he thought the movie's target audience was undemanding oldies. I wrote the novel to draw attention to exactly this sort of rampant ageism.

And so we are now at the nitty gritty. The murder charge.

Some of you may suspect that I am exaggerating: a little hyperbole to draw attention to a small problem.

You would be wrong if you thought that.

The fact is that throughout the world countless thousands of elderly patients with the coronavirus were thrown out of hospitals and dumped in care homes.

Now, let's pause a moment.

What sort of people are you likely to find living in care homes?

a) Fit young folk

b) Fit old folk

c) Sick old folk

Not difficult, is it?

You don't go into a care home unless you are elderly, frail and in need of some care and attention because you are probably suffering from a range of health problems.

And so hospitals sent patients with the coronavirus into care homes which were full of frail, elderly patients with health problems – the very people who often die of the flu. Every winter. No one would ever dream of sending a patient with the flu into a care home but hospitals sent thousands of coronavirus patients into care homes.

The staff in the care homes had no equipment or facilities for isolating the patients who came from hospital with the flu, sorry the coronavirus, from the patients who didn't have it but who were already ill with respiratory problems, heart problems or whatever.

And guess what happened next.

Golly, you really need a medical degree to work it out, don't you? Thousands of elderly, frail people in care homes caught the coronavirus and because no one would or could treat them they died in droves. Negligence in the care of the elderly in these homes has been widely reported – stories that would make anyone with a heart weep and feel a deep, undying fury. Thousands of older people died alone, with no family or friends allowed near them and with no spiritual support. The only people they saw were dressed as though for a spaceflight.

In Ireland, Norway, France and Belgium more than half of all the coronavirus deaths were in care homes. In the UK and Sweden, over a third of coronavirus deaths were in care homes.

Wasn't it an amazing coincidence that hospitals all over the world all did the same stupid thing. All dumped coronavirus patients in care homes.

For governments everywhere this had the bonus of pushing up the total death rates so providing some justification for the otherwise unjustifiable lockdowns and the utterly stupid and scientifically in-defensive social distancing nonsense. We all know that governments have been doing everything they can to push up the total number of coronavirus deaths by, for example, listing patients as having died of the coronavirus when they actually died with it – two very different things.

At this point we have to ask a simple question: were the old people with the coronavirus sent into care homes through stupidity and incompetence or deliberately to kill off lots of old people?

The answer to this question will only matter when the hospital staff responsible are taken to court and tried – as I sincerely hope they will be.

If they sent sick old people with the coronavirus into care homes through stupidity and incompetence then they will probably get away with a manslaughter charge. Even if they erroneously expected their hospitals to be filled with younger coronavirus patients that is still no excuse.

But if they deliberately sent old people with the coronavirus into care homes knowing that other residents would catch the bug and die then the charge will be murder, and we are looking at a mass murder charge of which even the Nazis might be ashamed.

The added bonus charge, by the way, is that most of the elderly people who were sent to care homes with the coronavirus had caught the bloody thing in hospital because as everyone knows, or should know, most hospitals are so badly managed these days that they are the one place in the world where you are most likely to catch a deadly bug.

In a way it doesn't really matter whether it was stupidity, incompetence, panic, a lack of care or homicide.

The fact is that umpteen thousand old people died before they should have died. And the hospitals which sent them to their death were largely left half empty because the expected hordes of coronavirus patients never turned up.

The hospitals, hordes of advisors and politicians who allowed it to happen and who recklessly created the circumstances, are all guilty and shouldn't be allowed to get away with their crimes – whether they be crimes of omission or commission. We live in rich societies and those responsible for caring didn't care. They dumped the elderly like bags of garbage.

The people who were responsible for this holocaust will probably whinge, wring their hands and say they were all just doing what they were told to do.

We have all heard that excuse before.

It didn't work then.

And it won't work now.

I'll be campaigning for all those responsible to be tried in court.

June 1st 2020

UK Government Now Only Six Weeks Behind Coleman

"Being black is a major risk factor for coronavirus," said Matt
Hancock, the UK Health Secretary, on 2nd June.
Brilliant.
I pointed that out on the web on April 13th. It's in my book 'Coming
Apocalypse' too – perhaps that's where Master Hancock saw it.
Time and time again the Government has been behind with seeing the
obvious.
Boris would do better to fire all the advisors and just read my articles
or watch my videos.

June 2nd 2020

Is This How They Plan to Steal and Sell Your DNA?

Governments everywhere are busy rolling out antibody testing programmes.

Antigen tests, which involve taking a swab from the nose or throat, simply show if someone actually has the coronavirus in their body. Antibody tests may involve taking a blood sample and looking to see if the body contains antibodies which respond to the virus. If you have antibodies in your blood then you have had and have overcome the coronavirus. The sample will be sent off to a laboratory to be tested. This will be a much bigger testing programme then the antigen testing. Governments are planning to do millions of antibody tests on their populations.

And the key words here are 'blood sample'.

Because when you take a blood sample you can, of course, easily take a DNA sample. (You can take DNA samples with other body tissues but blood is so easy.)

And if that thought doesn't strike terror into your heart then you really haven't been paying attention.

Since March of 2020, governments everywhere have been tearing up all the traditional values which we used to take for granted.

Freedom, democracy and privacy are now just a thing of the past.

Most people in the western world are now living in police states. The Emergency Bill which was passed by the British Government in March gave British politicians and civil servants much the same sort of power over the people that the Patriot Act gave the authorities in America. We all might as well be living in China or Russia for all the freedom we have these days.

And don't kid yourself that the governments will give back all that power in a few months' time. Governments never give back power they've taken.

So, to get back to your DNA.

If you trust your government to always do the right and decent thing then you can switch off now. I envy you your innocence and your faith. I suspect, however, that most people have by now lost what little faith they had in their government and its advisors.

I have shown in other videos how we have been lied to, tricked, manipulated and brainwashed.

I think I've had the coronavirus and if I have to have an antibody test I expect that the Government will also take my DNA.

And I expect them to store it.

Along with your DNA.

And everyone else's DNA.

The next big question is what will they do with it?

And this, again, is a question of trust.

Do we trust them to store our DNA so that they might be able to use it to help us one day?

Sadly, if we believe that when we are well into tooth fairy territory.

I think governments everywhere will take our DNA and store it.

And I think they will sell it.

Governments at all levels have a track record. They sell every bit of information they can collect.

They've been selling information about voters for decades.

They sell census information.

They demand private and confidential information.

And then they flog it to anyone prepared to pay the right price.

In the UK, the NHS has been collecting information about us all for years. To begin with, they promised they wouldn't sell the information. They actually gave us an option. If we didn't want them to sell our private medical information to drug companies then we could say so. And they wouldn't.

Well, that's what they said.

But I think they sold it anyway.

Look on the NHS website and you will see that they say that the NHS collects confidential patient information from all NHS organisations and all private organisations providing NHS funded care.

They then flog this information to researchers, to the medical establishment and, wait for it because this is the good bit, to drug companies.

They say that the drug companies won't use it for marketing or insurance purposes.

They presumably know that because the companies they sell it to tell them they won't.

There is still a get out clause if you don't want them to sell your information but it's got more holes in it than a colander.

The same is true everywhere.

Private medical information is sold to anyone prepared to buy it.

And this brings us back to your DNA.

I don't think they will be able to resist storing our DNA when they do antibody tests.

And they will sell it.

Of course they will. They'll say that since they took the sample then they own your DNA. And they'll flog it to drug companies, insurance companies and anyone else who wants to buy it.

Governments have already created biobanks with genetic material they took from screening tests. And now governments everywhere need huge amounts of money to pay for the coronavirus mess they have made of the world.

Does all this matter?

Well, I rather think it does.

Drug and insurance companies will know everything about your body. And they will be able to mix and match that with the information they buy from search engines, your bank, the supermarkets and everyone else. The last vestige of your privacy will be gone.

And they will use the information ruthlessly.

As an aside, let me just tell you that since my wife was diagnosed with breast cancer both she and I have been bombarded with utterly unnecessary and inappropriate online advertisements for funeral services, cancer charities and other goodies. I don't know who sold our information but it doesn't really matter where they got it, does it? To say that I find it intrusive is to be considerably politer than I feel.

I strongly suspect that we will have no rights over our DNA.

They will, of course, pass our DNA details onto all police and security services.

We can all trust them, can't we?

Drug companies will use your DNA to predict what diseases you might develop. And they will want to sell you useful drugs to stop you getting whatever it is they know you're going to get wrong with you.

Insurance companies will use your DNA to predict your future. You will, perhaps, find that your premiums suddenly soar because your insurance company knows something about your future.

Employers will doubtless see your DNA details and be unwilling to hire you if they see something in your future that doesn't appeal.

How many job candidates will find themselves being refused time and time again because prospective employers see that they are likely to develop Parkinson's disease or dementia or drug addiction.

Your DNA information will be used in conjunction with your credit card and bank information too, of course. And that will be so much easier when they get rid of nasty, grubby cash.

And they will mix it with all the information you've put on social media and which you cannot erase however hard you try. Anything you ever put on Facebook, for example, belongs to Facebook. Permanently, as in forever.

So, you will be standing at the check-out at the supermarket and the assistant will take the chocolate bar out of your shopping.

'What's the matter with that?' you will ask, puzzled.

'The system says you can't have that,' the assistant will say. She will look at the screen in front of her. 'You're going to get diabetes so you aren't allowed to buy chocolate.'

When you apply for a driving licence they will tell you that you can't have one.

'Why not?' you will ask.

'Because there is an 82% chance that you are going to develop epilepsy next year,' they will tell you.

You will have no rights over your private information. Companies everywhere will be able to buy it and hackers will be able to steal it. Hackers?

The woman in charge of Britain's track and trace system was in charge of a phone company called TalkTalk when hackers stole the personal information of 157,000 people. The company was fined massively for not looking after the information properly. Now she is in charge of the tracking and tracing system and the collection of vast amounts of personal information.

What can we do about it?

Well, until they make it compulsory I don't think I'll bother having an antibody test done thank you very much.

June 3rd 2020

Passing Observations (June 3rd 2020)

Why are so many doubtless well-meaning people doing odd things to raise money for the NHS? The NHS doesn't need money. It needs more common sense and more compassion.

There is much talk of a low slung wealth tax to make the middle classes pay for the crisis that has been created out of next to nothing. This would be truly stupid. Every country which has ever introduced a wealth tax has abandoned the idea because it always results in a fall in the total tax take. Those due to pay it either work less (and use up their savings to avoid the tax) or simply move to another country.

Who is paying YouTube to put promotional messages for the NHS underneath my videos? My videos are not monetised – which means that I do not allow advertising or sponsorship.

It has been obvious for ages that the people who need protecting from the coronavirus are not the over 70s but overweight, black diabetics. (They are the people most likely to die from the coronavirus.) But no one likes to say this. And no minister dares to put overweight, black diabetics under house arrest.

Shopping is, in future, going to require a good deal of standing about – waiting for someone to leave so that another shopper can enter the store. I intend to buy a shooting stick. It will be easier to carry than a folding chair.

Farmers don't have anyone to pick their fruit and other crops. We need a Land Army. Why not instruct fit people whose wages are being paid by the Government that they must become temporary fruit pickers for the summer?

The people who created this unholy mess (the politicians and the civil servants) are immune to pension problems – they all receive massive pensions paid for largely by taxpayers. Everyone else is pretty well buggered. The Government has instructed large companies to stop paying dividends and millions of pensioners (and those about to retire) will have to try to live on the world's smallest state pension.

June 3rd 2020

New Law – Everyone Must Now Hop and Wear Galoshes

It appears that the BBC was right when it recently appeared to warn that the coronavirus can be spread by footwear.

The British Prime Minister's team of scientific advisors, known as the Ministerial Intelligence and Notification Team (or MINT for short) has warned that this new threat must be taken seriously if the world is to be saved and drug company profits are to be maximised.

Professor Neil Ferguson of Imperial Mints and the Bill Gates Foundation for Jabbing Scared People with Chemicals has warned that if nothing is done then 300 million Britons will need to be hospitalised and at least 370 million of them will die.

When a journalist timidly pointed out that there aren't that many people in Britain, Professor Ferguson, known to his fan club as the Eddie the Eagle of mathematical modelling, replied that as a result of foot transmission he is expecting a second, third and fourth wave of the infection which will repeatedly wipe out 150% of the entire population.

To deal with this unexpected problem the Prime Minister's special advisor, Dominic Cummings set up a one man committee and has decided that the problem will be halved if everyone hops instead of walking.

'Hopping,' said Sir Dominic, 'will mean that only one contaminated foot will be in contact with the ground at any time.'

The Governmental Advisory committee known as MINT has also recommended that all citizens should wear disposable galoshes. These can be made at home out of old shoe boxes or, for those with smaller feet, old plastic detergent containers and some sticky back tape.

For the medium and long- term, Lord Cummings says that the Government has commissioned a factory in Hungary to manufacture three billion pairs of galoshes.

Laws to ensure that hopping and galosh wearing rules are carefully followed mean that those who do not obey will have one leg amputated. Those who break the law a second time will have a second limb amputated and so on until they have no more legs.

These rules will stay in force for 64 weeks, said the Prime Minister who added that citizens will also be expected to follow existing social distancing and lockdown rules at the same time. Two consenting adults can hop together in their own garden as long as they remain at least six feet six inches apart from each other.

A hopping hotline has been set up to provide advice for those who aren't sure how to hop satisfactorily.

Finally, citizens everywhere are advised to wash their feet in soap and water every twenty minutes.

'We must follow these rules very strictly,' said Lord Cummings. 'If people are careless then there could be a great many deaths among those who spend time walking on their hands or crawling on their hands and knees.'

In order to encourage people to follow the guidelines, the Government has introduced a new set of slogans:

Wash your feet

Wear your galoshes

Hop to it

In addition, every Wednesday at 7 p.m., citizens will be encouraged to stand on their doorsteps, on one leg of course, and to toss their unwanted shoes into the street while chanting Shoe, Shoe, Shoe as loudly as they can.

Concerned citizens who want to help the nation will be asked to hop around their gardens or up and down their stairs (taking great care as they do so, of course) to raise money for the Bill Gates Foundation for Global Control and World Government.

If you believe any of that you probably believe in the lockdowns and social distancing, which make just as much sense, you may have been permanently destabilised and I'm afraid there is little hope for you.

Finally, don't forget to brainwash yourself every day by repeating my special mantra:

Distrust the government

Avoid mass media

Fight the lies

June 5th 2020

Passing Observations (June 5th 2020)

Yesterday morning, YouTube took down my video about how I fear governments plan to steal and sell your DNA. I complained that the video contained facts and an assessment of the future – a prognosis. The only difference between my hypothesis and the hypothesis put forward by the seemingly hopeless Ferguson (the Eddie the Eagle of mathematical modelling) is accuracy. I don't think his was and I suspect mine is. That's why it was taken down. Ten minutes after I had complained, YouTube restored the video. This saves me making another 'Why Did They Ban My Video' tape. If you haven't already watched the first one please do. It's called 'Why Did YouTube Ban My Video', it's about free speech and the freedom of the press, and when I last looked it had received a respectable 258,000 views.

The demonstrations about the death of a black American are understandable and undoubtedly full of well-meaning people but I fear that those folk are doing what the authorities want them to do – they are distracting attention from our global fight for survival and freedom. If we don't all fight together then we will all be slaves for life. I'm not joking. The McCann story which hit the front pages of all the UK papers appeared to be another deliberate distraction. We only get one chance to win the big fight. Predictably, Lewis Hamilton, a racing driver, threw himself into the controversy about the killing of the black American. He said he was overcome with rage at the events following the death. How about a little rage at events which resulted in the deaths of thousands of British citizens (black and white) in care homes? If Mr Hamilton really wants to help improve society he could perhaps do more by moving back to the UK and paying income tax. The tax on his obscene earnings would pay for the hiring of many, many nurses or policemen. Mr Hamilton, who has lived in tax exile for years, is famous to many for even managing to avoid paying tax on the £16.5 million aeroplane he bought. He is alleged to have used a company in the British Virgin Islands and another one on the Isle of Man. In my view, people who are tax exiles and who work hard to avoid paying tax forfeit the right to comment on social issues.

Antoinette and I went shopping in a local supermarket. There were quite a few other shoppers around but I am delighted to report that I saw no masks and no gloves. There was no social distancing – we all just moved about as normal. Antoinette said there were some directional signs on the floor but I'm afraid I didn't see them. This was a pity because if I'd seen them I would have been able to ignore them. The Greens are demanding that if and when attempts are made to restore our economy, every effort should be made to do so along lines which will satisfy the looniest of the climate change nutters. If this happens then there is absolutely no hope for us, millions more will be unemployed for life and hundreds of thousands will die. The Greens have three qualities: they are arrogant, stupid and narrow minded. They also insist on wearing cameras on their silly cycling helmets.

Please do whatever you can to spread the truth. Share videos and ask people to visit this website. Try to convert those who are terrified and who believe that the coronavirus is the 21st century version of the plague. There are no subscription charges and no advertisements on my YouTube channel or this website and we promise not to try to sell them T-shirts or fancy mugs. But I will mention my books from time to time, when appropriate, so that, if you buy one, Antoinette and I can eat occasionally. (It's a bad habit we picked up.)

The BBC has reported (as though with surprise) that new car sales were down 97% in Northern Ireland in May. How could they be surprised? I am surprised that the sales were not down 100%. Who on earth managed to buy a car with all the showrooms shut? (We bought a new car about two days before the lockdown started. It's a dream vehicle and it has so far travelled a grand total of 175 miles in nearly three months.)

Although the lockdowns have been lifted a little, Antoinette and I hardly every go out. Our house and garden are big enough for us to move about and we live on a sort of island. When we do venture out through our gate it requires a good deal of effort. We are natural recluses and we are aware that if we aren't careful we will become complete recluses. I suspect there are several million more potential recluses in Britain alone.

Professor Ferguson (aka Professor Lockdown and Professor Pantsdown) is reported to have admitted to a House of Lords Select Committee that Sweden achieved much the same result as the UK in suppressing the coronavirus – but without a lockdown and the associated health, social and economic problems.

Sir Richard Dearlove, the former head of MI6 says he has seen a scientific report suggesting that the coronavirus was man-made by Chinese scientists. Donald Trump and the CIA have said the same thing. So why haven't we been shown this report?

Nearly half of all primary schools didn't open on 1st June as they should have done. Was this the fault of teachers or parents? And if parents didn't send their children to school was it because they were frightened of the virus or (more likely) that they refused to send their children into a scary environment where the teachers were likely to be wearing masks, gloves and plastic smocks.

The UK Government has introduced quarantine for travellers with absolutely no scientific basis for the decision. I suggested in March that if the Government were serious about the risk they should close our borders. The current quarantine plan is miles too late and useless. It will, however, destroy the tourist industry, the airline industry and much of the economy.

June 5th 2020

How the Hell Did We Get Here?

I am delighted that the German Government now agrees with my view, first expressed on February 28th on my website, that the fuss over the coronavirus was an exaggeration. They have not, however, gone far enough to agree with my view (expressed on the same date) that there were a number of hidden agendas.

I still stand by everything I said on 28th February and in my first video, recorded in mid-March and entitled 'Coronavirus Scare: The Hoax of the Century'. I wonder how many Government ministers and advisors can say that.

It is time, I think, to take a brief look at where we are.

Today, in Britain, we live in a country split in two. Some believe there is some dirty, hidden agenda and that the lockdown and social distancing are a nonsense. The others, now pitifully obedient and impoverished in spirit, are just waiting for the promised vaccine. When it arrives they will beg to be first in the queue – whatever the risks might be. I don't mean to be rude but I sometimes feel that a good many have been so terrorised, so overwhelmed with the Government's barrage of fake news that they have turned into zombies. If St Vitus turned up they would dance behind him to the ends of the earth. They would follow the Pied Piper of Hamelin anywhere if he promised them safety from the virus.

So, it is, I think, time to take a cold, hard look at where we are now and what has happened since the end of February during which time everything has changed and those of us who are creatures of habit are still desperately searching for new habits to which we can cling.

GPs all around Britain shut their surgeries back in March and many have been offering telephone or video only consultations. No one has yet managed to explain to me how it is possible to listen to a chest, look in a sore ear, palpate an abdomen or check a breast lump from the other end of a telephone. Maybe medical techniques have advanced a good deal since I was a GP. Or maybe a good many diagnoses will be missed and a good many GPs will be spending the next few years fighting in the courts to defend themselves against malpractice suits. Trying to diagnose patients through a video link isn't much better than using the telephone. GPs need to see their patients face to face. Looks, instinct, rapport and even smell are all important when understanding patients and making diagnoses.

Opticians and dentists are effectively closed, though dentists will be opening soon to try to deal with the huge backlog of patients needing emergency treatment. I wonder how many million teeth will be lost unnecessarily. I wonder how many people will lose their sight because of the lockdown. I doubt if anyone will ever know.

In the UK, hospitals are nearly shut and nearly empty. UK figures show that around 2.4 million cancer patients are now waiting for surgery, chemotherapy, radiotherapy, screening checks and mammograms. Patients who attend any medical facility, or ring 999 or 111, will be labelled according to whether or not they have respiratory signs or symptoms. Those who do have respiratory symptoms will be assumed to have covid-19 since it is the default diagnosis. They will be put into what hospitals think of as isolation and other possible diagnoses will almost certainly be ignored. There is no scrutiny or oversight of treatment programmes.

Hairdressers will open soon but the local hospital has announced that it has no idea when the physiotherapy department will open. And churches are still closed for the foreseeable future, which given the fact that few have a congregation that would threaten social distancing is downright cowardly and utterly shameful. Anyone seeking spiritual comfort or solace will have to manage without.

The rules about social distancing and the lockdown are so absurdly complicated that hardly anyone understands them. One of the Government's advisors said that if we all kept three feet apart we'd be fine (actually he said a metre but I haven't gone metric and don't intend to do so) but another two said we had to stay six feet six inches apart. The World Health Organisation which is supposed to know about these things said three feet would do nicely and so did the European Centre for Disease Prevention and Control. Keeping six feet and a bit apart will destroy cafes, pubs and restaurants, cinemas, theatres and most of everything else. There doesn't seem to be any science at all showing how far we should be advised to keep apart. The only real science is that which shows that coughs and sneezes can travel 24 feet but no one has suggested that. There is some evidence that the military like to keep people six feet apart because it makes identification easier.

The Government has said that up to six friends or neighbours may come into your garden unless they are over 70-years-of age. If you are in Scotland then you have eight friends or neighbours to visit. In Wales you may invite people from two households so two big families could produce a gathering of two dozen or more. But all this jolliness must take place out of doors. The visitors can only go through your house in order to get to your garden or, in extremis, to visit the loo. Visitors are warned that they should go to their own loo before visiting so as to reduce the likelihood of this being necessary. What if it rains? Well the rule is that you have to stay out of doors and so everyone will just have to get drenched and hope they don't develop pneumonia. Oddly, as far as I know, there have been no official rulings specifically banning guests from sheltering in a greenhouse, garden shed, log shed or coal bunker.

People coming into the country have to go into quarantine for a fortnight so that is the end of airlines, tourism and heaven knows what else.

If anyone takes notice of this nonsense then I fear for their sanity.

The confusion appears to be global. In one part of the United States it is illegal to sit on the beach but legal to swim in the sea but in another part it is legal to sit on the beach but illegal to swim in the sea. If anyone in the Government understood the rules they would doubtless produce an APP to help punters and Government advisors find out what is and is not allowed.

In Germany police arrested a man for not wearing a mask but the police who did the arresting weren't wearing masks.

It has been revealed that the mass media were bought with government advertising, and governments are now officially the main source of fake news. The wise will never again buy a newspaper (or read one online). We expect the BBC to betray us – but not the tabloids. I say this with great sadness for during two decades I wrote columns for four national newspapers and around 5,000 articles for magazines and newspapers.

Juries have been abandoned and criminals are now judged by establishment plants sitting alone. The Government is bringing in a law to make it illegal to reveal information about what is going on in Britain or to criticise anything that is happening. The punishments will be draconian.

School teachers are exhibiting remarkable ignorance in that the danger to them is not from children but, if at all, from other teachers. They have been seen dressed in the sort of protective gear you might choose if you were planning to remove six tons of asbestos from an old church. If they don't want to catch the flu they should just avoid other members of staff. Children, terrified and scarred for life, will never recover from this unnecessary trauma.

Shoppers have to wait outside, rain or sunshine, until someone leaves since most stores only accept a very limited number of customers. In some parts of the world shoppers have to go through a special shower cubicle where they will be sprayed with a light mist of a saline solution. (Spraying water in a mist is, of course, the way in which Legionnaires Disease usually spreads.) Once in a shop, potential customers aren't allowed to browse or try on items if it is a clothes shop. There will be no café and no loos.

On the internet the 77th Brigade of the British Army, which exists to fight information warfare seems to have turned its attention onto British taxpayers. There is now a special force of three to four thousand British soldiers engaged full time in removing material from social media. There are said to be around 20,000 keyboard warriors in reserve. The army is working with the Cabinet Office Rapid Response Unit to squash dissent. Goebbels and his chums were good at that sort of thing. I wonder whether we can thank the army for the distractions which have effectively changed the news recently.

Whether the army is deciding what to remove from the internet or obeying orders from somewhere else this doesn't seem an entirely democratic action but then we aren't living in democracy any more. We are paying soldiers to take down the truth so that the Government's lies will prevail.

This, we are constantly being told, is the new normal. What a hideous phrase. Is this how life is going to be? It certainly isn't a normal I'm prepared to accept. Normal is a world where honest, law abiding folk can speak their mind and say what they think without fear that they will be banned, demonised or imprisoned. What's normal about a world in which anyone who questions the Government is labelled a dissident, a subversive or a conspiracy theorist? What's normal about a world where thousands of soldiers, paid by us to protect us, spend their days censoring what we say and eradicating the truth so that the fake news spread by the Government can prevail?

Nearly half the people in the country are now being paid by the Government, one way or another, and when the Government stops handing out money many of them will be unemployed. Billionaires living in tax exile are being showered with taxpayers' money so that they don't have to spend their own money to keep their businesses alive. And that's all normal is it?

How bad has the infection really been?

Most doctors with brains now agree with me that governments, particularly the Government in the UK, have deliberately exaggerated the death total in order to justify their extraordinary response.

Whatever the death total is alleged to be today, you can take a third out of the total to cover the elderly people who died, needlessly and criminally, in nursing homes and care homes. And half to two thirds of those left would have died anyway of an underlying disease. Of the remaining deaths, a goodly proportion were wrongly labelled since they died with the coronavirus rather than of it. Most of the rest were over 80 years of age and very frail.

And whatever you are left with should be compared with the death rate from the ordinary influenza which, in a bad year, in the UK, can easily reach 50,000. The global deaths from flu can exceed 600,000.

As I've been saying for three months now, I feel safe in guaranteeing that the genuine coronavirus total will be nowhere near as high as that. So the only possible conclusion is that the coronavirus is no more dangerous than the ordinary flu – and possibly not as dangerous as a bad flu.

Even Ferguson, the serial dunce whose past record makes him the Eddie the Eagle of mathematical modelling (but without the sense of fun and patriotism) and whose sums were the trigger for the lockdown, now agrees that we would have been just as well off following the Swedish route and ignoring the notion of a major lockdown. I have to confess, by the way, that I can't believe that anyone who was looking for someone to give advice about how to deal with an epidemic, and who looked at Ferguson's past record, would put him in a short list of 60 million out of a population of 60 million. Is Ferguson the most incompetent scientist on the planet? I'd vote for him.

I've discussed his track record before. It is, I think, sufficient to say that I would find it embarrassing if it were mine.

Presumably, Comrade Boris knew of this when he hired him? If there are prizes going round for cocking things up then Comrade Boris would get the gold cup – unless, of course, he was acting under orders. I don't wish to be rude, I really don't, but you would have to be a moron to believe that the lockdowns, the social distancing and the fact that we are living in a police state have anything to do with a bug that would have a job to give a flu bug a run for its money. Only MPs, the BBC and assorted hack journalists, and a bunch of desperate celebrities and around 20 million assorted gullibles still believe that we are being threatened by the 21st century version of the plague.

The questions queue up to be answered.

Why are we still destroying the world when Dr Gupta, an epidemiology professor at Oxford University reported that the death rate from the coronavirus is between 0.01% and 0.1% – making it no more of a threat than flu?

Who is going to pay for the fact that the UK will have one of the highest death rates in the world and one of the worst social and economic results? Why do the experts seem unable to differentiate between assessing the number of people who will catch the disease and the number who will die if they do catch it?

Did Boris Johnson really have the coronavirus? It was a most convenient disease. Was he really as ill as we were told?

Is it true that everything is being done in order to sell a vaccine which will be compulsory and make gazillions for people not a million miles removed from the Government?

Is the sound we all hear at 8 p.m. on Thursdays now the sound of lawyers rubbing their hands with glee? If the lawsuits start coming then Ferguson and Imperial College will need even more money than Bill Gates has got in order to pay for this monumental series of disasters. Just think of all those thousands dying in care homes.

Are we going to see the biggest murder trial in history?

So, is the Government comprised entirely of morons?

I wouldn't say it was impossible. I certainly wouldn't want anyone in the Government, or any of the advisors, taking an IQ test for me.

Cummings is said by some to be the brains behind the Government and that says enough. The UK is now the most buggered country on the planet.

As we search for explanations, the questions just keep on coming.

Who bought the Government?

What's going to happen next?

It isn't about science and it's not simple politics.

So it must be about money and control.

Is the plan to force a civil war between those who are desperate for the lockdown to continue and those who are equally determined that it should end now? I have no idea. No one would believe what has happened if it were written as a science fiction novel.

There is nothing they won't stoop to and nothing I now consider impossible. We must now assume the worst of our Government at all times.

The only real certainty is that living through this is worse than living through a war. We aren't likely to be bombed, it is true, but in a war you do at least know who the enemy is, what is going on and what the end game is likely to be. Today, those of us who can see the truth look around and are bewildered by the lunacy of the grovelling masses; terrorised into obedience.

I no longer believe anything I am told by governments or the media.

Remember my three phrase mantra:

Distrust the Government,

Avoid mass media,

Fight the lies.

Paranoia is the only sensible, healthy, sane condition. Those who protest now regard themselves as being members of a resistance movement trying to rescue the last vestiges of freedom and democracy.

Britain used to be a wonderful place to live.

No more. We are now weaker than any other nation.

No one will want to come here.

And everyone who lives here will want to leave.

Eventually, someone is going to have to pay for all this.

Meanwhile, we must, can and will win this war – and we have to think of it as a war, the most crucial in our lifetimes.

June 6th 2020

Why We Must Fight To Keep Cash

I had an exciting moment the other day.

I popped into a shop.

I had to queue to get in, of course, because there were already two people in there.

And to be honest it wasn't too exciting.

It wasn't a bookshop or an antique shop or one of those lovely establishments that used to be called junk shops but which are now called something rather posher, depending upon the whim of the proprietor.

It was a greengrocer.

Cabbages, carrots, potatoes – the usual sort of thing. And walnuts. The squirrels who live in our garden and have their dreys in our trees love walnuts and now that cinemas, theatres, restaurants, pubs, amusement arcades and bowling alleys have all been forced to close we get a lot of excitement and fulfilment from watching squirrels crack open a walnut shell and enjoy the nut inside. We all get our thrills where we can.

So, there I was – in the greengrocers. I had no mask on because I wasn't planning to rob them but I was wearing a Panama hat which I consider far more useful protection since it provides protection against the sun, the rain and the seagulls.

I was standing behind a line painted on the floor, as they like you to do these days, keeping the legally acceptable distance from the till but just close enough so that I could just reach the counter if I stretched out. I put down my purchases, reached into my pocket, took out my wallet and removed a note.

The assistant behind the till looked at me as though I were about to hand her a grenade with the pin removed. She wore plastic gloves and a mask but no hat or goggles. I don't know about her feet. She may have been wearing galoshes.

'Cash?' she said.

'Yes!' I replied brightly. It seemed an odd question but these are strange times.

'People keep giving me cash,' she complained. 'You're the third in a row.'

'That's nice,' I said, handing her the note.

'You should pay with a card,' she said, sternly. She reluctantly took the note between finger and thumb, as though it might explode.

A bomb disposal expert would have accepted a pinless grenade with far less fuss.

She hurriedly stuffed the note into the till and threw some coins down as my change.

'They should make cash illegal,' she said, as I picked up my charge and my purchases. 'It's dirty and spreads disease,' she said. 'It kills people.'

I tried to offer her some reassurance. I pointed out that it has always been known that real money can carry bugs but that it's not really dangerous as long as you don't eat it. Washing your hands will get rid of any bugs.

She didn't want any reassurance. She had been terrified by the Government's brainwashing techniques and by the fake news spread by the mainstream media. I could have talked to her for an hour and not soothed her terror.

(There's an irony for you. The biggest source of fake news these days is the Government. The mainstream media spreads more dangerous, fake news than the internet. There was a story in the papers about a taxi driver who had allegedly caught the coronavirus from a note he had handled. How could anyone ever know that?)

Getting rid of cash is, of course, another of the Government's many hidden agendas. And their dream will soon come true; they are getting closer to achieving a cashless society.

An increasing number of councils are installing machines in their car parks which insist that motorists pay via an App – whatever an App might be. They don't want you to pay with cash anymore.

I hate council run car parks.

First, they insisted that you key your car number into the machine before you could pay. I can never remember our car number and I always have to trudge back to the car, write down the number and trudge back to the machine (where there is inevitably a queue) before I can pay. They want your car number for two reasons. First, so they know where everyone is and because they know you aren't at home they can send someone round to steal your television set. Second, so that if you have some time left on your ticket you cannot be a bit of a Good Samaritan and give the ticket to a motorist just arriving. Isn't that just the meanest thing?

I must stop rambling.

A cashless society won't be much fun. No sixpences under the pillow from the tooth fairy. No giving a few quid to a homeless person so they can buy a pair of second hand shoes, a charity shop jacket or a bottle of cheap plonk. No crisp note tucked into a birthday card. No saving coins in a piggy bank. No excitement from a half a crown tucked into a hot little hand by a loving grandma. No tips slipped into the gloved hand of a hotel doorman. No coins tossed into a hat for a busker who gives life to a dull street or underground railway station. No coins for an arcade machine. No coins in a wishing well. No three coins in a fountain.

A cashless society will be duller in a thousand ways. Giving money digitally is no fun. And if you don't know and trust the recipient it is risky too.

Cash helps children learn the value of money. Cash helps stop people getting into debt. Credit cards, on the other hand, encourage uncontrollable debt.

The woman in the greengrocer's, falsely terrified into believing that my plastic £20 note was going to kill her, probably didn't realise what she had been manipulated into wishing for.

Credit and debit cards enable governments to track our every move. And they enable the card holding companies to record everything we buy. Use a card at a supermarket and they know exactly what you buy. I know a woman who stopped buying tampons in her weekly shop. She was suddenly bombarded with advertisements for baby clothing and prams. Her husband wanted to know why he found that he was about to become a father through their shared email account.

Cash gives a sense of the reality and importance of money. Plastic encourages waste and unsustainable expenditure.

Cash can be stolen, they say.

Yes, it can.

But you can only lose what is in your wallet or purse.

Lose your plastic and you can lose everything you have and some you don't have. Bank fraud is growing and it is no fun. We had a bank account emptied by a thief through no fault of ours and it wasn't very enjoyable.

Finally, they can cut off your money in seconds with a few key strokes. If you speak out and cause trouble they can and will close all your accounts just to shut you up.

If you don't obey the social distancing laws they can turn you into a beggar overnight.

You think I am exaggerating?

You don't think they'd do that?

Let me tell you something about smart meters for electricity – those absurd little machines which the trusting and the innocent and the too honest have allowed their power company to install.

The UK's absurdly fashionable Department of Energy and Climate Change has boasted that if people have smart meters then energy supplies can be cut off if they are using too much electricity and only restored if their energy consumption becomes more conservative. (I have no idea who decides how much is 'too much'.) With a smart meter they can also cut off your power, and therefore your phones and Wi-Fi, if you put unauthorised messages on the internet.

They don't tell you this stuff when they try to persuade you to have a smart meter fitted. They just tell you that it will help you save nine pence a year.

So, next time you go into a shop and they don't want to accept cash, put your purchases down on the counter and tell them you will go somewhere else – where they do take cash. That's the only way we can fight back. Use cash as much as you possibly can.

June 7th 2020

Passing Observations (June 8th 2020)

Antoinette spotted a photo of a shop where the owner had put up signs saying 'No Masks, Handshakes OK, Hugs very OK'. Good for him. What a role model for shopkeepers everywhere.

Negative interest rates are almost here. This absurdity will mean that savers have to pay banks to store their money. Millions who have worked hard and saved will doubtless wish they'd spent their money. Is this another ploy to destroy our independence?

The hatred of those who question the value and safety of vaccination is so great (and so well organised by the pro-vaccine establishment) that my novel *The Truth Kills* has been attacked because one of the characters (a young female doctor) dares to question vaccination as part of the story. I find it rather worrying that people get demonically excited because of the views held by a fictional character.

The more a virus moves around the weaker it tends to get. And so locking people in their houses and shutting schools has meant that the virus hasn't been weakened. If more young people had been allowed to catch the coronavirus (a bug which doesn't usually do much harm to the young) then the number of older and more vulnerable people dying would have been dramatically reduced.

Shutting people in their homes and arresting them for sunbathing or sitting in parks was a criminal error. Our bodies need sunlight to boost vitamin D levels. Vitamin D provides protection against viruses such as those causing colds and flu. So preventing people from going outside contributed to the seriousness of the disease. The Government's absurd policy has, once again, killed people.

In Scotland, more people died from the coronavirus in care homes than in hospitals.

Synagogues have banned singing since singing can spread viruses. How long before shouting is banned? (Not a bad idea). And then how long before talking is prohibited?

Half of Britons increased the amount of alcohol they drank, or the number of days on which they drank, during their house arrest.

All the hand washing means that our water is running out. The consumption of water rose by a quarter during the mass house arrest programme. There will likely be water restrictions this coming summer.

Britain's mass house arrest led to a 42% increase in divorce enquiries.

Many shops (including bookshops) have announced that they will ban browsing. Here's a safe prediction: shops which ban browsers won't survive. They might as well close now and get it over with.

'Like many an oldie, he seems utterly baffled by the tech,' wrote Freddy Gray in *The Spectator* magazine. He was writing about Joe Biden, US Presidential candidate. Ageism just won't die, will it? Would Mr Gray have dared say: 'Like many a woman, she seems utterly baffled by the tech,'?

June 8th 2020

Face Masks – Ending the Confusion

Everyone in the world seems confused about whether or not we should wear masks to protect us from the coronavirus. The general consensus among politicians and the so-called experts quoted in the media appears to me to be that wearing masks does no good but that we should wear them anyway and that we don't need to wear them although they are very useful. This advice is given freely by commentators who are untroubled by facts or research or annoying things of that nature and conflicting pronouncements are regularly made by politicians who clearly know so little about medical matters that they probably couldn't even manage to spell technical medical words such as diarrhoea.

The World Health Organisation, which has loads of highly paid doctors and specialists investigating such matters, appears to lead the confusion. Indeed, their confusion seems to me so confusing that they have confused me. They initially said that healthy individuals only needed to wear a mask if they were taking care of someone suspected of having the coronavirus. The science doesn't seem to me to have changed but the advice from the WHO has changed. I'll come on to why that might be in another video.

Governments everywhere are collectively confused although individual politicians everywhere all seem to have firm views on the matter, usually derived from the bloke who cuts their hair or the woman in the corner shop who knows about these things.

Hospitals and doctors also seem confused. You find me 1,000 hospital staff who think that masks are a good idea and that we should all wear them all the time, even when we are in the bath, and I will find you 1,000 hospital staff who think they are useless or dangerous or both. The odd thing is that there don't seem to be any studies relating to the use of masks with the coronavirus.

Nevertheless, around the world the mask industry is booming. The people who aren't working on a new wonder vaccine are making masks.

There are videos and books explaining how to make your own mask out of unwanted bits and pieces found lying around the home. It is possible to make two excellent face masks out of the cups of an old brassiere, using the straps to fashion loops to go around the ears or the back of the head. Naturally, the size of the bra has a big influence on its suitability for turning into a face mask and a bra measuring 44GG is probably going to be a little on the loose side for most people. And if you need fresh masks every day you will need a large supply of bras. Despite the confusion, the British Government announced that from June 15th everyone in England must wear a mask when using public transport. You can travel on public transport on the 14th without a mask but on the 15th you will need a mask, presumably because the Government knows that the virus will suddenly become more dangerous then. I have absolutely no idea what the rules are in Scotland or Wales but they're bound to be different to England because both Scotland and Wales are desperate to prove that they are independent countries, but if they don't follow the English law then if you are on a train which crosses a border you can presumably remove your mask until your return journey. You may also have to wear a mask if entering a shop or a public building or an office though this doesn't appear to be a law. There doesn't seem to be much in the way of guidance for police officers but the Government says it doesn't expect there to be any problems. That's probably not quite the firm ruling that the police would have liked so we can presumably expect the confusion to spread into the courts.

In the UK, the Government that appears now to be only looking after England, has previously admitted that wearing a mask does not protect the wearer but it may protect other people if the wearer has the infection but doesn't know it. And the Government has added that you don't have to wear a mask if you are under the age of two, if you find it difficult to manage a mask properly or if you have a respiratory problem of any kind which may make breathing difficult. I take this to mean that anyone who has asthma, hay-fever, emphysema, bronchitis, a smoker's cough or anything else a bit chesty doesn't have to wear one. I suffer from hay-fever and get a bit wheezy from time to time so I'm afraid I can't possibly wear one. I'll write myself a little note saying that I have an intermittent chest condition and cannot possible wear a mask and if a policeman stops me I'll show him that. I should mention here that there is evidence that people who don't wear masks in public may be harassed and abused by people who are wearing them. I think that's a risk that I'm prepared to take.

No one with mental illness of any kind should be expected to wear a mask. Nor should anyone with dementia though I am not sure they are on the list of exclusions. No one seems to have worried much about this but the hearing impaired who rely on lip reading will obviously be badly affected if everyone wears a mask. People with skin conditions might find that wearing a mask causes eczema, dermatitis or other problems – particularly if the mask has been washed in a biological detergent. In my view, patients who are ill in hospital shouldn't wear a face mask, especially if they are in bed, because of the risk of them inhaling their vomit if they are sick.

The world is now awash with conflicting reports on how or when or whether to wear a mask to protect you against the flu, the lurgy or the embarrassment of having egg on your chin.

Some people, such as the Mayor of London, want masks to be compulsory though no one has provided evidence for the compulsion. Early on in this farce, Act 1 scene 2 I think it was, the Mayor allegedly threatened to order people to wear masks in London if the Government did not do so. In the end, I got so darned confused myself that I decided to put a cold compress on my forehead, settle down with some research papers and set out on an expedition to find the truth. In the end I came to a very firm, definitive conclusion which I shall now add to the mix. If the mayor of London, who was I believe trained as a lawyer, can have a view then I'm damned sure I am entitled to a firm view too. Maybe we can do a deal. I'll promise not to do any 'legal eagle' stuff if he'll promise to shut up about medical stuff.

Incidentally, talking of lawyers, I think Mr Khan can consider himself trumped because on 30th March, the former Supreme Court Justice Jonathan Sumption QC told us all that the police have no power to enforce Ministers' preferences and that there was nothing in the existing legislation which empowered a police officer to force a citizen of the UK to wear a mask on public transport or anywhere else.

Lord Sumption pointed out that even if the Government rushed through new legislation the laws would have to be justified and proportionate in order to avoid violating our human rights and civil liberties.

He went on to suggest that since masks may endanger the wearer, they are a contravention of Article 2 of the Human Rights Act.

'I hope,' he said, 'that UK citizens will unite in civil disobedience to the unlawful, unjustified and disproportionate violation of our human rights and refuse either to wear a mask or to pay the fixed penalty notice for not doing so. If enough of us take a stand against the further encroachment on our civil liberties, we can look forward to hundreds of thousands of court cases in which the Crown tries to prove the scientific validity of wearing masks to combat a virus that has been circulating in the UK for five months.'

That statement was made over two months ago, so it's seven months now.

I've been unable to find out if Lord Sumption still believes that but I'm really looking for medical facts so I offer his two month old views only out of curiosity and a sense of respect.

One thing I need to point out before I forget is that there is, as always, a good deal of fake news around about masks. In particular, some mainstream media outlets delight in dismissing the risks associated with face masks as fake news. The fact is that masks can be dangerous and need to be worn only when necessary. Anyone who denies that has either been bought or is woefully ignorant. There's a good deal of both around these days.

First, I want to give you some facts about face masks themselves which are, of course, much more complicated than they appear to be at first sight. Governments don't seem to bother differentiating between different types of mask and I think that tells us a good deal about why they want us to wear them – again, that's something I'll explore in another video.

The World Health Organisation recommends that disposable masks should be discarded after one use.

The WHO doesn't seem to have any guidelines for masks made out of washable material but it's a fair guess that it would recommend washing thoroughly at a high temperature after every use.

Unfortunately, washing cloth face masks makes them even less effective. The more you wash the mask the less effective it becomes. Masks are effective only when used in combination with frequent hand washing with soap and water or an alcohol based hand rub.

Fabric masks may allow viruses to enter and are not considered to be anywhere near as protective as surgical masks. A study I have seen entitled 'Optical microscopic study of surface morphology and filtering efficiency of face masks' concluded that face masks made of cloth are not very good at filtering out viruses because the pores are much bigger than the particulate matter that needs to be kept out. One study showed that facemasks may have pores five thousand times larger than virus particles. If this is accurate it means that the virus will wander through the face mask much like a mouse wandering through Marble Arch.

Masks are only really effective if they fit perfectly and if the wearer does not move their head while wearing them. Touching a mask appears to stop the mask providing protection. It has been suggested that you should put on a new mask if you have touched the one you are wearing.

Surgical masks are worn to stop bits of food or hair falling from the surgeon or nurse into a wound. They will stop some bacteria but will not usually stop viruses.

Much of the air we breathe in and out goes around the side of the mask unless it is very tight fitting. The effectiveness of a mask depends massively on the nature of the mask, how it is worn and how often it is changed. How long will it be before we are expected to attend facemask wearing classes?

So much for the masks themselves.

Next, I want to look at the serious health problems which might be associated with wearing a mask and which have been largely ignored or dismissed by politicians and the sort of media which has been bought by governments.

Does wearing a face mask reduce your immunity levels?

No one seems to know the answer for sure but it seems possible that if people wear face masks for long periods (months or years) then the absence of contact with the real world might well have a harmful effect on immunity – if the face mask works. Do face masks prevent us developing immunity to particular diseases? This depends on many factors – mainly the effectiveness of the face mask. But if the mask isn't preventing the development of immunity then it probably isn't worth wearing.

The two widely acknowledged hazards of wearing a face mask are first that the mask may give a false sense of security and stop people taking other precautions – such as washing their hands. Secondly, if masks aren't worn properly – according to the guidelines I have listed – they can do more harm than good.

There is no doubt that face masks can be dangerous. In China, two school boys who were wearing face masks while running on a track both collapsed and died – possibly, I would surmise, because the strain on their hearts by the shortage of oxygen proved fatal.

A report published in the *British Medical Journal* summarised some other risks.

First, when you wear a face mask some of the air you breathe out goes into your eyes. This can be annoying and uncomfortable and if, as a result, you touch your eyes you may infect yourself.

Second, face masks make breathing more difficult and, as I have already pointed out, anyone who has a breathing problem will find that a mask makes it worse. Also, some of the carbon dioxide which is breathed out with each exhalation is then breathed in because it is trapped. Together these factors may mean that the mask wearer may breathe more frequently or more deeply and if that happens then someone who has the coronavirus may end up breathing more of the virus into their lungs. If a mask is contaminated because it has been worn for too long then the risks are even greater. How long is too long? No one knows. No research has been done as far as I know.

Third, there is a risk that the accumulation of the virus in the fabric of the mask may increase the amount of the virus being breathed in. This might then defeat the body's immune response and cause an increase in infections – other infections, not just the coronavirus.

Another report, again written with medical authority, offers more problems.

Dr Russell Blaylock, a retired neurosurgeon, reported that wearing a face mask can produce a number of problems varying from headaches to hypercapnia (a condition in which excess carbon dioxide accumulates in the body) and that the problems can include life threatening complications.

The risk of side effects developing when wearing a mask depend to some extent on whether the mask is made of cloth or paper or is an N95 mask filtering out at least 95% of airborne particles.

One study of 212 healthcare workers showed that a third of them developed headaches with 60% needing painkillers to relieve the headache. Some of the headaches were thought to be caused by an increase in the amount of carbon dioxide in the blood or a reduction in the amount of oxygen in the blood. Another study, this time of 159 young health workers showed that 81% developed headaches after wearing facemasks – so much that their work was affected.

A third study, involving 53 surgeons, showed that the longer a mask was worn the greater the fall in blood oxygen levels. This may lead to the individual passing out and it may also affect natural immunity – thereby increasing the risk of infection.

An N95 mask can reduce blood oxygenation by as much as 20% and this can lead to a loss of consciousness. Naturally, this can be dangerous for car drivers, for pedestrians or for people standing up.

Dr Blaylock also pointed to a study entitled 'The use of masks and respirators to prevent transmission of influenza: a systematic review of the scientific evidence.' This study looked at 17 separate studies and

concluded that none of the studies established a conclusive relationship between the use of masks and protection against influenza infection.
'When a person has TB we have them wear a mask,' concluded Dr Blaylock, 'not the entire community of the non- infected.'
I wonder if our leaders know all this. If they do then why are they so keen to make face masks compulsory despite the dangers? And if they don't know all this then they should do.
The one remaining question is: why, when the disease is fading throughout the world, has the British Government decided that we should wear masks when there are so clearly very real dangers with wearing them.
I suppose they will say it is because the lockdown is being eased a little but they lie about everything so I don't believe that for a second.
I think they have another reason.
I'll discuss the psychological problems associated with the wearing of face masks in another article. And I will also explain how the Government is using masks to make us fearful so that we are easier to control.

June 9th 2020

Why Is the BBC Peddling Fake News?

Here are two recent headlines from the BBC website:
'We have a pandemic of black people dying every day'.
And
'Raheem Sterling: The only disease right now is racism'.
These are obviously absurd and seem designed to stir up discontent.
Of course there are black people dying every day. There are white
people dying every day too. It is a sad, inescapable fact of life that in
the end we all die.
But the headline from the BBC seems to suggest that black people are
the only ones dying. Are they suggesting that white people have found
the secret of eternal life but are hiding the secret from black people?
The second headline 'The only disease right now is racism' is
obviously nonsensical but it's worse than that – it is insulting to
millions of people who are struggling with real, physical disease which
threatens their very existence.
The BBC is quick enough to condemn people for what it calls fake
news but I doubt if there is any organisation more guilty of misleading
its audience than the BBC.
Here's a headline from the BBC website: Coronavirus: UK Exceeds
200,000 Testing Capacity Target
That sounds impressive does it not?
Go down to the sixth paragraph and the BBC admitted that only
115,000 tests had actually been carried out.
The BBC is, always, bending the way it presents the news to suit the
requirements of the establishment.
In another item on their website, the BBC printed a drawing of a man
walking through a tube train and leaving footprints behind him. The
suggestion was that it is possible to spread the coronavirus on your
shoes.
This is absurd fake news.
Is the BBC seriously suggesting that we wear disposable galoshes as
well as gloves and masks?
The BBC seems to delight in fact checking stories (though sometimes
rather comically I'm afraid) so maybe they'd like to check this story.
The BBC is always appalling as a source of news but it has excelled
itself during this bizarre, manufactured crisis.

You might have thought that the BBC would have invited one of the many doctors questioning the whole coronavirus hoax onto a radio or television programme to discuss things.

But as far as I am aware they haven't done so.

Maybe they thought it might upset the Government.

And with a review of the BBC licence fee they wouldn't want to do that, would they?

The truth is, of course, that none of this is new. The BBC has a terrible record when it comes to reporting things honestly and fairly.

It is, I think, now widely recognised that BBC journalists seem to have lost the ability to differentiate between 'news' and 'comment'. One independent think tank commented that 'the BBC pays lip service to impartiality but acts more like a political party with a policy manifesto.'

A survey of just under 40,000 people showed that 85% of Britons no longer trust BBC News to give unbiased political coverage and it isn't difficult to see why. Celebrities commonly speak out in support of the BBC and endorse its line on most things but it is difficult not to suspect that this is sometimes because they fear that if they don't then they will be ostracised and will no longer be offered well paid acting or presenting jobs.

Despite the celebrity endorsement, nearly ten million Britons cancelled their TV licences in recent years.

Many of them were disgusted by the fact that the BBC has been bought by the European Union. In one recent five year period, the BBC accepted 258 million euros from the EU. Over the recent years, the BBC has accepted huge quantities of EU money. I won't accept £5 from an advertiser or a sponsor or the EU because my independence is important to me. But the BBC has sold its integrity.

Inevitably, therefore, it is no surprise that the BBC is clearly biased in favour of the European Union. The BBC has for years been consistently pro-EU and before the Referendum it was clear that the Corporation regarded the very idea of leaving the EU as sacrilegious. Even though the Corporation is funded by a compulsory licence fee taken from a largely unwilling and often rather resentful electorate, the BBC has deliberately favoured the minority point of view in support of the EU.

In the months after the nation decided it no longer wanted to be ruled by a bunch of unelected bureaucrats living and working in Belgium, the BBC did everything it could to demonise Brexit and Brexiteers. On the relatively rare occasions when Brexit supporters were allowed into a studio, they were invariably labelled 'right wing' and treated as though they were in some way criminal. On the other hand, when Remainers were interviewed they were treated with great respect and introduced as though they were independent commentators.

It became quite well known that when the BBC arranged a programme with an audience then the audience would be packed with Remainers. Every piece of bad news was (sometimes laughably) blamed on Brexit and every piece of good news was accompanied by the phrase 'despite Brexit'.

Studies of the BBC have shown an overwhelming bias against Brexit. But this partisan approach to the news is not confined to Brexit and the European Union.

The BBC charter demands that the BBC is impartial and reflects all strands of public opinion. In return for this impartiality, the BBC is entitled to an annual licence fee (currently around £150). But the BBC is not impartial. On the contrary, it is a corrupt and traitorous organisation which has betrayed Britain and the British. I believe the BBC is in breach of its own Charter and no longer entitled to the annual licence fee. Far from being expected to continue paying money to the BBC, citizens of Britain are entitled to receive refunds for the money they have handed over in the past.

When Donald Trump was elected President of the United States of America, the BBC reported the event with sneery comments on his opinions, his political views and his personality. And when the BBC reported his policies on immigration, they did so as though they were eccentric and extreme although every poll showed that a majority of Americans and a majority of Europeans agreed with Trump's policies. Whenever Trump is mentioned, the disdain is almost palpable.

However, whenever the EU supporting Obama is mentioned, the BBC drools with affection – never mentioning the former President's crafty deceits and the broken promises.

Moreover, the BBC appears to have a deep contempt for populism; a movement which has become global and which worries the political establishment so much that they dismiss it in the same sort of tone which you might expect them to use for fascism or communism. Here again, the BBC's attitude is irrational for populism is defined as a movement that champions 'the common person' in preference to the interests of the establishment. Populism invariably combines people on both the left and the right and is invariably hostile to large banks, large multinational corporations and extremists of all kinds. You might think that an organisation which is paid for by the populace at large might have at least a little sympathy with their interests, needs and anxieties. But, no, the BBC has firmly allied itself with the ruling classes and the Europhilic establishment and has no time for licence fee payers who are concerned about mass immigration, overcrowding, relentless globalisation and absurdly ill-based 'green' policies which result in new laws which have pushed up energy prices so dramatically that millions of hard-working people have to choose between eating and keeping warm.

Most people now recognise that the BBC represents a minority viewpoint and gives absurd amounts of airtime and respect to the high priests and priestesses of political correctness. This may be because, as one senior BBC figure has pointed out, the BBC has 'an abnormally large number of young people, ethnic minorities and gay people' on its staff.

The BBC is not a broadcaster it is a narrowcaster; a propaganda unit for the elite.

Not surprisingly, the viewing figures for many BBC shows have sunk dramatically and in the last couple of decades the viewing figures for the BBC's news programmes have shown a decline that would have startled any broadcaster which did not have the State's authority to collect money from millions of unwilling citizens.

The position is now so bad that if the BBC loses its licence fee then it will die because it will be unable to find enough viewers prepared to subscribe to its services. If the BBC retains its anachronistic right to demand licence fees then the annual charge must rocket to counterbalance the fall in the number of people prepared to pay the fee. If you listen to or watch any BBC programmes do so with scepticism in your heart and mind.

Today's BBC is Biased, Bought and Corrupt.

Joseph Goebbels, the Minister of Propaganda in the Third Reich, would have been proud of the BBC.

The BBC now peddles fake news because it's the only thing the appalling staff know how to do.

June 9th 2020

Face Masks 2: The Reason They Want Us to Wear Them

In a previous video I summarised the scientific evidence and proved that wearing a mask is not risk free. There are very real dangers. I have no doubt that masks will kill some of the people who wear them. Indeed, there is evidence that people have already died as a result of wearing masks.

And yet, despite the very real dangers, and in the absence of any convincing evidence showing that masks are of value, a number of governments have made wearing them compulsory on public transport and in many public places. Around the world mask wearing is, or is about to become, compulsory in shops, public buildings, offices and even schools.

Are the politicians entirely stupid and reckless with the lives of their citizens? The bug has been proved to be no more dangerous than the flu bug but we are never forced to wear masks when there is a flu bug around. The WHO says that asymptomatic transmission is very rare. Or could there be some other reason for forcing us to wear masks?

Well, I wouldn't want to argue with you if you said that all politicians are stupid as well as crooked, they have certainly been working hard to give that impression.

But I think what is happening is beyond stupidity; there's a reason for the introduction of laws promoting the wearing of masks. And the reason has more to do with the fact that politicians are crooks, and are being controlled and manipulated by crooks behind the scenes, than the fact that they are all stupid.

Just remember that we know our politicians to be greedy and self-serving. Remember the British MPs expenses scandal? Well-paid men and women claiming for duck houses and endless packets of biscuits. Politicians everywhere are the professional group most likely to be sent to prison for fraud, embezzlement, telling big lies or stealing.

In Britain, the country I know best, there has been a coup.

And I suspect the same thing has happened in many other countries – particularly throughout Europe. I am not convinced that it has happened in the United States where the President's aims and objectives seem to be rather different to those of European leaders. But although this is a global problem it is nowhere as bad as it is in Britain. I am told, reliably, that a great many of the rich are planning to leave Britain as soon as they can. We will be told they are leaving because of the weather or the raised taxes – but they aren't. They are going to emigrate because they can see that the British are being turned into puppets, slaves. Comrade Boris and the rest of his ragbag Government can do whatever they like with the country. There is no effective opposition. The Emergency Bill which was passed days after the bug was officially downgraded to flu status has given Comrade Boris and his advisors the power to do whatever they like. Note the word advisors. It is important.

The coup didn't involve soldiers marching to Westminster or to Buckingham Palace but it was a coup and it did involve soldiers suppressing the people by deliberately taking down internet posts that were considered unacceptable.

You may think this sounds rather paranoid and three months ago I would have thought it was too.

But, as they keep telling us, nothing is the same, everything has changed forever. The only constancy, the only certainty, is that governments around the world, and particularly in Britain, have consistently and deliberately misled the voters.

In future videos, I intend to investigate what I think is behind everything that has happened. I fear it may all be worse than most people had imagined. I aim to try to unravel the complexities of a new world – where power and money are the only two driving forces.

Once again, I think there has been a coup.

Our country has been taken over without our consent, against our will. We are not alone. The same thing has happened elsewhere.

Saying this will, I know, immediately label me a subversive; a conspiracy theorist.

But the real irony is that it is the people who have taken over our world who are the conspiracy theorists.

As I explained in a previous video, a conspiracy theorist is someone who believes in something that the majority do not believe in.

And since thinking people in Britain no longer believe that our lives are being threatened by a deadly, plague-like bug, Boris Johnson's government and its advisors are the conspiracy theorists as, indeed, are those in the mainstream media who support them – and who have been bought for the price of some advertising.

Many are now too afraid to say that they no longer believe in the potency of the bug. But the word is spreading fast and I believe that those of us who no longer believe the Government are now in the majority. For weeks, the Government has taken advantage of the fact that the country has been divided into two; they have used the age-old trick of 'divide and conquer'. But I feel that they are losing that battle. I don't believe the takeover of our world was fortuitous or serendipitous and nor do I believe it was opportunism.

And so, as Sherlock Holmes might have said, when you have excluded all the possibles the only thing left is the impossible.

The whole thing was planned.

And it has, I suspect, been planned for a long time – for years.

Bit by bit our freedom and our privacy have been taken away. Gradually, almost imperceptibly, our rights have disappeared and the State has grown larger and ever more intrusive. I will deal with what I really think is happening in future videos, which I will intersperse with videos on other topics because it is going to take some time to unearth the truth and to find what is really going on.

But today I want to stick with why they want us to wear masks when there doesn't seem to be any need to wear them, when there is no medical evidence that they do any good but there is very real evidence that they can do harm.

The death rate from the bug has fallen considerably in recent weeks; most of the really vulnerable people have already died. The authorities have successfully cleaned out care homes and exterminated a good chunk of the population receiving pensions. I wonder how much that has saved the Treasury.

Moreover, the lockdown is now killing so many people that even if the number dying from the bug were to double in the next month, the total would still not come anywhere near to the total who die every year from the flu, when you add on the number who have died because of the lockdown.

Mental illnesses, anxiety and depression, will be the new pandemics. The Government admits that the number dying from the ordinary flu has fallen, what a surprise that is, but they cannot tell us how many have committed suicide since we were all put under house arrest.

They can, on the other hand, tell us precisely how many people died of their plague in Birmingham last Wednesday afternoon. And they are controlling the figures so precisely that they can probably tell us precisely how many people are going to die in Birmingham next Wednesday afternoon.

If there is a second wave of infections then we can be damned sure it will be deliberate. Bugs of this kind usually become weaker with time and far less virulent in warm weather.

Over recent years we have seen our privacy and our freedom gradually disappearing. Our rights have all but disappeared as the State has taken over responsibility for everything we do. We have seen the truth suppressed and we have seen those who dare to speak out demonised, monstered and silenced. We have seen the introduction of smart meters for electricity, so that they can cut off our energy supplies whenever they want to. The elderly have been steadily attacked and blamed for everything wrong with our society. Since I predicted that it would happen many weeks ago, it was no surprise at all to me that elderly folk are being found alone and dead in their homes. Some of them will have starved to death. We have seen the banks and the politicians pushing hard for a cashless society. Our broadcasters, particularly the BBC, produce an unending mixed diet of garbage and lies. The BBC produces dumbed down programmes and propaganda. Children have been brainwashed in schools, our history has altered to fit the requirements of the politically correct. The news we see on mainstream television has been dumbed down and controlled. Our hospitals have been closed, in whole or in part, for no reason other than to keep us afraid. And as I have shown in previous videos we have been brainwashed by experts with their slogans and trickery. All the things we used to enjoy, and look forward to, have been taken from us. We are told that sporting events, for example, may never again be possible with spectators. Theatres and cinemas will probably never reopen. Air travel has become extraordinarily complicated and will, no doubt, become prohibitively expensive. The closure of public loos means that town centres will die. We are told that churches are being closed and bishops are being sacked. We are being turned into a nation of drudges; broken and nervous and filled with uncertainties.

And that takes us back to the masks.

Why are we being told that we must wear masks – which will be especially uncomfortable in the hot weather?

Well, it is partly to weaken us. Wearing masks for extended periods will make us sick and will probably make us more vulnerable to illness. Wearing masks can damage the immune system. Fear and stress also weaken the immune system.

Don't believe anyone who tells you that is fake news, by the way. It may be inconvenient to the Government and their lackeys. But it is not fake.

In my first video about masks, I quoted the medical evidence proving that it is anything but fake news. The transcript of that video will, as usual, also be on my website.

It is partly to dehumanise us.

The process of dehumanisation has been slowly developing for some time. Our identities, our individuality, have been attacked in many different ways. Masks help to oppress us. They take away our personality and turn us all into faceless creatures; they keep us unsettled and they isolate us from one another. It is difficult to have a conversation when wearing a mask. There are no smiles to see. Good news is less exhilarating when delivered by someone wearing a mask. And bad news is far more painful when delivered by someone wearing a mask. There can be no sense of a real connection between two people both wearing masks. Hospitals, GP surgeries and dental surgeries will all be more frightening. Workplaces and public transport will be more depressing. Masks will create a whole range of psychological problems.

So does the Government really want us depressed and anxious?

Yes, they do. Because they are breaking us down. It is the next part of the brainwashing process which I have already described in detail in a previous video. Please watch it if you haven't already done so.

They want to keep us terrified.

Masks are scary in themselves. Robbers and bandits wear masks. But there is more to it than that.

The idea is to keep us aware of the danger that is alleged to be around us and to increase our sense of fear and our obedience.

By forcing us to wear masks they are making us more afraid, and so they can control us more effectively.

I don't believe we are being told to wear masks so that we will be safer.

But I do believe we are being told to wear masks to keep us weaker and more afraid.

June 10th 2020

Why I Resigned from My Job as a GP

Among the lies on the Web there is one claiming that I left the NHS after my first book, *The Medicine Men* was published. The book was about the relationship between the medical profession and the drug industry, and I'm not promoting it because it has been out of print for decades.

If those who make this stuff up bothered to do any research, or cared about the truth, they would know that this is nonsense.

The Medicine Men was published in 1975, and I received an advance of £750 to write it. The typist who worked on the typescript charged £800 and the insurers from whom I bought libel insurance charged me £700.

I had some money for foreign rights and paperback rights but the book wasn't going to take me off to the Bahamas on a huge yacht.

Besides, what the idiots on the Web don't realise is that I didn't resign as a GP until seven or eight years later.

Being a GP was the job I'd always wanted to do and one that I enjoyed a great deal.

In those distant days, GPs were responsible for their patients 365 days a year and 24 hours a day. So that we had some time off, most doctors worked in informal groups of four or five. Often the association was a very loose one in that individual GPs ran their practices independently and merely shared their out of hours' responsibilities. It all worked surprisingly well and easily.

If there were five doctors sharing their night time, weekend and bank holiday calls then each one of the five would be on call one night a week and one weekend in five. It wasn't particularly onerous.

At the end of the day, a doctor who was looking after a patient with a specific problem would ring the doctor due to be on call and tell him if he was likely to be called out. 'Mrs X has a bad chest infection but I think she is responding to the antibiotics. If her husband calls, you may have to fix a hospital bed for her.' That sort of thing.

I never particularly minded out of hours calls. Indeed, the best bit of being a GP was driving back home at 4.00 a.m. having spent an hour or two treating a patient at home. It might have been an asthmatic having severe trouble breathing and needing intravenous injections. Or a child screaming with pain from an ear infection.

Of course, the glow of satisfaction might dim slightly if, when getting back home, I found there was another call to be done. If there was then it would inevitably be to a house in the next street to the one I'd just left. There were no mobile phones in those days, of course.

After a night on call we still did morning surgery. And that was sometimes a little tiring. I wasn't the only GP to fall asleep in his consulting room.

So why, after just ten years, did I give up my dream job?

It was the paperwork, the bureaucracy, which defeated me.

One of a GP's tasks was to sign sick notes. And the law required doctors to put the diagnosis on the form. The patient then took the form to their employer. Inevitably, this meant that everyone in the office knew what the patient's problem was.

One of my patients was the manager of the local branch of a big chain store.

He came in to see me one day and it wasn't difficult to see the problem. He was severely depressed; worn down by demanding bosses and a difficult job. He needed time off work.

I reached for the sick note pad, scribbled his name and address and then wrote 'depression' in the box requiring a diagnosis.

'Do you have to put that down?' he asked.

I looked at him, puzzled.

'If my bosses see that then I'll be fired,' he told me.

I ripped up the form and wrote another. On this one I scribbled 'virus infection'.

A couple of days later, a young woman came to see me. She was pregnant and was suffering from morning sickness.

'Do you mind not putting down that I'm pregnant?' she asked. 'The girls at work don't know but I have to hand the form in to my boss.'

And so she had a virus infection too.

After that, all the sick notes I signed contained the same diagnosis: virus infection.

After a few weeks of this, I was hauled before a local NHS committee. They had a sheaf of sick notes I had signed. All the forms had the same diagnosis.

To cut a long story short, they fined me a couple of hundred quid and threatened to do it again and again if I didn't write down proper diagnoses. That was a lot of money in those days.

So I resigned from my job as a GP and became a professional writer.

Shortly afterwards, I'm pleased to say, the rules were changed and patients were allowed to write their own sick notes.

June 11th 2020

Why You Should Stockpile Food – Now

Food shortages are coming and the cost of food is going to rise even faster than it has been doing. And it isn't because of global warming or whatever other lies they tell you – it is however, partly a side effect of the coronavirus scandal; the biggest and most dangerous hoax in history.

All around the world, food is in short supply. The price of the world's most important staple food – rice – has risen by 70%. Food prices in the US have recently seen a historic jump and are destined to stay high and go higher. Countries which have good food production are halting their exports. Vietnam, for example, has stopped exporting because they need their food supplies at home. And you cannot blame them. The authorities condemn it as nationalism but all countries, all villages, all homes would do much the same.

And it is the absurd over-reaction to a bug no more dangerous than the flu that is causing the problem – and that will result in millions of deaths to add to the millions who are going to die as a result of the lockdowns. The total death rate from the coronavirus is let me remind you yet again just two thirds of the number who would have died of the flu in the same period. And the coronavirus figures have been artificially inflated.

But the global death rate from the side effects – accidental or deliberate – of what I now call the coronavirus scandal is going to be measured in millions.

So, how is the coronavirus scandal responsible for the food shortages that are coming?

That's easy to explain.

Processing plants and distribution centres all around the world have been severely disrupted by the massive over-reaction to this fairly ordinary virus.

If one worker on a farm or in a warehouse falls ill with flu-like symptoms then the authorities are often closing down the farm or the warehouse. Is this a panic? Or is it being deliberately orchestrated for some hidden reason?

Huge crops of vegetables and fruit are being ploughed into the ground. Millions of animals are being slaughtered and then buried or burnt because the supply chains have been shut down. America, almost unbelievably, is now importing beef because of the shortages there.

The world lockdown, and the mass house arrests that were engineered to keep us all subservient, mean that thousands of farmers cannot get their crops picked. Fruit in particular is likely to rot in the fields and tankers full of milk are poured away. Controls on transport have meant that it has been difficult to move food from where there is a glut to where there is a dearth. It would have been easy for governments to insist that furloughed workers should help pick the crops but they didn't do so. Or what about all those students locked out of their colleges?

And the unsurprising consequence of all this is that there are going to be massive shortages of fruit and vegetables, and so prices are probably going to rocket.

Inevitably, the most toxic of the Remainers, the fascist EU loving lunatics, bigoted, soaked in their own prejudices and consumed by ignorance will blame Brexit for the shortages. If they develop a bald spot or lose their keys they blame Brexit.

Sadly for them, the shortage is global not local to the UK.

All around the world there is a shortage of almost all foods.

And other factors are going to ensure that the shortage just gets worse.

If and when the economy is allowed to stutter into action again, the price of oil will doubtless eventually rise because the existing supplies are diminishing rapidly and most oil companies have pretty well given up exploration.

The rising price of oil will mean that farming and transportation costs will rise and that will also push up the price of food. I know oil is being made all the time but the current crop of oil in preparation won't be ready for another 50 million years at least and you'll probably want to eat before then.

I tell you this not to scare you but because when you know something is happening you can do something about it.

You may think it is worthwhile building up your stocks of long-dated food staples such as rice and pasta and bottled water (because that's going to be in short supply too) and maybe even an extra packet or two of loo rolls. Dried and tinned food with long dates are also good.

Governments tell us not to store stuff but the military don't buy bullets the day they need them, do they? If you have a garden and can grow your favourite vegetables or fruit that's probably a good idea but watch that no one climbs over your fence and steals them. I don't recommend having an allotment – the chances of you being able to harvest your own crops are too remote because they will be stolen. It might also be a good idea to stock up on vitamin and mineral supplements.

I rather suspect that we are going to have more alleged virus health calamities coming up. If it isn't the coronavirus in a pre-ordained second wave it will be something else. If they can make up one crisis then they can, and will, make up many more.

I've always been a bit of a contrarian, though I don't suppose anyone would notice, and I'm convinced that the time to panic buy is when there is no panic.

There are several other explanations for what has already happened and for what is going to turn this into a perfect storm of food shortages. Some of the explanations are short-term and some are long-term.

The next problem hasn't received as much publicity, largely because the newspapers and TV and radio stations have been too busy bombarding us with fake news authorised by government propaganda experts to bother with real news.

The problem is locusts.

Plagues of them have been travelling from Arabia into Africa. Most of us tend to think of a swarm of insects as being no more than a few yards across but locusts tend to think rather bigger.

A decent sized swarm of locusts can be as large as London and there can be lots of swarms. That's pretty scary but even scarier is the fact that a plague of locusts can in two days eat their way through as much food as would keep the whole of the population of the UK going for a day. A swarm can lay around 1,000 eggs per square yard of land. You can imagine what that will do to the world's food supplies.

Of course, we should be able to rely on the Food and Agriculture Organisation, a United Nations agency which is supposed to control problems like this. The FAO is a bit like the World Health Organisation so that's nice.

And so now there are swarms of locusts wandering across Africa, and each swarm can cover 20 square miles. All the locusts do is breed and eat. When they land on a tree, the combined weight will bring down large branches. Africans sometimes panic and fire at the swarms with rockets and anti-aircraft guns but when the enemy is numbered in billions just killing a few thousand doesn't make a lot of difference.

The FAO is crop spraying with chemicals but unfortunately the locusts seem to have developed immunity. In one area, locusts all fell off trees after being sprayed but three days later they all got up, shook themselves and flew away. A small swarm of locusts can strip 100 acres in minutes. Inevitably, the fake crisis that has been gripping the world has disrupted supplies of the chemicals for spraying, and the swarms of locusts are getting bigger and bigger and threatening food supplies in Africa, Arabia and Asia. The economies of those countries affected are going to be destroyed. Food will be scarce and what there is will be unaffordable. If the West hadn't been so busy looking at the virus hoax they might have been able to do something to stem the tide of the locusts.

But the locusts are munching away and the farmers are digging their crops into the ground and the food shortages which are coming will be biblical.

Is this why governments everywhere are determined to kill off old people as quickly as they possibly can?

Is one of the many reasons for the coronavirus being exaggerated the desire to close down farms and warehouses and distribution centres – apparently legitimately – when one worker tests positive for the coronavirus, or develops a mild symptom or two?

Maybe the advice here will help those who watch these videos: do a little food stock piling now so that you and your family will have a better chance to be strong and healthy. Countries look after themselves and we all need to do so. It isn't selfish. It's survival.

If and when your government finally warns you of this problem it will be far too late.

In my next video on food, I will deal with the other factors which are making this problem worse – and which may explain why governments and the people behind them have deliberately exaggerated the coronavirus crisis and have, with no exaggeration, turned it into the biggest scandal in human history.

June 11th 2020

The Coming Global Food Shortage – A Perfect Storm

In my first video about food, I explained how the coronavirus scandal had led directly to the closure of farms, warehouses and distribution networks – and had created a massive, global food shortage.
I described how a plague of locusts was eating its way through food crops on at least two continents.
And I promised to discuss other factors which have led to the coming global food shortage.
Here they are:
First, there has been recent massive rising demand from emerging economies. The people of China and India can now afford to buy food and so they that's exactly what they are doing. Twenty years ago, most people in the world subsisted on 1,600 calories a day. Now they want to eat like the Americans and the British. India produces 70 million tons of wheat a year and is the second largest wheat producer on the planet. But India became a net importer years ago.
The people of China and India want to eat western foods. They want to eat meat. No longer satisfied with a bowl of rice they want to dine on burgers. The consumption of meat in China is increasingly rapidly.
But there are problems. One is that with so much land being used to grow biofuels there is very little land left for growing food for animals. And so the cost of hay has rocketed. Moreover, turning vegetation into meat is grossly inefficient and costly.
Next, the world's population is exploding – particularly in Asia. Just to cope with the population growth the world's food production will need to increase by 50%.
And there are more problems leading to the perfect storm.
As populations grow, people want to live in nice, suburban houses with neat little lawns. As this happens, so the amount of land available for arable use falls. Every year for the past decade, China has lost fertile land equivalent in size to the area of Scotland. To feed its growing population it needs to be increasing its land area by the equivalent of Scotland. Whoops. Things are the same in India.
And, of course, encouraged by brain dead politicians, vast quantities of the world's crops of corn, soy bean and so on, are being used to make biofuels so that motorists can continue to buy cheap petrol for their motor cars. A while ago a list of 51 things you and I can do to prevent global warming was published. Number 1 on their list was headed 'Turn food

into fuel'. This, they claimed, would have a 'high impact' on the global warming problem. It was suggested that ethanol is the alternative fuel that 'could finally wean the US from its expensive oil habit and in turn prevent the millions of tons of carbon emissions that go with it.'

This is dangerous nonsense. When more land is used to grow biofuels, so that green motorists can drive around feeling virtuous, there is less land for growing food and an increase in the number of people starving to death.

The demand for biofuels has been soaring for years (despite the knowledge that, as a result, people are starving) and the increased use of biofuel is a major force behind the rise of food prices.

If greens keep promoting biofuels then there is going to be a global shortage of food and millions are going to die.

Here's another problem: big American seed companies have been busy patenting the rights to many individual seeds. They have done this so that they can force farmers around the world to buy their products. One result has been that small farmers in India are no longer allowed to grow seeds from crops that their families have been planting for generations. If they do, then lawyers for American multinationals will smother them with writs, injunctions. The incidence of suicide among small farmers in developing countries is terrifyingly high.

Finally, large modern farms are remarkably (and surprisingly) inefficient. When the fuel used to build tractors, make fertilisers and pesticides and so on is taken into account, it turns out that the energy cost of a kilogram of corn has actually risen in the last few decades. Soil erosion, the loss of pollinators (such as bees) who have been killed by chemicals, evolving chemical resistance by pests and numerous other environmental problems have also reduced farm crops.

The result of all this is that food is becoming scarce and prices are rising. This is not a cyclical change (with prices falling next year due to better weather and better crops). It is a structural change which has been exacerbated by the coronavirus scandal. I fear it is, in other words, permanent.

As far as food prices are concerned, the conditions really are optimum for a 'perfect storm'. Things really couldn't get much worse.

Actually, they could. American genetic engineers have been 'modifying' food for years to make it more profitable. No one knows what effect their modifications will have on the safety of food for human consumption. No one knows what other horrendous side effects there might be. The risks are unbelievably dangerous.

For those in Europe and America all this is not yet critical.

But for those in many parts of the world this is already an outright disaster. In some countries nearly half of all children are malnourished. And things are getting worse and will continue to get worse. Rising prices and falling quantities of food available for eating (as opposed to filling petrol tanks) will result in massive starvation around the world. The fake coronavirus hoax, and the consequent economic problems which will devastate economies everywhere, will exacerbate the problem and, as a result, the incidence of global starvation is set to rocket. It's no good saying that the planet isn't overcrowded or that there is plenty of food. The inescapable fact is that five million infants and small children die each year – in a good year. That figure is set to rocket in India, Nigeria and the Congo and elsewhere. The number of people in extreme poverty around the world could double to over 160 million. The UNs World Food programme predicts that by the end of 2020 the number of people facing acute hunger will double to 265 million – as a direct result of the economic chaos caused by the lockdowns in the developed world. Increasing agricultural production enabled the world to grow from 1.7 billion people to nearly 7 billion people in just a century. But when the oil runs out, the world will not be able to feed that many people. The oil is needed for farming as well as for transport.

How many people will the planet feed?

Well, it's a safe guess that it will support around as many people as there were before oil changed farming. So we've already got five billion people too many – and the population is growing fast.

If we don't voluntarily reduce the size of the global population (and there are no signs that any nation will choose this route) the answer will be famine, plagues and war.

Welcome to the future.

Is this why governments everywhere are determined to kill off old people as quickly as they possibly can?

Is the coronavirus being exaggerated so that farms and warehouses and distribution centres can be closed down – apparently legitimately, when one worker tests positive for the coronavirus, or shows mild symptoms? Or could it be that big corporations want to kill off traditional farming so that they can sell us fake foods made in their factories. Controlling the oil used to be the way to control the planet. Controlling the food supply will give big corporations control of everything and everyone.

Maybe the advice here will help those who watch these videos: do a little food stock piling now so that you and your family will have a better chance to be strong and healthy.

Countries look after themselves and we all need to do so. It isn't selfish. It's survival.

Remember: if and when your government finally warns you of this problem it will be far too late.

June 13th 2020

Have the Lockdown Laws Caused Vitamin D Deficiency and Increased the Number of Coronavirus Deaths?

Right from the start of the lockdown I have argued that forcing people to stay indoors would lead to millions of people suffering from vitamin D deficiency – and all the associated health problems.

It was pretty obvious – though apparently not to governments and their highly paid medical and scientific advisors.

Vitamin D is an essential substance which most of us get when sunshine hits our skins. Inevitably, most people are deficient in vitamin D towards the end of the winter season. In the Northern hemisphere that means the months of February, March and April.

So people living in the Northern Hemisphere were being forced to stay indoors just when their vitamin D levels were at their lowest.

Vitamin D shortage can lead to many problems. It is necessary for the human body to absorb calcium and phosphorus – required for making strong bones and teeth. Individuals who are short of vitamin D are likely to develop osteomalacia – a serious condition in which the bones become brittle and more likely to break. In children, a shortage of vitamin D leads to rickets. How many children will now grow up with rickets?

Oh, and vitamin D shortage can increase the risk of cancer developing. Moreover, it has also been known for some time that people with vitamin D deficiency are more likely to develop upper respiratory tract infections.

And, more specifically, there is now some evidence appearing which suggests that individuals with vitamin D deficiency may be more likely to suffer badly if they catch the coronavirus. How many people died of the coronavirus because they were vitamin D deficient? I doubt if we will ever know.

And how many people will suffer from osteomalacia or rickets because of the lockdowns? I doubt if we will know that either.

Incidentally, as I was the first to point out many weeks ago, dark skinned individuals are more likely to die from the coronavirus than light skinned individuals – and this could well be because people with dark skins are often deficient in vitamin D.

I have two conclusions.

First, the idiotic lockdown laws will undoubtedly lead to widespread vitamin D deficiency and much illness. Many of us get most of our vitamin D from sunshine.

Second, many individuals will need to increase their intake of vitamin D – either by increasing their intake of the appropriate foods or by taking supplements. It is important, however, not to take too much vitamin D since excessive quantities can damage the body by encouraging deposits of calcium in places where calcium shouldn't be. This is yet more evidence that the stupid and unnecessary lockdown laws (supported by the local authorities and police forces which stopped people sunbathing and exercising out of doors) have done infinitely more harm than good.

June 15th 2020

Why There Will Be A Second Wave (They Need One)

They have done very well so far, with the aid of wildly inaccurate predictions made by a bunch of mathematical modellers who have never diagnosed or treated a patient in their lives, they have succeeded in putting much of the world under house arrest, closing down the global economy, shutting schools, exterminating vast numbers of older folk, sentencing millions of untreated patients to death and more. There was never any reason for any of it, of course. We knew that and they knew it too. The virus which was the subject of all this legalised mayhem was never more dangerous than the ordinary flu. The number of people killed by the prescribed treatment, the lockdowns and the social distancing, will, far, far exceed the number killed by the coronavirus.

The big question of the moment is: 'will there be a second wave?' And the questions which follow are: 'will there be a third wave, a fourth wave and a fifth wave'.

In reality, I don't believe there should be one.

Viruses don't usually behave that way. In my experience, the same flu doesn't keep coming round and round again.

But that doesn't mean there won't be one, of course. Indeed, they seem pretty certain, don't they?

The people who are in control of the coronavirus crime want a second wave because they need to keep us subjugated but they know that reality is against them. Too many people are immune, the virus is probably weaker, the weather is warmer and most of the vulnerable are already dead. In the UK, the hospital bosses have murdered tens of thousands of elderly folk by dumping them, tested or untested, into care homes. It's as if they were deliberately trying to recreate a Typhoid Mary situation without Typhoid Mary.

There are already signs of dissent. A relative of one man who died is suing the Government and although I loathe litigation I wish her luck. Everyone involved should sue the Government. They forced the elderly and the lonely to stay in their homes but they deprived them of food and medical care. It was a domestic version of the murderous Liverpool Care Pathway. As predicted we are now finding the decaying bodies of lonely, elderly folk – many of whom probably died of simple starvation. They weren't allowed to go to the shops and they couldn't arrange food deliveries and, despite all the politicians' promises, no one helped them out. Still, the Government won't mind. They'll save hundreds of millions a year in pensions and health care costs.

People are getting feisty. They are ignoring the laws and questioning what is going on. There is some concern about the vaccine that is promised. Or should that be threatened. People are becoming edgy about the brainwashing, the deliberate creation of fear, the conditioning techniques, the tracking and the enforced isolation. More and more people understand that we don't usually have a global reset, as some are calling it, whenever there is a touch of the flu around.

Governments, however, want a second wave. Everything that has happened is about control, power and money. And it will be very easy to prove that there is one. Indeed, news reports are constantly warning us that second waves have been spotted emerging in some parts of the world.

It will be remarkably easy for them to prove that there is a second wave. (And if there was ever a 'them' and 'us' situation, this is it.) They will merely test more people. Many of those who are tested will have the disease but be asymptomatic. It doesn't matter. Was this the reason that they didn't test more people months ago when the information which testing would have provided, would have doubtless helped us avoid the lockdowns? Were they keeping the testing until when they needed to prove a second spike of the infection?

They will repeat the threats until we are fully cowed and ready to accept whatever they order us to do; until we beg for the vaccine they promise, or threaten us with, depending upon your point of view.

They have sold the vaccine to the populace at large as a cure. But they don't want the cure too soon. They want the fear to continue. Having said that, it is worth noting that a drug company called AstraZeneca has started making two billion doses of a coronavirus vaccine although tests for safety and efficacy have not been completed. That shows confidence and a determination to be first if nothing else. Even Bill Gates, the world's self-appointed spokesman on all medical matters, admits that it usually takes at least five years to prepare and test a vaccine.

Eventually there will be a vaccine because it is the perfect way to force us to accept ID cards (they will call them certificates) or tattoos (they will call those implants) or apps (they will call those apps). And the vaccine will be compulsory even if they cleverly manage to avoid that word.

If there is a second wave it will be deliberately created. They can blame the street demonstrations which the police allowed to take place – even though they were breaking lockdown and social distancing laws. This will add to the divisions in our society and it will increase racism. Evil governments want divisions.

Back in the middle of March, I described this whole thing as a hoax – my first video, published on 18th March, used that very word – the title was 'Coronavirus scare: the hoax of the century'– but since then it has become abundantly clear that none of this happened accidentally or through simple incompetence (though there has been a good deal of that) – this is all about control, money and power. It seemed to be a hoax, then it became a scandal and now it's a crime. Nothing is impossible, anything goes and if you aren't paranoid then you aren't paying attention.

And the people who want those three things are using the threat of a second wave to keep us cowed. It enables them to excuse every new lunacy – such as the forced wearing of masks. It's a constant threat. If you don't eat your broccoli you won't have any ice cream. Wait until your father gets home. If you don't behave you won't be allowed to play outside. If you make a noise you will be in detention. If you don't obey the social distancing laws and the lockdown laws then there will be a second wave and the social distancing and lockdown laws will be stricter than ever. If you dare to doubt our forecasts, if you speak the truth, we will bludgeon you to death with propaganda and abuse. And if we need to introduce a second wave we will make sure that some of the blame lands on your shoulders.

The track and trace system is a way to keep people locked up permanently. If they stop us paying by cash, they will know where we are all the time. And if you visit a shop or a park or a petrol station it will be easy for them to say that you were near to someone with symptoms and therefore you must go into lockdown for another fortnight.

Oppressing the public is a time honoured way of managing the public. The Soviet Union kept people obedient with shortages and queues. We have been subjugated with pictures of huge, purpose built mortuaries filled with empty coffins to show us a glimpse of our future.

Our world now looks a little like a communist State. But in reality our State is slightly different. We are rapidly acquiring a system with complete State control, forcibly suppressed opposition, close links with and heavy regulation of large companies, the elimination of small companies and the disappearance of democracy. There are elements of nationalism and racism and slavery of the people. All around the world changes are being made. The EU, for example, has waived the rules forbidding individual countries from supporting their industries. The result is that the multinationals are now receiving truck loads of taxpayer billions. In 2008, it was the turn of the banks. Today it is the turn of the airlines and the car manufacturers. Companies which saved a little money and were sensible will not enjoy this bonanza, of course. And small companies will lose out – inevitably. But the multinationals which have received 'free' money will be tied closely to the State which handed out the money. At the same time big companies have been ordered to stop paying dividends – thus impoverishing the elderly who rely on private or corporate pensions. They want us all to build up big debts. People with debts are vulnerable and can easily be pushed around. Interest rates are probably about to go negative, wages will fall, property prices will fall and unemployment will soar.

(As an aside, small companies have long been targeted by the European Union and, indeed, individual governments everywhere because they are considered too much of a nuisance and too difficult to control. Government loans made to small companies, in an unprecedented loan sharking exercise will enable tax inspectors and bureaucrats to delve deep into each company's accounts and they will end up being virtually owned by the State. And these days the word 'virtually' is pretty much synonymous with the word 'reality'. Politicians, bureaucrats and tax office staff have yet to realise that large companies were once small companies and that if you crush all the small enterprises then, in a decade or two, there won't be any large ones.)

And all that is the precise definition of fascism – which is, of course, the close cousin of communism but in truth rather different.

The last few months have been among the darkest days in the planet's history, and when you look at it coldly it's been an impressive job. The soul of the world is now drenched in darkness; for many the light of hope has been extinguished. You don't hear many people laughing these days. Smiles have been crushed – either by fear of the oversold flu-like virus or anger at the way such a modest threat has been deliberately turned into utter chaos. Any smiles which are there are hidden behind masks. Our economy is going to be reset (whatever that means – and I have some ideas) and we are going to be controlled by apps on our smart phones. Those who don't have smart phones, and the obligatory apps, will become non-citizens.

Neil Ferguson of Imperial College, the mathematical modeller who appears to have led us down into this doom laden hell fire scenario is about as convincing as that little Swedish girl who was all the rage a few months ago. They seem to me to have much in common: arrogance, ignorance and a yearning to be in the spotlight. Maybe the two of them could join up as a joint entry in the next Eurovision song contest. They could put together a rousing performance of 'Puppet on a String'. Picking the Eddie the Eagle of sums to front the scam shows the level of contempt in which we are held by the people who have planned this takeover of our lives.

Although he resigned after breaking his own lockdown rules, Ferguson recently told a Parliamentary Committee that the number of UK deaths could have been halved if the UK had gone into lockdown a week earlier. He admitted, however, that he had no proper scientific basis for this extraordinary claim. It is bizarre that anyone still listens to Ferguson. If he were a child at school no one would bother to copy his homework because it would be wrong. The only thing he seems to be really good at is selling himself.

Ferguson originally forecast that there would be 510,000 deaths in the UK (not 509,000 or 511,000 but 510,000) and 2,200,000 deaths in the US. As I said at the beginning of this whole farce his estimates were, of course, always absurd.

It is worth noting that South Korea, which has a population of 50 million, has had around 300 deaths nationwide. And South Korea had no lockdown.

The organisers of all this mayhem are doubtless well pleased with themselves.

They have disrupted billions of lives and created terror and global chaos. No terrorist group has ever been as effective. But then this scam was organised by people who already had unlimited supplies of money and power. Populations everywhere have accepted the story that we are fighting a war against a plague like virus that threatens the entire planet. It's science fiction but it's been presented as news in the way that Orson Welles presented the War of the Worlds on American radio, terrifying the millions of listeners who believed the story. Britain is now the worst governed and least democratic state in the Western world. The rich who are not in on the scam are quitting the UK in droves. The loss to the Government in terms of tax take is going to be phenomenal. Government ministers who don't know what is going on (and I suspect that's most of them) are blundering around, struggling to understand why everything is going wrong and putting all their energy into attempting to cover up their ignorance and their incompetence. Early on, the specialist scientists (as opposed to the mathematicians) knew this wasn't a new version of the plague. The bug was downgraded to flu level before the lockdowns began. It was clear from the start that lockdowns and social distancing laws were not necessary. But just look at how successfully governments have terrorised their voters.

School teachers and parents are scared out of their wits and if the absurd social distancing laws are maintained there is a very good chance that schools and colleges will never open again – certainly not in any meaningful way. A generation of children, who should now be at school, looking forward to their summer holidays, will be frightened for their lives. They will be so consumed with in-grained fear, so scarred psychologically, that they will never be able to form proper, close relationships with other folk outside their immediate family. If and when the schools reopen, they will never be back to anything resembling normal. There is a good chance that many children will never finish their education. Is this a government plan? Providing less education will cost less money, and young people who are illiterate and innumerate are, of course, easier to control and far less likely to be troublesome. Besides, there won't be much need for skilled workers in the future. Unemployment is going to stay and millions are going to be entirely dependent upon the Government for their daily bread. This is no accident. In whatever sort of future we have, robots will do most of the tricky work. Robots are being trained as baristas and waiters and nurses and doctors and cooks and anything else you can think of. If you have a job, a robot can probably do it. And probably will. Though, come to think of it I doubt if they'll programme one to be a dissident. Anyone who wants to study will be told to take advantage of distance learning software. Parents who work will be working at home and students who study will be studying at home.

Shops have been closed for so long that many will struggle to survive as absurd social distancing rules mean that they cannot operate normally – or anywhere near normally. And in closing public loos the councils have done their best to ensure that by Christmas, High Streets everywhere will be decorated with nothing more festive than estate agents' boards. We will be doing all our shopping over the internet.

Those who don't have access to the internet will simply starve to death – as they have already been doing.

Reports show that people are killing themselves because they are frightened that they have the bug or frightened that they might catch it. It's just like the terror that was falsely created over AIDS in the last century, when for a while the number killing themselves because they were terrified exceeded the number dying from the disease. The curious thing is that the people who are panicking over the coronavirus, handle their recycling bins every week with bare hands – apparently not caring that the dustmen, sorry consultant recycling experts, who pick up their recycling bins have also picked up several hundred other recycling bins, and so the bins are smothered with all the bugs from all the hands of all the people who have touched them. I would estimate that recycling bins and wheelie bins cause more infections than railway loos and £5 hookers.

Thousands of GPs have virtually shut their surgeries. Convinced by the lies, rather than by the evidence, they are so terrified that they deal with patients by telephone and on the rare occasion when a face to face meeting is unavoidable they wear the mask, the visor, the gloves and the smock. They clean their surgeries between patients and they never touch patients without wearing gloves. It does not seem to have occurred to doctors that such a deeply unpleasant experience is for most patients so scary that they will avoid visiting their local family doctor not because of some perceived risk but because the process is severely forbidding.

Dentists' surgeries were shut for months, and now 40,000 people a day are joining waiting lists for urgent treatment. Like GPs and hospitals, the dentists say they cannot get hold of hospital quality surgical masks and so on but you can buy the stuff, properly approved, on the internet. Millions are so scared that they will accept facial recognition, iris scans, implanted vaccines and slavery with enthusiasm. They want a cashless society and they are happy to be zombies, living half lives, if they can be promised that they won't die from the plague. If the scientific advisors tell them that the only way to survive is to stand on their heads in a bucket of horseshit they will do so with enthusiasm. And the scientific advisors will, of course, happily provide the horseshit. A fifth of the population are so consumed by fear that they wash their cash with soap and water or disinfectant wipes but never dream of washing their wheelie bin handles or the sides of their recycling bins. At least that gives a whole new meaning to the term 'money laundering'.

Since April, I have been warning that there is going to be a global food shortage and although this is inevitable as the oil runs out it is difficult to avoid the conclusion that this has been engineered to keep us fearful and obedient.

The electric vehicle enthusiasts will claim that it is possible to make combine harvesters which run on electricity and that may be true – but where is the electricity going to come from to keep huge pieces of farm machinery running for hour after hour? And the production of modern fertilisers will be impossible too.

Big companies, spotting an opportunity, want to get rid of farms so that they can take over food production in their robot managed factories – with food such as fake meat made from chemicals. And there will be more genetically controlled food. When we are hungry enough we will eat anything. This is all part of the attempt to control the planet.

We need to start planting and growing our own food if we want to eat well. Meanwhile, stockpiling food is like buying insurance. You just hope you won't need it.

In poor countries the effects of the economic collapse of the Western world will be devastating. The coup and the lockdowns and social distancing will result in far more deaths than even I originally feared. Tens of millions will die of starvation every year as a direct result of this massive hoax.

The coronavirus hoax, scandal, crime is going to kill more people than the most evil despots in history.

They want to take our freedom.

We want to keep it.

Wanting to keep our freedom is a stronger emotion.

They're just fighting out of greed.

We're fighting for our survival.

And that's why we will win.

June 17ᵗʰ 2020

The End of Dentistry?

I doubt if anyone really looks forward to going to the dentist. Most of us find it a slightly unnerving experience at the best of times.
But when dentists open their doors after many weeks of shutdown, the experience will be considerably more unnerving than it ever was before.
The Government and the dental governing bodies in the UK have together created a nightmare scenario which will scare the living daylights out of even the most robust of patients and put most dentists out of business well before Christmas. Dentists will have to spend a fortune obeying the new laws and they will be forced to see around a third of the patients they saw before. More expenditure and less income doesn't sound like much of a business plan to me – especially when dentists have been shut for months. There will not, I suspect, be any time for preserving teeth or for the dental and gum care we have, for so long, been warned is essential. Long-term – dental care in Britain is about to hit a bad few decades. If international travel ever becomes possible again everyone will be able to spot the Brits by their rotten teeth.
Most of us don't spend much time feeling sorry for dentists. But it's time to start.
Here's the plan; these are rules that dentists have been told they must follow if they plan to reopen their practices on the 15th June.
And if the barking mad quartet from that wonderful movie the Dream Team had sat down with the Marx Brothers they could not possibly have dreamt up a dafter, more absurdly chaotic scheme than the one which dentists say will be their new normal.
I hate that phrase. New normal. It may be new but there is nothing normal about it. Nothing at the moment is normal and it never will be.
Apparently dentists are going to have to follow official government advice from the Chief Dental Officer. I honestly didn't know we had one but I'm told there are individual Chief Dental Officers for all the UK's regions and I have no doubt they are all well equipped with Deputies, Assistants and the usual platoons of administrative staff. The formal advice hasn't been issued yet or hadn't when I recorded this, though there is only a week to go before opening day, but the guidance available, predictably entitled Standard Operating Procedures for

Return to Dental Practice will give dentists enough information on policies and procedures for them to start planning.

So, here is what I am assured will be the new normal as far as dentistry is concerned.

Could the administrators who've thought up all this crap be unaware that dentists have for years been accustomed to using procedures which protect them and other patients from infectious diseases such as AIDS and hepatitis? Of course not. But then this is the new flu.

Back in May I reported that I'd heard a rumour that the Government was going to force dentists to see no more than one patient an hour.

And now it appears that the rumour was true. Dentists working in the NHS have to see a huge number of patients to make a living, and I honestly cannot see any NHS dentists managing to survive these rules and regulations. I suspect that getting rid of NHS dentistry was part of the deliberate, planned reset of our society.

And unless they quadruple their fees, I can't see many private dentists surviving either. Those who obey all the new rules simply won't be able to see enough patients to earn a living. Those who don't obey the laws will doubtless be defrocked de-smocked or whatever they do to naughty dentists these days.

To start with, of course, dentists will give priority treatment to patients who have had untreated dental emergencies during the last three months. Unfortunately, dentists have been told that they cannot use procedures which generate aerosols so they can't use the drill. This means they can't do fillings or use ultrasonic scalers to clean teeth. One assumes, therefore, that teeth with enough decay to be painful will have to be removed. The tooth fairy is going to have a busy future and the denture making industry is set to boom.

Patients who are in the high risk groups are advised to delay routine dental treatment as long as possible. I'm not sure what the high risk groups are today but they have, at various times, included transplant patients, anyone over the age of 70, anyone living with someone over the age of 70. Male, black, diabetics who are bald and overweight should be top of the at risk groups but no one likes to say that in case it sounds racist, fattist or some ist.

So here's the protocol, as they love to say these days.

First, you ring and make an appointment. This won't be easy and you will see why in a few minutes.

Three days before your appointment date the dentist will email you a medical history questionnaire, a covid-19 screening questionnaire and a consent form which you have to fill out and return via email so that all your private information goes online and is readily available for hackers to steal.

If you don't have access to email you're stuffed but no one ever said life was fair. No one seems to understand that several million people in Britain don't have a computer, a mobile phone or any idea what an email is.

Pigeon keeping and pigeon racing is, however, one of the most popular sports and pastimes in Britain, so it did occur to me that maybe dentists could be persuaded to allow patients without computers to use pigeon post. It would make as much sense as anything else. But then I realised that no one is allowed bits of paper anymore so the pigeons are out.

Dentists may also carry out a video consultation prior to their appointment. If the dentist doesn't receive all the completed forms on time then they will almost certainly cancel the appointment and you'll have to go to the back of the queue.

The day before your appointment, you will be contacted again to discuss the forms you have completed. If you or anyone in your household has any of the 3,937 symptoms so far thought to be associated with the plague, sorry the flu, sorry the coronavirus, you will be asked to postpone your appointment but if you have a real, real emergency and you can convince someone that you will kill yourself if you aren't treated, you will be referred to an Urgent dental Care hub which will probably be 600 miles away and shut but hey ho no one ever said life was fair and this is, after, the new normal in the toothless land of Comrade Boris.

You'll be asked to pay in advance for your treatment because you won't be able to pay with cash because cash is dirty and kills people and the banks don't like it. If you don't have a suitable means of paying over the internet or by telephone then it's hard luck and you'll have to resort to the old piece of string and a door handle solution. Things now start to get exciting.

Before you leave home for your appointment you are advised by the Government to ensure that you have cleaned your teeth, drunk plenty of fluids and been to the loo. This assumes, of course, that everyone lives next door to the dentist. Anyone unfortunate to have to travel for an hour to reach their dentist will probably find it impossible to be fully hydrated and not need the loo on arrival.

As you set off on this adventure, you should take only essential items with you and you should attend your appointment on your own unless you can't stand without support. You should make sure that you wear extra layers of clothing because the surgery will be colder than usual as air conditioning is used to replace the air in the room at regular intervals. The dentist and his nurse, who have to spend all day in cold air will presumably wear thick sweaters and overcoats under their protecting clothing but will, nevertheless, be for ever falling ill with colds and having to take two weeks off work. It is of course well known that air conditioning causes breathing problems, dry skin and constant tiredness. It also tends to exacerbate all existing illnesses. The dentist's front door will be locked and when you arrive you'll have to telephone and let the receptionist know that you've arrived. If you don't have a mobile phone or your battery is dead then you're buggered. You could I suppose just shout loudly and hope someone hears you.

But no, that won't work because when the dentist is ready for you as you wait outside in your car, they will telephone you to say that there are no other patients in the reception area and so you can safely enter. If you are travelling by public transport then you have to let the dentist know in advance so that special arrangements can be made for you to wait inside the building safely.

I am not, I promise you, making this up.

Once you have been telephoned to confirm that Elvis has left and that you can safely enter the building, a receptionist or nurse will unlock the door and let you in. She or he will be wearing personal protective equipment including a mask and a visor. Don't jump out of the car and expect to be let in soon however because there will have to be a delay after the departure of one patient and the arrival of another because the staff will have to disinfect all common areas including door handles and all surfaces.

Once you get into the now sterile surgery premises, floor markings will enable you to make sure that you obey social distancing requirements. You will be asked to put all your belongings including your coat and any bag you are carrying into a large box in the reception area and you will be asked to sanitise your hands. If you aren't already wearing one you will be offered a mask to wear.

You will then be taken into the surgery which will have been thoroughly disinfected and cleaned after the last patient – you are I suspect beginning to see why dentists aren't going to be able to see quite as many patients as before and why, if this farce continues much beyond the summer, most of them will be planning to emigrate or looking for some other form of employment.

In the surgery, the dentist and the dental nurse will both be smothered in protective equipment. There will be no shaking of hands. You will be asked to keep your mask in place until the dentist is ready to start sticking his gloved fingers into your mouth.

As soon as the treatment is completed, you must sanitise your hands again and replace your mask. There won't be any jolly little chats afterwards. If you need to discuss anything, the dentist will telephone you later when you are safely separated by some distance.

All things considered, I wonder how many will bother going to the dentist in the future?

And I wonder how many will choose to resort to the old trick of tying one end of a piece of string to the painful tooth and the other end to a door handle. Slamming the door half a dozen times to yank out the tooth will seem to some to be a darned site easier than this crazy charade.

Finally, as we trudge reluctantly into the Government's carefully designed new normal where the entire nation becomes slowly edentulous, we can perhaps take some small comfort from the knowledge that when we have lost all our teeth, we will be able to hide our empty mouths behind a mask.

Perhaps that, after all, is what mask wearing is all about.

June 17th 2020

Passing Observations (June 17th 2020)

Why did it take so long to show that a simple, cheap steroid might help treat patients with severe covid-19? Steroids have been the drug of choice for severe breathing problems for decades. Could the answer lie in the word 'cheap'?

When a shop assistant insisted that I had to pay for my purchases with plastic, I had great joy in pointing out that the British 'paper' currency is now made out of plastic.

I wonder how many people will be eager to climb into aeroplanes when they realise that the same air commonly constantly circulates within aeroplanes – with the result that if one traveller on a plane has a bug (whatever it is) then everyone will catch it. The risk is not, of course, unique to the coronavirus. Tuberculosis, anyone?

We had a car serviced the other day. The garage added an extra fee for sanitising equipment. I think this could be commonplace now. I hear that dentists are adding an extra sum to their fees for their sanitising costs.

I now understand why millennials never have any money. While lighting a bonfire the other day I noticed an article in the newspaper I was using which extolled the virtues of 'gardening clothes'. It appears that when millennials buy their first home with a garden, they rush out and buy special gardening clothes – special jacket, special trousers, special hat, special shoes and for all I know special underwear too. I suspect I am not alone in always retiring old, frayed clothes for gardening work. The idea of buying a special pair of trousers for digging, mowing and pruning never occurred to me.

A dear friend of mine owns some shops. I am trying to persuade him to put up a sign saying: 'No more than 700 people in the shop at one time, please'.

People who are living in care homes but who are able to look after themselves and just need support with food and laundry and so on, might consider moving into a hotel (when hotels are allowed to open). I fear that if/when there is another lockdown hospitals will once again use care homes as dumping grounds. And the number of deaths will again be terrifying.

For years now there has been a massive, global water shortage. Water use has gone up six-fold in the last century and is rising by 1% a year. But the amount of drinkable water is limited – and much of that which is available has been polluted. The United Nations estimates that global demand could outstrip supply by 40% by the year 2030. And that, you will note, is just a decade away. Water shortages and water wars are coming. Meanwhile, encouraging people to wash their hands in running water for twenty seconds, every twenty minutes seem rather unnecessarily wasteful.

The widespread depression caused by lockdowns and social distancing is having powerful effects everywhere. A friend of ours who has breast cancer has talked of stopping her daily drugs because she cannot see any point in trying to stay alive.

There are two sorts of mental illness rife today. First, there is the fear of the coronavirus. Second there is the rage at the way 'they' have exaggerated the fears and destroyed the world and killed untold numbers of people for absolutely no good reason at all. I suspect this rage is doing even more harm than the fear of the virus. Antoinette and I are so devastated by what is going on that we are both depressed and neither of us can sleep properly.

I heard the other day that Obama, the beloved hero of the liberal left, bombed five more countries than George W. Bush. Indeed, he did so much bombing that at one point America ran out of bombs. Still, his fans will no doubt point out that Obama got the Nobel Peace Prize.

The fall in investment in energy will drop by 20% this year – that's a $400 billion fall. The result is going to be a greater reliance on fossil fuels and, since the big oil companies are not doing any exploration, the price of oil is likely to rise considerably.

I was delighted to see reports boasting that 80% of commuters in London had worn masks on buses and tube trains. The other side of that is that 20% had not worn masks. Good for them. Let's hope it's 30% by next week.

The Treasury in the UK is considering suspending the State pension triple lock. This will dramatically reduce pension payments. The UK already has the worst State pension in the Western world. A large army of civil servants will, of course, be able to look forward to huge pensions – largely paid for by British taxpayers. None of this will come as a shock to those who have read my book, *Coming Apocalypse*. Many are rightly worried about the future for young people but I am afraid that the future for pensioners is bleak, indeed.

I tend to get most of whatever credit is going for the articles on this site and for the videos on my YouTube channel. But that's not fair. Antoinette has ideas and does a great deal of the research. She is the only one who knows how to put stuff on the website and all I do for the videos is sit in a chair and read my script. She does all this with equipment that most Web people would laugh at.

June 17th 2020

Why We Are Fighting for Our Future – and Why We Will Win

Huge changes have taken place in the way countries round the world are run.

As I predicted would happen many weeks ago, governments everywhere have been taking full advantage of the manufactured crisis. The Hong Kong government extended its covid-19 regulations banning gatherings of more than eight people until 4th June – coincidentally covering plans to commemorate the anniversary of the Tiananmen Square massacre which took place on 4th June 1989. And the coronavirus has given the Chinese a tough new national security law. In the UK, legislation is on the way which will remove the right of shareholders to attend the annual general meetings of the companies they co-own. They will not be able to challenge company directors. The change is said to be temporary but these days the word temporary appears to be synonymous with the word permanent. Meanwhile, those same directors are taking huge loans from the Government. The Government may well then take shares in those companies turning them into state owned, nationalised zombie companies. When governments subsidise big companies, the end result is rarely a happy one. It is scandalous that company owners should lose control and everyone with a pension will be affected by this.

Everything that has happened is about 'them' taking control and turning us into slaves. This is not conspiracy theory stuff; it isn't paranoia, it's very real. The baddy from all those James Bond movies, the one who wants to rule the world, is well on his way to taking control. Actually, of course, there isn't just one baddy – there are a number of them.

Doctors have spoken out and have dared to point out that this is not a plague bug and that the dangers have been exaggerated. But they have been quickly punished. I have seen evidence that one eminent doctor was, just a day or two ago, struck off the medical register in the UK for twelve months for daring to voice his doubts about the official line on social media. Whatever happened to free speech and human rights? Article 6 of the Human Rights Act gives us the right to a fair trial and Article 10 allows Freedom of Expression. Long gone. I doubt if he will be the last doctor to learn that silent obedience is now as essential as a stethoscope and illegible handwriting.

From the moment I first spoke out about this fake crisis I have been demonised, monstered and traduced all over the internet by lies and clever distortions.

I have been writing about international drug companies for half a century and I'm accustomed to their methods but things have got far worse than they have ever been before.

When a government suppresses information or opinions then the end result is inevitably oppression and tyranny. And we are seeing a good deal of that.

The advice being given by the experts is laughably inconsistent. They say you can catch it from people with no symptoms but they say you can't. They say you don't get immunity when you've had the disease but they say you do. They say there will be a vaccine by the summer but that it takes at least five years to make one.

People have been advised by experts to leave the loo seat up all the time so that it is touched less frequently. Unfortunately, the experts don't seem to know that when you flush the loo with the seat up, the atmosphere is filled with an aerosol spray full of bugs which will spread dangerous infections in the area and on all the room's surfaces.

Every time anyone with a little independence offers a sliver of hope, that sliver of hope is crushed by paid for mouthpieces who invent facts to fit the official agenda. Governments are busy creating fake news and then blaming the truth tellers for spreading fake news. It's a classic misinformation process.

And, of course, they say that you must wear a mask even though it is perfectly possible that the wearing of masks will kill more people than would have died if they had caught the coronavirus. Anyone who says that masks are perfectly safe to wear forever is probably a fool or a liar or working for the BBC. Two boys died in China when wearing masks while exercising. Masks dehumanise us and make us both fearful and falsely confident. We associate masks with surgeons, dentists and robbers. Masks also fit in nicely with the modern gender neutral philosophy which is being used to damage our individuality.

A good number of hospital departments all over the world are closed to patients with cancer, heart disease and other potential killers even though the storm of patients with covid-19 never materialised. The UK government wasted £200 million building temporary Nightingale hospitals which lay empty. And the irony is that a fifth of all the patients in the UK who contracted the coronavirus, caught it in hospital. Another indictment proving that hospitals are still not good at preventing the spread of infection.

The average age of those dying of the coronavirus was over 80, and this is not surprising since 25,000 elderly hospital patients were dumped into care homes to make way for the tsunami of covid-19 patients which never came. Those patients were discharged without being tested to see if they'd picked up the coronavirus while in hospital, and so the care homes, full to the brim with patients who were aged and ill, became the killing fields. Care homes in England and Wales contain only 3% of pensioners but 29% of covid-19 deaths occurred within their walls. Governments everywhere will save huge sums of money as a result of all these deaths. Although we are bombarded with statistics, it is difficult to get hold of accurate figures but my conservative estimate is that in the UK the Government will save £200 million a year as a direct result of those early deaths of elderly patients.

In the UK, there are 2.4 million cancer patients waiting for treatment. Many of them will die before they get it. There will be ten million people on waiting lists by Christmas. Many of them are now in agony and they too will be dead before they get half way up the waiting list. People wake up every morning crying in pain and despair, and some hospital departments still stay shut. Pubs and hairdressers are opening but some hospital departments are staying shut. Thousands will die unnecessary from asthma, diabetes and coronary heart disease. The only bright spot on the mortality figures will be that very few will have died from the ordinary flu. They were all put down as having died from covid-19.

And charities won't be able to help. The big charities in the UK are facing a shortfall of £10 billion this year. They will want government bailouts. Many smaller charities will go bankrupt.

There is little solace to be found in our institutions. Churches, mosques and synagogues are closed, although pubs and hairdressers and zoos will be open. Our church leaders have betrayed us and abandoned us to our fate. And the royal family, particularly the Queen, will be tucked away out of sight for their safety because all icons can be a comfort and a centre point for protest and revolution.

But although it is claimed that schools and churches and hospitals cannot open because of the social distancing laws, the police condone mass demonstrations which threaten to disrupt society and therefore suit the aims of those who would like to be in charge.

The resultant damage will be extraordinary. The Bank of England says that the UK economy is set to fall by 14% this year – the biggest decline since 1706. In the US, joblessness is on the scale of the 1930s. Around the world, the laws are getting tighter and more intrusive. There are laws about lockdowns, social distancing and mask wearing and in the UK the police in London even used the excuse of a demonstration to introduce a curfew.

There are signs that the social distancing will be permanent. Cities and towns are already widening pavements so that pedestrians can safely keep their distance from one another. Cycle lanes are being enhanced too and the result will be less space for motor cars, more congestion, slower speeds. How long will it be before there are special traffic lanes for the important people to use? That was common in the Soviet Union and it was tried in England for the London Olympics.

Confusion about which is, and is not, allowed has reached absurd levels. One German state has abandoned plans to reopen brothels because they are worried that hookers and punters will rush to the state from neighbouring areas where the brothels are closed. Jonathan Sumption, a former Supreme Court judge, who, it's reasonable to understand, understands the law as well as anyone in the UK, has pointed out that sex with a person from another household is classified as 'a gathering for the purpose of social interaction'. This means that it is now legal providing that it happens in the daytime and not at night and that the sexual activity takes place in the garden and not in the house. Unless a sex worker is involved, in which case the sexual activity can take place indoors and at night because it will be necessary for work purposes.

The mass market media, bought and paid for, enthusiastically spread whatever lies they are told to spread. They ramp up the fear with new horror stories. I have no doubt that BBC dramas will make social distancing and lockdowns seem normal and essential.

It is now possible to discern a pattern and a purpose in all this.

Look around the world and you can see what they have planned for us. In 2017, the Chinese gathered DNA and iris scans to create a massive data base. The Chinese police were also gathering blood types and fingerprints. There's not much left. By June 2019, the Chinese required mandatory face scans for all would-be phone users. Buy a new phone and you wouldn't be given a number until or unless your ID had been verified with a face scan. Consumers were reported to have welcomed all this new technology.

In Russia people who are self-isolating have to take photographs of themselves on their mobile phones, using a special App, to prove that they are in their homes.

In Ohio in the United States, when 4,800 schoolchildren eventually return to school they will wear electronic beacons to track their locations through the day. The beacons will enable the authorities to record where students sit, who they meet and so on. Naturally, all this is to prevent another outbreak of the coronavirus. If the technology works, it will doubtless spread faster than the coronavirus itself.

Small businesses have been destroyed in their thousands and, at the same time, big businesses have been enriched and strengthened with huge grants; the money handed over by politicians without the knowledge or the approval of the taxpayers.

There are still plenty of vulnerable people, the elderly, the frail, the disabled, who are still alive, still costing money and still weakening the gene pool. They have to be exterminated.

This was always part of the plan.

And I have no doubt that things are going to get worse.

If we don't stop it soon then it will be too late. The plan will be unstoppable. We are destined to become slaves in a society where freedom and democracy are no more than words in dictionaries that will doubtless be banned.

Why did governments deliberately destroy their own economies? So that they could rebuild them. This is a battle for control, money and power, and it was triggered by a minor virus that just happened to be handy at the right time. A division four virus leapt into history through timing. The British economic downturn is forecast to be the worst in the G7; the British will be the hardest hit of all the major economies. The cause? Not even Boris and his fellow buffoons are this incompetent. It must have been planned.

If there isn't a second wave of the coronavirus, or a new infection from a new deadly virus, it will only be because they are scared that too many people know and have shared the truth about their attempted takeover of our lives.

They need to shut us in to weaken us. Masks will, despite their lies, make us weaker and more vulnerable. Locking us in will deprive us of vitamin D. Our immunity to other infections will fall as we are kept locked indoors and away from other people. The brainwashing will continue – in exactly the way I described in a previous video called, 'You've been brainwashed, here's how they did it'. If you haven't watched it please find it and watch it. They are using every trick known to the behavioural psychologists. They want to create the circumstances for war so as to frighten us with that. They want to divide us from our friends and our neighbours – to weaken us, to break us up into separate factions, black and white, believers and non-believers and so on, so that we are busy hating one another rather than hating them.

But if they can get away with a second wave then afterwards there will probably be a third wave and a fourth wave until the zombies are begging for their vaccines and their subcutaneous implants.

We are fighting for our present, our future and our children's future. And it is going to be a difficult fight. Trillions have been borrowed from future generations, who will, having been kept out of school, probably not be numerate or literate enough to realise what has happened to their world.

Our real problems are not the mad scientists or the madder politicians but the zombies – the people who accept the lies they are told without question, who dutifully wear their masks and step off the pavement to maintain their social distances. (I don't like to call them sheep, by the way. I have kept sheep and they are very intelligent animals. In my experience, they are far brighter than Ferguson, for example. None of my sheep ever put the country into unnecessary house arrest.)

They are using what is called the spiral of silence to oppress us, too. Many people now fear that what they are thinking is not what the majority is thinking. They don't believe that the virus merits taking away all our human rights but they are worried that the majority believe the politicians and the State scientists, and so they stay silent through fear.

We have to encourage those who are nervous about speaking out. We have to awaken those who are still frozen with fear.

The James Bond baddies, the people who want the control, the power and the money, are talking about a global reset. This is, they say, a good time to reorganise the economy.

That's why they desperately need a second wave of the coronavirus. They need to keep us down, they need to keep us oppressed, fearful and cornered.

They want to introduce vaccines and identity certificates and intrusive apps tracking our every movement. They want to impoverish us and they want total control over the internet. They want to restructure the monetary order. Their aim is social engineering that will lead to a world government with unelected billionaires sitting around the table. They want to introduce eugenics on a big scale – getting rid of the sick and the weak and the frail and the elderly and the vulnerable. They want to remove health care from the masses so that more and more of us die.

If you don't believe me about the seriousness of what is happening then I am afraid you haven't been paying attention.

This is war.

We're on one side.

On the other side there are the governments of the world, the mass media including the major broadcasters and the professional censors; the fascists who are doing their best to control the internet with lies and propaganda and fake news.

But take heart: it's not a fair fight.

They have a great deal to win. Money, power, control.

But we have more to lose: our freedom and our individuality.

They want us to be slaves.

We want our freedom and our human rights.

And so we have more power than we think we have.

At the moment they cannot manage without delivery drivers, supermarket workers, factory staff, shop assistants, hospital staff and so on. If we stand up to them and refuse to accept their lies then they will lose.

And we have to laugh at their insistence that we wear masks and follow their stupid rules.

We have more power than we think we have.

They want to take our freedom.

Wanting to keep it is a stronger emotion.

They're just fighting out of greed.

We're fighting for our survival. So we will win.

Remember the mantra: distrust the government, avoid mass media, fight the lies.

And if you visit a mass media website, leave polite messages expressing your disgust at their failure to expose the dishonesties.

June 18th 2020

Have You Been Put On A List to Be Left to Die?

What I am about to reveal is, perhaps, the most shocking evidence I have come across in 50 years of writing about health matters.

To say that I am horrified is the biggest understatement of all time.

You will be shocked too.

It started a while ago.

The internet has, for months now been full of stories of patients being asked to sign 'Do Not Resuscitate Forms or having Do Not Resuscitate forms signed on their behalf. They are known as DNR forms or DNAR forms – for Do Not Attempt Resuscitation.

GPs all over the country have been contacting their elderly patients, and those with chronic health disorders, and asking them two questions.

Are you happy for us to put a DNR on your file?

And

Are you happy for us to put on your file a note that you won't be admitted to hospital if you become unwell?

Note the clever wording, designed to elicit a positive response. It's the sort of trickery used by crooked pollsters and insurance salesmen – knowing what answer they want and shading the question in such a way as to ensure that they get it.

One GP surgery sent out a letter to a home catering for autistic adults saying that the carers should have plans to prevent their patients being resuscitated if they became critically ill.

Other GPs sent out similar letters to establishments caring for the elderly and the disabled. Blanket decisions were made for care homes and residential homes caring for patients with learning difficulties.

This isn't entirely new, of course, and it wasn't all a result of the coronavirus nonsense.

A 51-year-old man with Down's Syndrome was given a DNR because of his disability, and instructions were left that there was to be no attempt to resuscitate in case of a cardiac arrest or a respiratory arrest. No consent form was signed and there was no agreement with the patient or his relatives. The Medical Director for the relevant part of the NHS said that their policy complied fully with national guidelines from professional bodies.

The boss of a large charity said that they believe that DNR orders were frequently being placed on patients with learning disabilities – without the knowledge and agreement of their families.

This was, of course, illegal.

Back in 2015, the High Court in the UK ruled that carers for patients with mental illnesses should be consulted before DNR notices were applied.

But the coronavirus nonsense has resulted in a flood of such cases.

A man in his 50s, with sight loss, was issued with a DNR notice giving 'blindness and severe learning disabilities' as the reason.

A man with epilepsy was issued with a DNR notice, and at the end of March this year a GPs' surgery in Wales urged high risk patients to complete a DNR form if they contracted the coronavirus. The letter said, 'you are unlikely to receive hospital admission'.

A woman in Bristol received a phone call from her GP asking if it were OK for her medical records to be updated to say that if she contracted the coronavirus she wouldn't go to hospital or receive any medical treatment.

And on my website and in my book about the coronavirus, I have provided more evidence of this.

But is all this really legal?

Well, yes, it is if permission is obtained.

In the UK, the National Institute for Health and Care Excellence, known as NICE, is the official advisory body to the health care world. And the NICE ruling is utterly crucial.

NICE classified people in nine categories. If you are in category 1 then you are very fit. If you are in category 9 then you are terminally ill (though, when it suits them NHS staff sometimes devise another category of 'terminally, terminally ill').

On 29th April 2020, NICE issued amended advice to NHS staff about its resuscitation guidelines, saying that doctors should 'sensitively discuss a possible DNAR with all adults with CFs of 5 or more'. This was issued in response to the coronavirus hoax.

Doctors and nurses were instructed that they should review critical care treatment when a patient 'is no longer considered able to achieve desired overall goals'.

So, what the devil does this mealy mouthed nonsense mean?

And what is a CF? What does a CF of 5 mean?

Well the letters CF mean clinical frailty and there are several stages.

A CF of 5 means that a patient is mildly frail and may need help with heavy housework, shopping and preparing meals.

A CF of 6 means moderately frail – people who need help with bathing.

A CF of 7 means severely frail – people who are completely dependent for personal care.

And so on.

Now you could, I suppose, argue that if a patient is clearly dying then it would be cruel and pointless to continually attempt resuscitation. That was why DNR notices were devised. They were originally for patients who had only hours to live and it was considered not fair to those patients to continue to 'strive to keep officiously alive'.

But that's not what is happening now.

Today, in the UK, in the National Health Service a patient considered unsuitable to be saved or treated is now considered to be a patient who needs help with the heavy housework and who may have difficulty preparing meals or going to the shops.

I could manage a bit of light dusting, I suppose, but more than that would require more effort than I have available to spend on such matters. I would have great difficulty in preparing a meal and I hate going to the shops. So, presumably, I'd get dumped into the CF5 category and so there is no hope for me, and the NHS would recommend that I be denied antibiotics, painkillers or surgery if I fell down and broke an arm.

The post-coronavirus hoax NHS doesn't want to save anyone who is disabled and all patients in care homes are, by definition, suitable for murder by omission.

Originally NICE told doctors that they should assess patients with autism as scoring high for frailty. I am, I confess, still rather confused about when or whether this advice was removed.

I checked around with other bodies.

I didn't find the BMA website much help, though it did have a useful commercial webinar for doctors wanting financial advice. The BMA is, after all, a trades union which exists to look after doctors not patients.

And the General Medical Council, rather bizarrely, got in on the act by defining 'approaching end of life' as patients who are likely to die within the next twelve months.

This, of course is the sort of dangerous rubbish one might expect from the overpaid bureaucratic form shufflers at the General Medical Council because it is always impossible to say that a patient is going to die within twelve months. It may be possible to say that a patient might die within twelve hours but not twelve months. Only arrogant doctors and ignorant bureaucrats claim to know that a patient might die within twelve months. When I was in general practice a couple of centuries ago, I knew many patients who were given months to live but who lived many, many years. Two, I remember well, had young children to look after and although they had been given only months to live they both lived for years – simply refusing to give up and surviving on sheer willpower as much as anything else. If the GMC rule had been applied, they'd have been allowed to die. Or, the way things seem to be going, they would have been quietly euthanized in case they fell ill and needed care.

While digging around I also found this statement:

'Physicians have been empowered to grant a mercy death to patients considered incurable – the mentally ill and the handicapped.'

And then I looked a little closer and realised that the date of that policy statement was October 1939, and the author was a well-known 'medical expert' known as Adolf Hitler.

Hitler's policy, which seems to me to bear an uncomfortably close relationship to the official policy of the UK's National Health Service these days, was created in 1920 in a book written by a psychiatrist and a lawyer (what a deadly combination) who argued that the economic savings justified killing those with 'useless lives'.

The policy was to kill the incurably ill and the physically or mentally disabled and the elderly.

Hitler's policy was officially discontinued in 1941 when it seems that even the Nazis found it a bit much.

But the advice from NICE is still valid. And the NHS is still prepared to refuse life-saving treatment for the elderly, the disabled or the frail. Refusing treatment to patients solely because of their age or fitness is a form of eugenics. It seems that social cleansing is alive and well in Britain today. If you aren't saving people (when you could do so) then you are killing them. There doesn't seem to me to be all that much difference between the thinking behind the policy of Matt Hancock's NHS and the policy of Adolf Hitler's Germany.

If you slap a DNR form on a patient, with or without their permission, you are condemning them to death. If you trick someone into agreeing to one then that's just as bad.

In my view, the NHS has been Nazified.

There are many good doctors and nurses working for it. But there are many who are so bad they are evil.

Obedient souls have been witlessly clapping the NHS and all the time the NHS has been deliberately delivering death notices, DNR forms, to the frail and the elderly.

The British shouldn't have been clapping – we should have been clicking our heels and snapping off fancy Heil Hancock salutes.

Which of us gave doctors permission to behave like Nazis and to deny treatment to people considered unimportant, expensive or expendable? In my view, every single doctor or nurse or administrator who has put a DNR notice on a patient under these regulations should be fired, arrested and imprisoned. I don't know what for. There must be something. How do these people sleep at night? Don't they feel anything for the people they are supposed to be looking after? I am prepared to believe that not everyone in health care can have a genuine vocation. But the people who were scattering these DNR notices around were paid to look after people. And they have betrayed those people. Do Not Resuscitate notices were devised to ensure that the genuinely terminally ill were allowed to die with dignity – without being dragged time and time again from wherever they were heading. DNR notices were originally a necessary part of medicine – to avoid General Franco type situation.

But now we have a thousand Dr Mengele clones working in the health service. That sounds as if I'm exaggerating but the sad thing is that I am not. Dr Mengele would have thrived in today's NHS. He'd have liked the clapping and the adulation too.

NICE should be disbanded immediately. We'd all be better off without it.

And while we are it, we should get rid of hectoring Hancock who should be hung, drawn and quartered.

Meanwhile, if you think you, or someone you know could be rated C5 or worse, it might be a good idea to ask your GP if you've been put on the 'suitable for dying' list.

June 18th 2020

Advice for Anyone Not Wanting To Be Stuffed

Note: This is a word for word transcript of the video on this subject. I used the word 'stuffed' instead of 'vaccinated' in a (successful) attempt to prevent the video being removed – at a time when using the words 'vaccine' or 'vaccinated' was pretty well guaranteed to result in censorship. As time went by, the attention of the censors was moved over to words such as 'masks' and 'social distancing'.

This video is what I believe the IT specialists refer to as a multi-media presentation. So we are all going to have to concentrate hard – especially me, as I struggle to cope with the technology.

I have been around for a long time – I know you'll be surprised by that but it's true – and I have learned that there are two words which cannot be uttered in public without causing a tremendous amount of trouble. Indeed, I am confident that if I use those two words on this video it will only be a matter of hours before the video is removed. The Chinese Government banned all my books because of a column on this subject which I wrote for a Chinese newspaper.

So I am going to use alternative words.

For the purpose of this video I shall use the word STUFF (hold up paper A) when I mean VACCINE (hold up paper B) and I shall use the word STUFFING (hold up paper C) when I mean VACCINATION (hold up paper D).

This little bit of sleight of hand should keep this video on air until one of the Army censors working for the Government bothers to listen to the whole thing instead of deleting it because the title or the key words are in breach of security regulations.

The full text of this video will of course be available on my website with some suitably positioned asterisks to ensure that the censors are not troubled.

So, that's the introduction over with.

Now for the nitty gritty, as they say.

Some years ago I wrote a book about stuff and about stuffing programmes. I filled the book with information that I had collected from medical journals. I have been studying stuff for half a century or so.

I ended the book by pointing out that my view is that stuff is unsafe and worthless and that I would not allow myself to be stuffed again.

I added that this was a purely personal view and since I was determined to be completely fair to the other point of view, I stressed that mine is not a view shared by the majority of doctors, nurses, health visitors, journalists and war criminals.

I suggested that readers should make their own judgements based on all the available evidence, and I strongly recommend that anyone contemplating being stuffed discuss the issue with their own medical adviser.

The bottom line is that I do not advise anyone not to be stuffed, or not to have a child stuffed because I am merely an author: it is not my job to tell people what to do.

My role, as a writer, is merely to provide information (which isn't provided by the Government or the medical profession) and to give some idea of the sort of questions which readers may like to ask when considering a stuffing programme.

So, before you allow your doctor to stuff your child (or yourself), you may like to ask her or him these essential questions which I wrote for my book.

I wrote these questions in 2011 but they are as valid now as they were then:

1. How dangerous is the disease for which the stuff is being given? (Exactly what are the chances that the disease will kill or cripple?)
2. How effective is the stuff?
3. How dangerous is the stuff? (Exactly what are the chances that it will kill or cripple?)
4. What side effects are associated with the stuff?
5. Which patients should not be given the stuff?
6. Will you guarantee that this stuff will protect me (my child)? If not – exactly what protection will it offer?
7. Will you guarantee that this stuff will not harm me (my child)? If not – exactly how risky is it?
8. Will you take full responsibility for any ill effects caused by this stuff?
9. Is the stuffing essential?

Finally, I suggested to readers of my book on stuffing that they should ask their doctor to sign a note confirming what he or she had told them.

'If your doctor or nurse wants to stuff you,' I wrote 'ask him or her to confirm in writing that the stuff is both essential and safe and that you are healthy enough to receive it.'

You may, I warned, notice his or her enthusiasm for the stuff (and, indeed, your company) suddenly diminish.

'Ask your doctor or nurse to give you written confirmation that he or she has personally investigated the risk-benefit ratio of any stuff they are recommending,' I suggested, 'and that, having looked at all the evidence, they believe that the stuff is safe and essential.'

How could any honest, caring, well-informed doctor or nurse object to signing such a confirmation – effectively, accepting responsibility if things go wrong?

Similarly, I suggested that parents who are worried about having their children stuffed should ask their doctor or nurse to sign a form taking legal responsibility for any adverse reaction.

I pointed out that they might find doctors and nurses slightly reluctant to do this.

It is important to remember that most of the doctors (including nearly all GPs) who write and speak in favour of stuffing are making money out of it.

On the other hand, doctors who oppose, or even question, stuffing, do not stand to gain anything but are, on the contrary, putting their careers at risk.

It is true that I've written a book about stuff. Writing books is what I've done for a living for many decades. But to be honest I wish I hadn't written this one. Although I did my best to make it a fair book – albeit with a conclusion – it has brought me considerable amount of trouble and abuse. I have often thought about taking it off the market but decided that doing that would not stop the abuse I receive.

Daring to question the value of stuffing has led to all my books being banned in many countries. For example, my books are now not available at all in China where they had once been bestsellers.

In my book, I suggest that readers ask the doctor responsible for the stuffing to tell them the batch number of the stuff. And I suggested that they keep the name of the doctor, the date and time and the batch number of the stuff. And the surgery or clinic address. Lawsuits against doctors, drug companies and the Government usually fail because people don't have this information.

I am very well aware that there are two sets of opinions about stuff. I am also aware that as someone medically qualified who does not believe that the stuff has been proven safe or effective I am a member of a disappearing minority.

By giving my point of view about stuff, I have attracted a phenomenal amount of abuse. I've lost count of the number of websites containing lies and blatant misinformation about me. My doubts about stuff and the fact that I have pointed out that there is no evidence proving them to be both safe and effective have made me very unpopular and have resulted in my being widely vilified. Governments around the world have, in recent years, made a real effort to silence the critics of stuffing.

I strongly suspect that none of those critics has ever read my book or articles about stuff. Some of my fiercest critics have boasted that they've never read anything I've written.

I have always based my views on solid facts and I have never tried to persuade anyone to accept my opinions without considering both points of view.

However, the supporters of stuffing tend to take a very one-sided view: they are right and that's an end to it. They aren't interested in facts or evidence.

I would add that on many occasions over the years, I have offered to debate the subject of stuffing live on network television or radio with the Government's chief medical officer. Indeed, I offered to debate with any twelve medically qualified stuffing supporters all at once.

These offers have always been rejected.

The medically qualified supporters of stuffing are adamant that they are right.

But they are not adamant enough to be prepared to argue or to defend their point of view in public.

I find that strange.

I would have thought that if they were confident in their position, they would have welcomed the opportunity to try to shoot me down and to prove that the stuff they advocate so enthusiastically is both safe and effective.

After all, their confidence is so great that their constant instruction to the public is that everyone should get stuffed a good many times by their doctor.

June 18ᵗʰ 2020

How Many Coincidences Make a Conspiracy?

In the old days, when you went to the theatre, the orchestra would play a bit of music before the main play or opera started. It was called an overture. Well, you will be relieved to hear that I'm not going to play music because I don't have my harmonica with me but in order to help keep this video online for as long as possible I'm going into the realms of high tech information technology again.

Throughout this video when I say STUFF I mean VACCINE and when I say STUFFED I mean VACCINATED.

OK?

Right, the overture is over.

Oh, and two other things.

If you put a comment underneath this video please don't use the word VACCINE.

And if you want someone to find the video give them a link or the title because the word VACCINE does not appear on any of the tags.

Down to business.

Ever since this fake crisis began, doctors and governments have been pushing us all in a single direction. Once again, much of the information relates to the UK – but it is, I think, valid for just about every country on the planet and it is fair to say that the global medical profession has hardly covered itself in glory during the last few months.

It is difficult to avoid the suspicion that everything that has been done has been directed towards preparing nations everywhere for mass, mandatory stuffing programmes. It seems that nothing else matters. And it seems that the stuffing is being done not to protect but to control.

Just the other day, the New York State Bar Association said it should be mandatory for all Americans to have a covid-19 stuffing – including those who don't want it for religious, philosophical or personal reasons.

They don't give medical reasons as an exclusion possibility but they presumably wouldn't allow that as a let out either.

Now I don't know about you but I'm a bit wary about being given medical, religious and philosophical instructions from a bunch of lawyers. I just hope the American public feel the same way. Let the lawyers have the jabs if they want them.

In the UK, it was pretty obvious back on the 3rd March when the Government introduced its Coronavirus Action Plan that its focus was fixed firmly on the development and distribution of some stuff.

A lot of nonsense has been spoken since then and some strange things have been happening. As I mentioned in another video, I know of at least one doctor who has been struck off the medical register – for twelve months no less – for daring to question the coronavirus story.

They cannot strike me off the medical register because I'm no longer on it. The GMC introduced a complicated and stupid but doubtless profitable scheme which pretty well ensures that retired doctors can't retain a medical licence. So yah boo sucks to them.

There have been a good many coincidences recently. I want to tell you about just a few that I've noticed.

For example, I was astonished when I saw a fuss being made the other day about using a simple, cheap steroid to help with the breathing problems suffered by coronavirus patients.

When I first started wielding a stethoscope in anger it was commonplace to use steroids for breathing problems.

Where was the surprise in this? I'll answer that if you haven't already beaten me to it.

The surprise was that a drug company controlled government actually dared admit that a cheap, readily available drug might be a good remedy for the coronavirus and mean that the over promoted jabs might not be necessary after all.

They've been so desperately promoting the stuff they want to sell that governments and the medical establishment everywhere have suppressed or demonised cheap and effective remedies.

But eventually, the good old steroid broke through and got an honourable mention.

Here's another astonishing story.

You will have no doubt heard of hydroxychloroquine – the drug that Donald Trump has been taking to help keep him free of the coronavirus.

Hydroxychloroquine has been used for years and early research showed it was very useful. You might think that governments everywhere might have been excited by this.

Not a bit of it.

Eminent researchers who had shown that the drug was incredibly useful at preventing covid-19 were attacked by the media who said it was dangerous. They were told it was dangerous by politicians who

193

had heard it from a bloke who doubtless gave them the news in a brown envelope. The WHO didn't want any trials. The French Government suddenly classified it as a poison. In the UK, government agencies didn't want any clinical trials. They all wanted to concentrate on the stuffing.

But there were many demands for some tests, and eventually work was done by researchers who had funding from a bloke called Gates.

And before you could whisper the word 'conspiracy' a journal called *The Lancet* published a study which claimed that the drug could cause nasty side effects such as heart trouble and death.

And so the research was immediately stopped.

Phew, thought the stuff lovers. That was a close one.

But then doctors around the world flooded *The Lancet* with letters and no doubt emails and so on pointing out that the research they had published was so badly flawed that it was, well, useless and dangerous. The research, by the way, had allegedly and in my view rather bizarrely been based on some mathematical modelling and you'll have heard that phrase before.

Other research, done responsibly, showed that hydroxychloroquine worked well, cutting the risk of infection by 80% in people who didn't have the coronavirus. No wonder Donald Trump was taking it. What a pity residents in care homes weren't given it. Thousands of them would still be alive. The drug is as cheap as chips because it's been around forever and is out of patent.

If you want to know the details of the crappy research that *The Lancet* published, I recommend that you go to the excellent UK Column website where there is a brilliant article by Iain Davis detailing exactly what was done.

Eventually, *The Lancet* withdrew the paper, blaming the researchers instead of taking responsibility for publishing the rubbish.

Now, by another of those astonishing coincidences with which we are becoming familiar these days, when it comes to stuff and stuffing, I cannot think of any medical journal which has quite the enthusiasm of *The Lancet* for encouraging doctors to stick needles into people and pump drugs and chemicals into their bodies.

In March 2019, an editorial in *The Lancet* reported that parents who refuse to have their children stuffed are often required to attend a course on the risks of not stuffing their children.

They did not suggest (though it would have made far more sense to me) that those who have their children stuffed should be required to attend a course on the risks of stuffing their children.

(My own philosophical belief is that parents who have their children stuffed are guilty of child abuse and should be charged accordingly. I recognise that this is not a view widely held within the medical profession.)

It is, I think, worth pointing out that *The Lancet* is a commercial journal which makes a good deal of money from advertising.

The last time I looked, a full page advert in *The Lancet* could cost over £10,000.

And who buys the advertising?

Well, if you guessed that most of it was paid for by drug companies then you probably would not be far off the mark.

And who makes stuff?

Well, drug companies of course.

Am I being unfair in fearing that there could be a conflict of interest here?

Let's just call it a coincidence.

So, anyway, that's the story of hydroxychloroquine.

A cheap, readily available but out of patent drug was available and far, far more useful than a jabby thing but serious attempts were made to block its use.

I wonder why.

This whole story gets more staggering by the minute and I confess that sorting it out is rather like sitting on a swing and trying to do a jigsaw with your eyes shut.

However, I have put together a lot of the facts and gathered together some more curious coincidences.

For example, at one point, the WHO announced that people who had had the coronavirus would not be immune and would still need the stuff. No one ever tried to explain how stuff for a disease could provide immunity if the disease itself couldn't provide immunity but it was also suggested that we might all need to have two doses or, possibly an annual dose to keep us topped up. Boy wouldn't that bring in the billions.

But we must not be cynical about this. Nor must we be cynical about the fact that the drug companies appear to be negotiating zero liability for themselves. In other words if some stuff should kill or maim then the company wouldn't be responsible. I don't think that has ever happened before in any sphere of human activity.

By coincidence, the Bill and Melinda Gates Foundation give more money to the WHO than the British Government. Only the American Government gives more.

Bill Gates, the billionaire software chap, and former chum of that Epstein fellow who might have killed himself and who certainly died in prison, pretty well controls the WHO. And he has tentacles everywhere. In his clear desire to control the world he looks more and more like a James Bond baddy though I think that is being unfair to the James Bond baddies.

Incidentally, you might think that if one of the world's greediest and most ruthless men suddenly wanted to save millions of lives he might build roads in poor countries. Set up farms and good water supplies. Those are things which are proven to save lives.

But not our Bill.

Gates is, it seems, obsessed with stuffing everyone on the planet, and the Bill and Melinda Gates Foundation has its disgustingly filthy fingerprints all over everything.

By the way, Gates and UK Prime Minister Boris Johnson have been speaking a good deal recently, and at a stuffing summit which raised £7 billion to spend on stuffing 300 million children, Comrade Boris handed over £1.65 billion of UK taxpayers' money, making the UK the biggest donor. Boris, who has apparently acquired medical qualifications since we last heard from him, said that up to eight million lives would be saved but he didn't mention how many children would be killed or brain damaged and he didn't say how he knew that eight million lives would be saved but these rash judgements seem to come easily to anyone who has dealings with Mr Gates. Maybe it's some sort of infection. Maybe someone could invent stuff to stop it.

One other thing you should know: Gates has for years argued that the world is overpopulated. He reckons that if you stuff people then the world's population will fall. I don't think there is any scientific evidence for Mr Gates's claim which I would describe as baloney. Actually, I can think of an explanation for why the world's population would fall if you stick stuff into them all.

And I expect you might be able to do so if you think about it.

Now, the word 'foundation' suggests charity and kindness and generosity but I think it would be a mistake to assume that is the case here.

Gates has given over $4 billion to something called the GAVI stuff alliance which exists to create 'healthy markets for stuff'. The GAVI alliance is a mixture of WHO, World Bank, drug companies and Gates. This whole thing is a mixture of public policy and corporate profits but, hell, if Mr Gates is going to save us all from the plague he and his chums deserve to make a few bob don't they?

That $4 billion is no problem for Gates because during a decade of apparent generosity his wealth has increased from 50 billion to over 100 billion. I'm not sure whether that is in dollars or pounds but who cares. And I'm not sure whether it's from flogging his overpriced software (it must be overpriced for him to have become so rich) or from his drug company connections but what the hell, money is money, eh?

Gates, who somehow manages to combine medical knowledge which is clearly unsurpassed with arrogant, arbitrary, rash and entirely unscientific garbage, has stated that it will take eighteen months to create the stuff against the pesky virus and that if we go back to normal before then, we will be putting lives at risk. Gates is almost on a par with Ferguson when it comes to making arrogant and unsupportable predictions.

Of course if there never is a stuff then we'll never be able to go back to normal, will we?

And then there is the United Nations.

If you look at the UN's 'Sustainable Development Goals' you will find this:

'Currently the world is facing a global health crisis unlike any other – covid-19 is spreading human suffering, destabilising the global economy and upending the lives of billions of people around the globe'.

No, that's wrong on two counts.

First, it is the absurd over reaction to the coronavirus which is causing the problems. Not the bug itself.

Second, covid-19 is a minor killer compared to tuberculosis, malaria and, indeed, the common flu. The United Nations should know that. And, incidentally, the 12-year-old fact checkers at the BBC and so on might like to look at the facts if they get excited about that.

So, what is the UN doing?

Well, it is accelerating the research and development of stuff.

Gosh.

Are you ready for another coincidence?

Here's another one.

The United Nations is a partner of the Bill and Melinda Gates Foundation. And it's that way round too. The UN is lucky enough to be a partner of the Bill and Melinda Gates Foundation.

Would you like some more coincidences?

You're going to get them anyway – unless you switch off.

Here's one or two.

The UK's Chief Scientific Advisor is a bloke called Sir Patrick Vallance.

Before becoming the UK's Chief Scientific Advisor, Sir Patrick worked for a company called GlaxoSmithKline.

And, be sure you are sitting down for this, GlaxoSmithKline makes stuff.

And do you remember that Dominic Cummings, the man who pulls the strings at 10 Downing Street, broke the lockdown and drove up to Durham and while there drove to a place called Barnard Castle to see if his eyes were working?

You do?

Well, guess who has offices at Barnard Castle?

No?

It's our friends GlaxoSmithKline.

And here's another coincidence.

Guess what happened two days later?

GlaxoSmithKline signed an agreement to develop and make a covid-19 stuff.

Next, you will remember Neil Ferguson of Imperial College of course. (Incidentally, I'm fed up with the Government listening to Neil Ferguson who has been serially discredited, and at the end of this criminal enterprise, I would rather like to see him locked up for helping to cause more global deaths than Hitler. Add in all the people who will die of starvation as a result of this unholy mess and the Hitler notion is not too far-fetched.)

We all know that Ferguson and Imperial College received huge amounts of loot from the much rightly cursed Bill and Melinda Gates Foundation but I wonder if everyone knows that Professor Whitty, the Government's chief medical officer, worked at a place which received 40 million dollars from Gates for a research project.

I'm exhausted by all these coincidences. That'll do for today.

Oh, there is this one.

Gates is treated like some wonderful saint by the BBC.

And he has given loads of money to the BBC.

And Gates and *The Guardian* newspaper, the world's most sanctimonious and hypocritical publication work together. That might have been a waste of money, however, since *The Guardian* will hopefully be closing soon by the way because of its links with slavery. So, how many coincidences do you need before you have a conspiracy?

What else is there?

Oh, yes, the British Government tells us proudly that one big company is already making a stuff that has not yet passed any tests. It appears that they have bypassed the usually necessary animal experiments, presumably because they have listened to me and now accept that animal experiments are unnecessary and misleading, and they are going straight into manufacture though they are giving the stuff to a few people – presumably to see how many of them die. I bet the research paper gets published in *The Lancet*. This is, I feel safe in saying, the first time that a drug company has started to make something before any tests have been done. Have they been guaranteed permission to use the stuff whatever the results? Is it pre-approved whatever the danger? Or have British taxpayers underwritten the costs? The one absolute rock bottom certainty is that you cannot safely fast track the production of anything you intend to put into human bodies. This plan to inject everyone on the planet with an experimental stuff is, I suspect, going to be the most dangerous experiment in the history of the world. But still, we are going to give legal immunity to the researchers, the drug companies and no doubt the Government. Gates, I should mention, has a history of being involved in some pretty dodgy medical goings on. Just check out what has happened in India, for example. And take another look at my video entitled 'Advice for anyone not wanting to be stuffed'.

And this, remember is all for a virus which is known to be less deadly than the flu – and if anyone tells you different they are lying.

Oh, and another day I must talk about Gates and his determination to have us all eating his fake food, and is that the reason we have to get rid of farmers. And there's his enthusiasm for reducing the size of the world population that is worth more time. And the way he made his money. Oh there's so much to talk about.

One thing is for certain.

The world would be a damned sight safer if Master Gates went home and used his money to hire someone to improve his rotten software.

Finally, here is another coincidence.
I hope they won't take it personally, or feel offended, but not one of the people I have mentioned here appears to me to have the morality of a walnut.

June 22nd 2020

The Stupidities Keep Coming but Lockdowns are Finished

Every day I see more horrors that shock me and then enrage me. It has at last been announced that churches, synagogues and mosques may open on 15th June, together with hairdressers and some shops, but only for private prayer. They say that places of worship will remain shut for services until Christmas and maybe longer. Maybe forever.
Why? What rational reason can there be for this? They cannot open places of worship even if social distancing is observed? Why?
There is no scientific reason for it. If they are worried about people singing and blowing out extra air then just ban singing, though as far as I know there is not, as yet, any law banning signing in the street.
The only conceivable reason for this is to suppress religion and prevent people obtaining comfort and solace from the expression of their beliefs.
When are the clergy going to find the courage to defy this stupid and oppressive law, defy the governments and open up places of worship?
To keep them closed is a betrayal, an act of supreme cowardice by religious leaders at a time when people need the comfort of religion more than ever. My congratulations to those clergymen in the US who have opened up their churches and been arrested.
Then I saw that children in school playgrounds have been told that they are allowed to throw a ball but they aren't allowed to catch one.
Think about this for a moment.
Children in the school playground, standing in a chalked square or a hula hoop laid upon the ground can throw a ball but they cannot catch one.
So the child stands there, alone and silent and terrified and throws their ball.
That's it.
No one can throw it back. Or if they do, the child cannot catch it. They stand there along, and silent and terrified that a bug laden ball thrown by someone else might hit them.
What a stupid, criminal and cruel ban.
What do they think children are going to catch from catching a ball?
By and large the coronavirus is not a bug which usually does much harm to children.
The world has gone stark raving mad and the lunacy I described in a previous video in which people were told to hop so that they halved the

non-existent risk of carrying the virus on the soles of their shoes, gets closer to reality by the day. Some might say that countries are now run by homicidal psychopaths determined to destroy every generation – present and future. I couldn't possibly comment.

The prospect of there being any sort of recognisable world left at the end of this stupid, pointless, criminal lockdown is now remote.

In the US, it has been estimated that unemployment is as high as 36% and nearly half of the job cuts will never be restored. A quarter of restaurants say they will never reopen. And hundreds of thousands of small businesses are probably finished.

Next, there is the wretched R number that our supremely ignorant politicians keep bandying about as though it were important.

The R number, they insist, must fall because it measures the rate at which the disease is likely to spread.

Well, I'll tell you something about the R number.

I think it's irrelevant – it doesn't matter a damn.

What matters is not the number of people who catch the disease but the number of people who die from it. And we know that that's lower than the number who die from the flu.

They have, after six months, managed to get the global total number of coronavirus deaths up to 400,000 by cheating. And crumbs weren't they excited by that. But the World Health Organisation says that in the same sort of time period the flu can kill 650,000.

So, ignore anyone who goes on about the R number.

And ignore the promises to reduce social distancing in Britain from six feet six inches to three feet three inches. If they do that we will be expected to rejoice and to accept the shorter distance as permanent. And they will tell us that we will also have to wear masks permanently.

And ignore too the weasly promises not to make their damned wonder vaccination compulsory. They will be too frightened to make it compulsory by law so they will make it compulsory be default. Unless you have your vaccination certificate or perhaps your vaccine number tattooed on your arm you won't be allowed to use the health service, have a bank account with a credit card, have a passport or a driving licence. And since they will get rid of cash, without a credit card you won't be able to buy food. But the vaccination won't be compulsory.

My big concern about the recent Black Lives Matter demonstrations is that the demonstrators, many of whom dutifully wore masks, and who obviously care about people, have not been demonstrating about the hundreds of thousands of elderly folk, black and white and every other colour, who have been murdered in care homes and nursing homes by the incompetence or criminal actions of hospital administrators.

Why not demonstrate about them?

Celebrities have been joining in the Black Lives Matter campaign – showing how caring they are.

But I haven't heard or seen many celebrities speaking out about the mass extermination of care home residents – how many would bother to shout 'Old Folk Matter'?

However, some good has come out of the demonstrations.

The police support for those demonstrators has made it impossible for the police to stop anti-lockdown demonstrations. They cannot possibly arrest anti-lockdown demonstrations now without making it very clear that the police have become blatantly political.

And by the same token, the police can no longer arrest anyone who breaks social distancing laws. They didn't arrest the thousands who protested as part of the Black Lives Matter campaign, and so how can they now arrest those who choose to break social distancing laws on the streets, in parks, on beaches, in pubs or in their homes?

The Black Lives Matter protestors didn't realise it but they marked the end of the lockdown and social distancing laws. The police who knelt during those demonstrations must now shout out, 'Stop the lockdowns' and 'End social distancing'.

If our politicians and police try to continue with these absurd laws we can all point the finger and accuse them of hypocrisy, and we will have proof of what we have known for a long time: that the lockdown and social distancing laws have nothing to do with a virus and everything to do with money and power.

June 23rd 2020

This Couldn't Possibly Happen. Could It?

I want to start with an extract from a book that was written and published in the UK in 1977. I think you will find it important.

'For over a century, doctors have known that if wires are poked into the brain and an electric charge passed through them, there will be different responses from different parts of the brain. A wire poked into one part will cause a leg to move, the same wire poked into another part of the brain will cause an arm to twitch. Fifty years ago, we knew that with the aid of electronic stimulation, doctors could induce pleasure, eradicate pain and recall memories previously lost.'

'With electrodes in position, the patient can be controlled quite effectively from a distance. He can be made to eat, to sleep or to work. His appetite, heart rate, body temperature and other factors can also be monitored and controlled.'

'Researchers have shown that gentle cats can be transformed into aggressive beasts if certain parts of their brains are stimulated. In one dramatic experiment, Dr Delgado of the Yale University School of Medicine in America wired a bull with electrodes and then planted himself in the middle of a bullring with a cape and a small radio transmitter. The bull charged but was stopped by Dr Delgado pressing a button on his transmitter. The bull screeched to a halt inches away from Dr Delgado.'

'Dr Delgado reported that 'animals with implanted electrodes in their brains have been made to perform a variety of responses with predictable reliability as if they were electronic toys under human control.'

'Similar experiments had even then been performed with human beings. The patients selected had all proved dangerous and had shown that they had uncontrollable tempers.'

And that's the end of the quote.

I don't have to get permission to read that extract because it was from my second book which was called, *Paper Doctors* and was published in 1977 by Maurice Temple Smith in London. There are some reviews of the book on my website under the 'biography and contact' button. Incidentally, I gather that a website on the internet has published old email addresses for me. I'm afraid those addresses haven't worked for ten years so please don't use them.

Sadly, 'Paper Doctors' has been out of print for years. And for the record, I loathed animal experimentation as much then as I do now. I am delighted that the British Government now appears to accept experiments on animals are pointless.

Although I wrote all that in the 1970s, Delgado was working in the 1950s and 1960s and his work was just the beginning of a very complicated story that is only now coming to its final chapters.

Most people – and in that I include most doctors and most scientists – have never heard of Delgado's experiments and do not realise just how significant they now are.

But it was Delgado, and people like him, who started the long, slow journey towards the control of the human body and human mind.

There have, of course, always been two essentials for controlling people from afar.

First, you need a way to implant some sort of receiver in the human body. Over the years the receivers available have got smaller and smaller. People still think of microchips as being little things you can pick up and hold between your fingers. The sort of thing you might find in a mobile phone for example.

But some microchips are now way, way smaller than that.

You can get a pile of the things on your fingernail. You could get one in a syringe and through the needle. You could get one in a spray and blow it up your nose. That small. Not that anyone would want to inject a microchip into themselves, of course, though other people might, I suppose, like to do it for them.

The second necessity is for a transmitter.

And that's not difficult at all. You need a tall post of some kind, a flagpole or a tall building, or a pylon of some kind, and then you stick your transmitter on the top so that it can send its messages out over a wide area. That bit's easy. Something like a radio transmitter. Or, I suppose, like those things that send signals to mobile phones. It would have to be a bit more sophisticated than the old mobile phone signals, of course.

So, that's all the equipment you need.

A little chip in the body of the person you want to control.

And a transmitter to send messages.

If you were a mad doctor and you wanted to control an individual it would be a doddle.

You'd just tell them you were giving them an injection to protect them against the flu or something like that and in the syringe there would be a little receiver. And then you'd stick a transmitter on the roof of the house across the road from where they lived.

And then you could send messages to make them do whatever you wanted them to do. You could make them sad or angry or happy or contented. You could make them run or fight or just spend all day in bed.

Remember, that's what Dr Delgado was doing over half a century ago. It's nothing new.

Of course, if you wanted to do the same thing for lots of people you'd need a whole lot of people to help you.

Say you were a really bad person and you wanted to control a whole population, for example. You could make people do whatever you wanted them to do. You could make them go shoplifting or commit murder or all vote for somebody or commit suicide or anything you wanted them to do. If you wanted a smaller population, you could make everyone stop wanting to have children. It would be terribly easy. Remember Dr Delgardo was doing this over half a century ago. It's just that his receivers and transmitters were a bit cumbersome.

If you wanted to do this you'd need someone very rich to start with. Someone with loads of money and contacts. A billionaire really. And someone without much in the way of morals.

And you'd need something to inject into people. A medicine of some kind for example.

And then you'd need someone good at software to help with all the transmitting and the receiving, and you'd need people with access to lots of tall poles or roofs where they could put the transmitter things. But none of that would be any good unless you had a reason for injecting people. You can't just go around injecting millions of people for no reason.

Ideally, you'd need them all to be frightened of something so that they were keen to let you inject them. And then you could put your tiny receivers into the stuff that was being injected. Or squirted up their noses or whatever.

But that would be the tricky thing to organise because you'd ideally need a threat of some kind.

You could tell everyone that they were going to get the plague or something if they didn't let you give them their wonderful antidote. That might work.

But for that you'd need to have a really big scare about something.

And that wouldn't be possible because you'd need some experts to say that there was a big scare coming when really there wasn't. So they'd have to make up something or find something and then exaggerate it. Or you find someone not very good at what they did and get them to make a forecast that terrified the life out of everyone.

And then you'd have to keep people really scared.

You could, I suppose, make them so scared that they were happy to put up with all sorts of rules and restrictions. And you could tell people that if they didn't do what you told them to do then the scary thing was going to get worse than ever.

And you'd need experts and advisers who had links to the companies making the stuff you were planning to give people. And you'd have to promise them all sorts of things. And you'd probably need some greedy and compliant politicians too.

So it really wouldn't be possible to arrange all that.

And anyway there's another problem because you would need to keep people separated so that you could make sure the messages you were transmitting reached the individual receivers. You'd have to have people standing several feet apart all the time and there's no way that people would do that.

So it couldn't possibly work, could it?

Even if that's what someone wanted to do.

June 24th 2020

Rage Against the Zombies

When I go out I don't wear a mask, of course, though I do own a rather snazzy Zorro mask which I can fish out if requested.

I don't follow those 'this way round' signs either. Indeed I never see them. The other day I was asked if I thought the one way system in our local supermarket was easy to follow. I don't follow them, of course, not since I got shouted at by an apprentice Nazi storm trooper in a supermarket. I had to admit that I hadn't even seen any signs.

Apparently they had signs painted on the floor. Who, apart from cheapskates looking for dropped coins, walks around with their eyes looking at the floor?

And I don't do social distancing because it's stupid and about as necessary as doing the cancan in public which I have always tried to avoid since an unfortunate experience I had in Birmingham in 1964 and which will doubtless appear on Wikipedia now that I've mentioned it.

Almost inevitably I get the frosty looks from the morons wearing masks.

They stare at you, goggle eyed and disapproving and so I always grin back like an idiot. If they don't look away I give them my best 1000 yard stare and they usually hurry off.

But I am having more and more trouble with the cretins who are following the social distancing rules.

Earlier in the week I was about to enter a department store which had decided to open, and a woman at the door stopped me to give me instructions about how and where I could go and so on. And she told me they were following strict six feet six inches social distancing rules. (She said two metres of course but I don't do foreign stuff like metres.)

'You're not six feet away,' I pointed out, since she was about two feet away at the time.

The lock of horror on her face was a wonder. She leapt backwards and very nearly went through one of the plate glass windows. I thought she had done this in jest but I was assured that it was done in earnest.

And today, I was merrily wandering along in the garden centre when a woman coming towards me suddenly did an amazing leap to her right. I swear she leapt four feet in one bound. When they introduce an event for the social distancing leap in the Olympics, which they no doubt will, she will win the gold, silver and bronze medals.

I used to be sympathetic and understanding towards these people. But I've decided I've had enough.

I'm fed up with the sanctimonious, empty headed idiots who say, 'oh its bit far-fetched thinking this is all about compulsory jabs or population control or a cashless society or getting rid of the elderly'. And the ones who say: 'Oh I know the politicians and that nice master Ferguson have made a few mistakes but they all mean well'.

What do they think Bill Gates and Prince Charles are talking about when they and the rest of the World Economic Forum sneer and brag about a global reset of the economy, health care and everything else important? What is Soros planning? In simpler times there were just four horsemen of the apocalypse, today there's a cavalry regiment of them lining up to inject us and suck us dry of our very humanity.

And I am fed up with the 12-year-old self-styled fact checkers who say that the claims about Gates and sticking needles into people are wrong. There are widespread claims, for example, that 496,000 children were paralysed in India from the polio jabs from Bill bloody Gates. It's no stretch for me to claim that Pablo Escobar did far more good for the world than Bill Gates. If and when Gates dies they will need to drive a stake through the bastard's heart – though they will need to find it first. The WHO – which is partly funded by Gates of course, as is just about everything else including the BBC and that pompous, sanctimonious, hypocritical newspaper *The Guardian* (which was founded on money from slavery let us never forget) – has allegedly admitted that the global polio explosion is predominantly the Gates strain of polio. By 2018, three quarters of global polio cases were said to be derived from Gates. Indian Government investigators claimed that Gates's people were guilty of pervasive ethical violations including bullying, forging consent forms and other bad, bad stuff. Yards of it. But fact checkers say these claims are untrue because 'the Gates Foundation has debunked the claim'.

That's like saying Stalin didn't kill anyone because he said he didn't. And it's the standard way that amateur fact checkers work.

They go straight to Gates or one of his paid for organisations or publications and they think that's fact checking.

Children, fact checking means going back to source.

Talking of amateurs reminds me of Wikipedia where the entry with my name on it was changed dramatically and beyond recognition the day after I recorded my first video. Anything notable was removed and really old, old stuff inserted.

For example, I am said to have been banned by an organisation called the Advertising Standards Authority. Well, the ASA is a private, organisation largely funded by big advertisers, which can't ban anyone from anything and which has itself been reported to the Office of Fair Trading. Decades ago, the meat trade complained to the ASA about an advert for a book of mine which proved that meat causes cancer. I offered the ASA 26 scientific papers proving that eating meat causes cancer. The ASA refused to look at any of the scientific papers and found for the complainant – the meat trade. It is of course a coincidence that the meat trade buys a lot of advertising. Exactly the same thing happened with another non statutory organisation, now long gone, called the Press Complaints Commission. Details of some of the scientific papers which the ASA refused to look at are on my website.

Incidentally, I wish the Wikipedia editor who keeps writing to me offering to improve the page for a hefty fee would stop bothering me. It could be a good scam, though, couldn't it?

Wikipedia is edited by amateurs but they could make quite a lot of money. One editor demonises me on the page and then another editor puts back my achievements and charges me £500. I wouldn't bet against there being some Wikipedia editors making a good living doing that. A pair of editors could do well out of it.

Now that I know how it works, I never use Wikipedia at all – in my experience it seems to be too easy for editors with a personal grudge to make changes to damage a reputation. And living individuals aren't allowed to correct errors or misleading material on the page with their name.

Another claim about Gates is that his foundation arranged for people to be given tetanus jabs laced with human chorionic gonadotrophin – to stop them getting pregnant. It is said it was part of a population control plan. Reducing the population is one of Gates's pet projects.

The laced stuff was found in Mexico, Nicaragua and the Philippines and the project was funded by two Gates funded organisations – the WHO and the World Bank, and if the fact checkers are interested they should just look at the National Library of Medicine in the US.

Incidentally, suspicions about these jabs organised by the population control people at the Gates Foundation were allegedly aroused when the anti-tetanus campaign was apparently promoted only to women of child bearing age and excluded men and children. Gosh, I wonder why anyone found that suspicious.

Gates, who has medical qualifications like I'm a nuclear physicist, reckons that jabbing people stops them having more children and will reduce the world population. The theory is that if they have two or three children living then they will stop having more. I don't really see how this would reduce the global population but Gates says it would, and so half the world's press merrily prints it and says how clever he is to just know this. Gates is so rich he didn't need to go to medical school he just made loads of money flogging software, which I have always regarded as crappy and overpriced, and appointed himself the world's most important doctor.

It's the mask wearing, social distancing zombies who are helping to wreck our lives. By putting up with the garbage dribbling out of the mouth of Hancock they are encouraging the nonsense and making things worse.

In the UK, it's the school teachers refusing to go to work even though everyone with a bit of brain tissue knows the biggest danger they'll face will be falling off their bicycles or puncturing a finger while buckling up their sandals. A statistician has worked out that the risk of a child under 15 dying from the coronavirus is one in 5.3 million. Even teachers admit that the rules are to protect them rather than children but they don't seem to have read the evidence showing that adults don't seem to catch the bug from children. Research published by the Royal College of Paediatrics and Child Health found that children under the age of ten do not transmit the virus. A joint commission by the World Health Organisation and China could not find one case in the entire solar system of a child under ten infecting an adult.

If they are really worried, however, why not put plastic screens around the teachers?

Millions of children are going to be permanently damaged in every conceivable way because of these school closures. And there is absolutely no reason for schools to be closed.

Mind you, it's not just the teachers who want to keep schools closed. A poll showed that only 36% thought it was safe for schools to open on 1st June, and so 64% of the population are completely moronic. Worse still, 22% don't think it will be safe for schools to open in September. One possible conclusion is that none of those people should be allowed to vote, drive cars or leave their homes without adult supervision.

But another interpretation is possible.

Maybe all those who want to keep our schools closed realise that teaching has deteriorated so much that children are better off staying at home. For years now children have been indoctrinated rather than taught. They have been told about the bureaucratic wonders of the fascist EU super-state and force-fed all sorts of pseudoscientific garbage about global warming. Like so many geese being fattened up, pupils are filled up with bizarre sex education studies, and history teaching appears to have been designed to replace all the truths with politically correct dogmas.

If schools are going to stick to absurd, cruel and damaging social distancing nonsenses then many parents will want to home school their offspring – and who can blame them. Maybe we would all be better off if schools stayed shut permanently.

I'm fed up with demonstrators wearing masks while they are doing it – apparently not realising that the mask is today a sign of slavery to a corrupt system. The funny thing is that it used to be illegal to wear a mask at demonstrations because it made it difficult for police cameras. I daresay some of today's demonstrators use their masks as a disguise. But why bother? The police don't care because, although the demonstrators don't realise it, the demonstrations suit the Government's sinister purposes.

The evidence proving that mask wearing is pointless just grows and grows. The *New England Journal of Medicine* recently published an article concluding that 'we know that wearing a mask outside health care facilities offers little if any protection from infection' and 'in many ways the desire for widespread masking is a reflexive reaction to anxiety'. In other words, people are wearing masks because they are ignorant and stupid. I suggest that all those 8-year-olds writing 'it's fake news' websites for their paymasters might consider learning how to do proper research before sharing their brainless opinions with the rest of the world.

And what about spectacle wearers? They often find that their lenses steam up when they're wearing a mask. That'll be handy for motorists and bus drivers.

Talking of fake news inevitably reminds me of the BBC where I have just seen a headline which reads: coronavirus – social media spreading virus conspiracy theories'. I fell out of my chair laughing when I saw that. Has anyone at the BBC ever heard of black pots and black kettles?

The one jolly fact the BBC produced was that there have been just 3.5 million visitors to the widely promoted and undoubtedly expensively advertised websites run by the UK Government and the NHS. This modest figure seems to prove that no one trusts the Government or the NHS about anything these days.

I am fed up with banks taking advantage of this fake crisis to try to force us to use internet banking. When things go wrong and all your money is stolen they'll turn the other way, of course, and it will be your fault. Why are banks still only working part-time when zoos and hairdressers can open? Hairdressers have to get a damned sight closer to their customers than bank tellers. This 10 a.m. to 2 p.m. nonsense couldn't possibly be to force us to go online could it? So that they can say no one is using high street branches so they might as well close them.

The fact is that you'd have to be half-witted to think that this so-called crisis was anything other than a conspiracy. As I have been screaming for months our lives are being destroyed not by a pesky virus but by the absurd and quite deliberate over-reaction to it. They need to keep us terrified so that we're wound up nice and tight when they're ready to tell us that the jabby thing is ready. By then the zombies will be on both knees begging to be injected with something – anything.

Zombie leaders of the medical establishment are apparently warning of a second wave. Since the medical establishment warned that we would all be dead or dying of AIDS by the year 2000, we can safely ignore them. (I got into terrible trouble at the time for saying that the risk was exaggerated.)

The unthinking, unseeing zombies are making things worse by helping crooked governments and stupid scientists to destroy our lives for a pesky virus.

So in future I am going to take a pro-active role in my dealings with the zombies. I intend to carry a bell with me, and if they leap to one side follow them shouting 'unclean, unclean' until they race away in terror.

I have decided to wage war on the zombies.

I'm fed up with being understanding and sympathetic. They're too bloody stupid for words. And it is partly their fault that our lives are so miserable. Without the compliant zombies we would not be living in an upside down world. And why would anyone want to live the way the zombies are content to live? It isn't living, it's enduring.

The coronavirus, as you all know, is no more dangerous than the flu. That's been my opinion since this whole fiasco started. But I'm not alone in thinking that.

Here's another scientific paper I found in the *New England Journal of Medicine* (which is, unlike many medical journals, magazines and newspapers very decently making all its covid 19 articles freely available). The paper is called, 'Covid-19 – Navigating the Uncharted' and one of the three authors is Dr Anthony S Fauci. The paper was published on March 26th

The authors conclude: 'the overall clinical consequences of covid-19 may ultimately be more akin to those of a severe seasonal influenza (which has a case fatality of approximately 0.1%)'.

The significance of that paper is, of course, is that Dr Anthony Fauci is one of the lead members of the Trump Administration's White House Coronavirus Task Force. He is the doctor usually seen on the TV alongside Trump.

Nothing in the scientific journals could have changed that point of view. Indeed, the statistics prove that it was an accurate prediction. Fauci's attitude since he wrote that paper has been puzzling to say the lease. But his paper in the *New England Journal of Medicine* is there for anyone to read.

I don't mind betting that the *Daily Mail* and the BBC missed that paper. It was a proper scientific paper in a proper scientific journal and so the juvenile fact checkers would have missed it too. There were some long words in it so no one at the BBC would have been able to understand it.

Finally, here's my message for the day.

Next time you see a zombie in a mask, or social distancing, regard them as the buffoons and half-wits they are because through their ignorance and their stupidity they are helping to destroy everything that is valuable in our world.

The zombies are enabling the deceitful bullies who are, I believe, destroying our society for their own gain; the empty headed zombies are endorsing the malicious wickedness which will result in millions of deaths and appalling poverty for decades.

The time has gone for patience, sympathy and understanding: the zombies are our enemies as much as the people pulling the strings.

June 25th 2020

Climate Change is a Lot of Hot Air

Pronouncements from the climate change, global warming spokespersons are greeted as though they are holy relics – far too important to be questioned. The surprise is that they are not handed down from mountaintops, carved on tablets of stone.

Three people appear to have become the poster-children of climate change mythology. Prince Charles (a prime candidate for Hypocrite of the Century), David Attenborough (a television presenter) and a schoolgirl called Greta Thunberg who is famous for playing truant from school, and seems to be regarded by millions as a new Joan of Arc. All of them, and their supporters, spend a good deal of time travelling around the world to address meetings and conferences. A decent sized climate change conference can bring 20,000 enthusiasts flying in from all over the world.

The problem is that politicians and journalists are now too frightened to ask proper questions or to deal with the issue of global change in a robust scientific manner; interviewers never ask the celebrity global change stars the questions which really need to be answered. The result is that the climate change believers get away with a good deal of pseudoscientific gobbledegook which does not bear close examination.

The first point is, of course, the unavoidable fact that the climate change spokespersons have very large carbon footprints. Although Greta famously travelled to America by boat, it was widely reported that the boat's crew had to make at least one journey across the Atlantic by plane. It would surely have been better for the planet if she had simply flown across the Atlantic – but that wouldn't have gathered quite as much publicity. The world would have lost all those photographs of little Greta braving the elements to save the planet. All the climate change personalities travel a great deal to conferences and meetings – but all travel requires energy and trains, and electric cars rely on electricity which is largely produced by burning fossil fuels. It isn't difficult to argue that the world would be better served if they all stayed at home.

There would, unhappily, have been problems with that since between 5% and 9% of all electricity used around the planet is used by information and communications technology. Aviation only produces as much carbon dioxide as the world's computer data storage centres. All those banks of servers, upon which social media campaigners share their global warming nightmares, burn up vast amounts of electricity and hysterical climate change protestors probably use up as much energy as the world's aeroplanes.

Oh, and the climate change enthusiasts who insist on cycling everywhere should realise that bicycles are a major cause of pollution. As cyclists pedal along, the traffic queuing up behind them burns up far more fuel, and emits far more pollution, than would otherwise be the case.

The climate change mythmakers have made many claims about the future of the planet.

For example, back in 1989, a United Nations environmental expert stated that whole nations would vanish if global warming was not reversed by the year 2000. In 2009, Gordon Brown told us that we had 50 days to save the planet. Eleven years ago, Prince Charles stated that we had eight years to save the planet. In 2017, the United Nations revised their prediction and said that we had three years left. A while ago, an American politician called Alexandria Ocasio-Cortez stated that 'the world is going to end in 12 years if we don't address climate change'. Swedish teenager Greta Thunberg recently wrote that: 'around 2030 we will be in a position to set off an irreversible chain reaction beyond human control that will lead to the end of our civilisation as we know it'. In 2019, she stated that we have eight years left to save the planet.

Climate change campaigners have forecast that 'life on earth is dying, billions will die and the collapse of civilisation has already begun'. They have also compared global warming to the Holocaust but 'on a far greater scale'.

None of these predictions is ever supported by any scientific evidence, and I have been unable to find one credible scientist who has ever claimed that climate change threatens the extinction of the human species or the collapse of civilisation. I can find lots of 12-year-olds who say it but 12-year-olds think and say lots of silly things which don't usually get given headlines in the world's press.

Talking of children, two things come to mind.

First, in the UK half of all children under the age of 10 are driven to school every day – or at least they were in the distant days when they went to school and people tried to teach them things. If they really wanted to save the planet and help improve the quality of the air, it would help if they walked to school instead.

Second, a group of British psychologists have reported that children are suffering from anxiety caused by the frightening predictions made by those predicting that climate change will affect our future – and may result in the death of mankind. The self-publicising celebrities who travel the world spreading doom and gloom might like to reflect on that.

The fact is that the global warming campaign is led by people who grew up in rich countries and who travel easily and comfortably. They have enough to eat. They have wonderful phones and computers and television. All those things require a good deal of electricity – most of which is produced with the aid of oil, gas and coal. Now those campaigners, whose lives were enriched by fossil fuels, want to stop poor people in Africa and Asia from improving their lives. The fact is that oil and coal will give them their only chance to catch up.

The campaigners who want to stop the world using fossil fuels are suppressing the world's poor and condemning them to starvation, malnutrition and early death. That seems to me to be rather selfish – and a hell of a price to pay. Climate change campaigners want to deny poor countries the right to use cheap energy sources from fossil fuels – but they, and their countries, became rich by using such fuels. If the climate change nutters are looking for a slogan it should be 'hypocrisy rules'.

There are lots of things which annoy me about the pseudoscience which is climate change and the ignorant pseudoscientists who jabber away about the climate as if they understood anything they were saying.

First, consider renewable energy. Well, the biggest source of renewable energy is said to be biomass – the 'green' word for wood, and we have to remember that although wind farms and solar panels get a great deal of publicity, they produce a marginal amount of electricity. The greater part of the energy which is said to come from renewables comes from burning wood pellets – biomass – and in the UK, most of the biomass is imported from America. So the trees which the planet needs are chopped down, chopped up and shipped to the UK in big ships driven by diesel. And once the trees get to the UK, they are renamed biomass and burned to produce clean electricity. Climate change campaigners want to stop funding so that oil companies will not find more oil. They want us to stop using oil. However, the International Energy Agency has stated that by the year 2040, our planet will still obtain only around 5% of its energy needs from renewable sources (including burning trees or 'biomass'). So if we give up using fossil fuels, we will have to cut back a good deal. No heating, no cooking of food, no lighting, no television and definitely no laptops and mobile telephones. If that's what Greta and company really want then that's fine. But they should, perhaps, understand what they are asking for.

Second, the climate change nutters are forever claiming that global warming will kill off all sorts of animals. The most popular claim seems to be that climate change will result in koala bears becoming extinct. Well, the last time anyone counted there were around 300,000 koala bears living in the wild. And the main threat to their existence is the destruction of their habitat – often as a result of farmers requiring more land upon which to grow biofuels. And biofuels, remember, are the fuel of choice for climate change nutters. It's also worth pointing out that the stuff known as biofuel, crops such as corn, is known to much of the world as food. By encouraging the use of biofuels, the climate change nutters are condemning much of the world to death by starvation. Incidentally, the climate change campaigners claim that many people will starve to death if the global temperature rises. There is, of course, no evidence to support this claim.

The United Nations Food and Agriculture Organisation say that crop yields will rise by 30% by the year 2050. The planet's poorest countries will see their yields rise by 80-90%. But the increase in yields will depend on the use of tractors and heavy machinery which will, of course, require oil. Rural areas of poor countries will not be able to afford electricity and charging points until they are richer.

If the climate change campaigners get their way, poor countries will be forced to stay poor and the people living in them will remain hungry.

Third, climate change campaigners claim that forest fires are a result of climate change. But experts in both Australia and America have concluded that climate change has had little or no impact on the development of forest fires – which are, in any case, less frequent than they used to be. The average annual acreage of American forest burned is now around 6.6 million. Back in 1928, the average annual acreage of American forest lost to fires was 41.7 million. As a mathematician, I wouldn't put myself in the same class as Neil Ferguson but I am pretty confident that 41.7 is a bigger figure than 6.6.

Indeed, between 1931 (the peak) and 2020, there has been a 99.7% decline in the death toll from disasters around the globe?

Then there is the economy.

The Intergovernmental Panel on Climate Change (IPCC) predicts that a global warming of 2.5 degrees centigrade to 4.0 degrees centigrade would reduce global GDP by 2% to 5% by the year 2100 but that the global economy will, by 2100, be between 300% and 500% larger than it is at the moment.

So, that's another worry we can forget about.

We can also forget all that rubbish about the sea rising up and swallowing millions of square miles of land.

The IPPC's estimate is that sea level could rise by two feet by the year 2100. How much of a crisis do you think this is, given that one third of the Netherlands has always been below sea level –some of it over 60 feet below sea level.

The fact is that there isn't any scientific proof that if the planet is getting warmer then the warming is man-made.

You'd think that if there were any, the climate change nutters would make it available, wouldn't you?

I apologise if all these facts rather spoil a good story.

But the fact is that the whole climate change malarkey is just another piece of propaganda. And it perhaps says a good deal about the whole thing that the three best known spokespersons for climate change are a little Swedish girl who didn't go to school, a British prince who is better known for his habit of talking to flowers than for his intellectual abilities and who forecast that the world would end in 2017, a television presenter who has made a number of programmes with the BBC, some of which should, perhaps, have been categorised as drama rather than documentaries.

To those we can add an assortment of slightly hysterical priggish children who are enjoying the freedom to join a campaign about which they know absolutely nothing, the usual crew of luvvies and what seems like the entire editorial staff of the BBC, who seem happy to give airtime to any minor celebrity or pseudo-scientist who is prepared to enthuse about the dangers of climate change while denying any airtime at all to scientists who bravely refuse to follow the official BBC line.

Climate change enthusiasts have promoted their cause by throwing bombs at policemen, by holding demonstrations designed to block the traffic and pollute the air and by forging documents purporting to give their spurious arguments some sort of a scientific basis.

I'd love to interview Greta about climate change.

Perhaps the BBC would set it up.

219

Or perhaps they wouldn't.

June 26th 2020

Would You Trust these People with Your Life?

My first book, written in the early 1970s, was largely about the hold the drug industry has over the medical profession. I was a young doctor when I wrote that book and although I was absolutely shocked at the way drug companies lied and cheated, I was even more shocked at the way the medical establishment had allowed itself to be bought by the drug industry. When I investigated the parts of the medical establishment which were supposed to protect patients, I was astonished and horrified to discover that every single member of the medical establishment that I could identify was receiving drug company money.

And I'm not talking about free television sets, expensive holidays, wonderful weekends away in posh hotels and very pricey meals in good restaurants – all those were freebies enjoyed by many doctors. I knew doctors who ate lunch every day in lovely restaurants at drug company expense.

Most of the doctors running the profession were being paid as advisors and consultants. I found it impossible for me to find a doctor overseeing drug safety who hadn't been on the payroll of at least one drug company.

Even I was once offered money by a drug company. My book, *The Medicine Men* , now out of print, attracted a good deal of publicity nearly half a century ago when it first came out, and one drug company offered to pay me to go on a nationwide tour to promote it to doctors everywhere.

Can you imagine?

This was a book attacking their industry. And they were prepared to pay me to attack them.

Why would they do that?

So that they could buy me.

I obviously laughed at them and said no and they've never tried since then. I promise you all the drug companies in the world haven't got enough money to buy me or buy my approval or my silence. I earn my living writing books and that's it.

Anyway, when I talk about drug companies I know what I am talking about.

All this background is important because I want to write about two big drug companies which are said to be among those companies preparing coronavirus vaccines for the British government to use on the British population and – indeed – on the populations of other countries.

First, let's deal with GlaxoSmithKline, which is known to its friends and it has no doubt bought a good many of those, as GSK.

GSK is one of the world's biggest pharmaceutical companies, and in my view if it made toasters you'd never buy a toaster from them.

In 2014, for example, GSK was fined $490 million dollars by China after a Chinese court found it guilty of bribery.

The court gave GSK's former head of Chinese operations a suspended prison sentence and they gave suspended prison sentences to other executives too.

GSK published a statement of apology.

The BBC said that GSK had said it had learned its lessons, and the BBC added that one of those lessons was 'clearly that foreign companies need to keep a close eye on China's fast changing political and regulatory weather if they are to prosper'.

Sadly, that misadventure in China wasn't GSK's only mistake. Here are some other recent ones.

In 2006, GSK paid out $160 million for claims made by patients who had become addicts.

In 2009, GSK paid out $2.5 million to the family of a three-year-old born with severe heart malformations. And in Canada, a five-year-old girl died five days after a H1N1 flu shot, and her parents sued GSK for $4.2 million. The parents' lawyer alleged that the drug was brought out quickly and without proper testing as the federal government exerted intense pressure on Canadians to get immunised.

In 2010, GSK paid out $1.14 billion because of claims over a drug called Paxil. And they settled lawsuits over a drug called Avandia for $500 million.

In 2011, GSK paid $250 million to settle 5,500 death and injury claims, and set aside $6.4 billion for future lawsuits and settlements in respect of the drug Avandia.

In 2016, GSK paid out $6.2 million in Canada.

In 2017, GSK were ordered to pay $3 million to a widow.

In 2018, GSK faced 445 lawsuits over a drug called Zofran.

There's a quite a list of drug recalls too but that's a bit dull so let's just also look at the accusations of fraud, misbranding and failure to report safety data.

In 2012, GSK pleaded guilty to federal criminal offences including misbranding of two antidepressants and failure to report safety data about a drug for diabetes to the FDA in America. The company admitted to illegally promoting Paxil for the treatment of depression in children and agreed to pay a fine of $3 billion. That was the largest health care fraud settlement in US history. GSK also reached a related civil settlement with the US Justice Department. The $3 billion fine also included the civil penalties for improper marketing of half a dozen other drugs.

Oh, and there are a couple of other things you should know about GSK.

First, GSK is one of the top earning vaccine companies in the world. And in 2010, there were reports of narcolepsy occurring in Sweden and Finland among children who had the H1N1 swine flu vaccine. It is reported that not all the safety problems were made public. I have seen a report that by December 2009, for each one million doses of the vaccine given about 76 cases of serious adverse events were reported though this was not made public. A paper published in the *British medical Journal* in 2018, reported that GSK had commented that 'further research is needed to confirm what role Pandemrix may have played in the development of narcolepsy among those involved.'

The writer of the BMJ article commented: 'Now, eight years after the outbreak, new information is emerging from one of the lawsuits that, months before the narcolepsy cases were reported, the manufacturer and public health officials were aware of other serious adverse events logged in relation to Pandemrix.'

In Ireland, the Irish Government kept inviting people to get vaccinated even when it was clear that the pandemic was on the wane and it was nowhere near the catastrophe portrayed by influenza researchers, governments, industry and the media.

Clare Daly, a member of the Irish parliament, called the adverse effects after Pandemrix a 'completely avoidable catastrophe'. She told the then Prime Minister. 'The Health Service Executive decided to purchase Pandemrix and continued to distribute it even after they knew it was dangerous and untested.'

It is perhaps worth noting that Professor Neil Ferguson, the Eddie the Eagle of mathematical modelling though perhaps without the charm, had predicted that the swine flu could lead to 65,000 deaths in the UK alone. In the end, the swine flu killed 457 people and had a death rate of just 0.026 per cent of those infected.

Second, Sir Patrick Vallance, is the Chief Scientific Adviser in the United Kingdom and, I suspect, a key figure in dealing with the coronavirus in the UK and the plans for a vaccine. Vallance worked for GSK between 2006 and 2018. By the time he left GSK, he was a member of the board and the corporate executive team. All of the fines and so on which I have listed took place while Vallance was working as a senior figure at GSK.

Still, I suppose it's nice for the company and for the Government to have someone in common; someone who knows both sides of the coin as it were.

What are they going to do next? How about making the Yorkshire Ripper the Home Secretary? Or why not dig up Mussolini and make him the next Pope?

Oh, and when Dominic Cummings went for a drive to test his eyesight, after his drive up to Durham, he went to Barnard Castle which by coincidence is where GSK has big offices. And two days after he went there, GSK signed a vaccine contract.

And then there is Astra Zeneca.

In 2014, Astra Zeneca agreed to pay $110 million to settle two lawsuits brought by the state of Texas, claiming that it had fraudulently marketed two drugs. The Texas Attorney General, when he announced the settlements, said the company's alleged actions were 'especially disturbing because the well-being of children and the integrity of the state hospital system were jeopardised'.

Astra Zeneca said it denied any wrong doing. So it paid out $110million for not doing anything wrong which was generous.

That wasn't the only little problem for Astra Zeneca.

The company had to pay $350 million to resolve 23,000 lawsuits.

The company was also charged with illegal marketing, including corrupt data in studies for marketing a drug to children, a sex scandal and a poorly run clinical trial that could have compromised patient safety and data reliability.

The study for this drug was financed by Astra Zeneca and originally included 30 children – that's not particularly small for a drug trial by the way – but only eight children completed the trial and the researcher who conducted the trial concluded that it was inconclusive. The researcher was paid at least $238,000 in consulting fees and travel costs.

However, the study was published anyway and led to a national recommendation that the drug be used as the leading choice for children.

Other studies which showed that the drug produced harmful results were never published and were covered up. A company email revealed: 'Thus far, we have buried trials 15,31,56. The larger issue is how do we face the outside world when they begin to criticise us for suppressing data.'

After years of investigations, Astra Zeneca paid a $520 million fine in the US and paid $647 million to settle global lawsuits.

In 2014, there was another scandal. After a trial described as sloppy, which resulted in a third of the participants dropping out because of side effects, results published in the American Journal of Psychiatry showed the drug as a promising treatment. The head of a psychiatry department was paid more than $112,000 for speaking and consulting fees and other payments.

That, incidentally, is a common trick these days.

It's similar to the technique used to buy politicians.

The company has had a number of other lawsuits but you've probably got the picture.

If these companies were human beings they would be described as recidivists. They didn't make one mistake. They are both guilty of systemic deceits.

So GlaxoSmithKline and AstraZeneca appear to be among the main contenders to make the coronavirus vaccine which governments are so excited about and which we are told will be the answer to all our prayers. And drug companies, let us not forget, are going to be given indemnity so that they cannot be sued if they do something bad.

Astra Zeneca is so confident that its vaccine will receive authorisation that it has already started making billions of doses. The WHO says it is the leading candidate for the billions in profit that lie ahead.

I shan't be allowing anyone to jab me with any of the rubbish made by either of these disgraceful companies – or, indeed, by any other drug company. As a doctor I have no doubt in my mind that whatever vaccine is produced will be rushed into production and will be inadequately tested.

In my view, we should not be doing any business with these companies, or any other drug companies which put profits way above human health. These companies are serial cheats – how else would you describe companies which have enormous responsibilities but which regularly deceive, maim and kill – all for profit. And why the devil was Vallance appointed Britain's Chief Scientific Advisor after working in a senior role for GlaxoSmithKline – which, among many other sins, admitted to committing federal criminal offences? I suspect that Vallance, with his experience at one of the world's top vaccine companies, will be part of the process which decides whether we have a vaccine and which company makes it.

Please, please ask anyone you know who thinks vaccines are wonderful or essential to watch this video. I cannot stress this enough. If enough people watch this video then I believe there will be no coronavirus vaccine and certainly no mandatory vaccination.

It is absolutely no exaggeration to say that all our lives and our futures are at stake.

June 27th 2020

The 'Banned' Plays On

My original video about food shortages was censored, banned and taken down by Mr and Mrs YouTube. Although I do not think it breached any of their guidelines it obviously upset some important people and I suspect it was taken down because it is full of truths that some people would prefer remained hidden away in some dark corner. I fear the video embarrassed Mr and Mrs YouTube and the 77th Brigade of the British Army, whose members do such wonderful work in helping to edit the internet and keep it strong and healthy and free from truths. It is always a delight to see their witty and informative jottings, accompanied by their little golden lion, scattered around the internet. Rock on Brigadier. It's so good to know that my taxes are being used to keep Britain safe and profitable for Mr Gates and his billionaire chums. Without their help Mr Gates would probably not manage to become the world's first trillionaire.

And, of course, my video doubtless embarrassed the world's governments who have worked tirelessly to keep us all protected both from uncomfortable truths.

What a pity.

Sadly, I'm afraid that my original video on food, which was entitled 'Why You Should Stockpile Food – Now!' is, thanks to kind viewers, still available on other platforms and the script is available in full on this website www.vernoncoleman.com.

In order to avoid upsetting Mr and Mrs YouTube, the 77th Brigade of the British Army, the World Health Organisation, the BBC, Bill Gates and Matt 'call me Matt' Hancock you should obviously do everything you can to avoid reading the script or watching the video.

June 28th 2020

Your Government Wants You Dead

I first wrote about the coronavirus crime back in February, and on the 28th February I suggested that there were hidden reasons for the way the coronavirus was being exaggerated.

I suggested that the scare might have been orchestrated to persuade us to travel less and use up less of the world's disappearing oil supplies. I also suggested that the plan might have been to prepare us for a compulsory inoculation programme.

'There will doubtless be stuff in a syringe available within a few months,' I wrote, 'and if the scare is big enough the authorities will be able to introduce laws forcing us all to be inoculated. And once one type of inoculation becomes compulsory then the same will happen with other stuff from syringes.'

That was back in February of 2020.

'Am I being paranoid?' I asked myself. 'No,' I replied. 'I don't think so.'

And then in my first video for YouTube, which was published on 18th March and entitled 'Coronavirus scare: The hoax of the century', I predicted that the hoax had been designed primarily to do two things: to prepare us for a mandatory jabbing programme and also to demonise and marginalise the elderly population.

As the outrageous piece of criminal enterprise known as the coronavirus hoax got going in earnest, governments everywhere pretended that the lockdowns and social distancing they were introducing were designed to protect the elderly – and health services which would soon be overwhelmed.

It was one of the biggest lies in history.

There was never any need to protect hospitals because there was never going to be a tsunami of patients needing treatment. Right at the start it was clear that the coronavirus that was the centre of attention was not going to be any more of a threat than a fairly bog standard flu bug. Anyone with more than two brain cells to rub together could see that. For the record, it is worth remembering that the ordinary flu can, in a single flu season, kill 650,000 people globally. Keep that number in mind when politicians and scientists and the mass media keep reminding us of the total number of global deaths from the coronavirus. The coronavirus has killed nowhere near that many – even though many doctors now agree with me that the coronavirus death total has been wildly exaggerated.

Right at the start, one of the mathematical modellers responsible for this mess remarked, rather sniffily, that the coronavirus is nothing like the flu.

Well, he was absolutely right.

The evidence shows quite clearly that it isn't as deadly, and if YouTube takes down this video because I have said the unsayable it won't change the truth. You can't banish the truth just by hiding it.

Incidentally, if you haven't already watched it you might be amused by my video entitled, 'Everything you are allowed to know but I can't tell you what about'.

What I didn't expect was that governments and health officials around the world would use the coronavirus to trigger a mass extermination programme.

Today, I don't think anyone not working for a government or the mainstream media can doubt that the elderly have been marginalised, targeted and eliminated.

It now clear that the aim all along was not to protect the elderly but to get rid of them.

Horrifying as it sounds, I firmly believe that an essential part of the coronavirus crime was to murder as many old people as possible.

The same thing happened all around the world.

Hospital administrators sent elderly patients who had the coronavirus into care homes where they knew there were lots of frail, elderly patients.

So either the world is stuffed to overflowing with utterly brain dead administrators who know absolutely nothing about how bugs are transmitted and who threw patients out of hospital and into care homes through plain callous stupidity, or else it was done according to some devious master plan.

To begin with, I wasn't sure which it was.

But it is the fact that it was global that gives it all away.

I can believe that there might be a bunch of administrators in one country who are so stupid that they have difficulty telling the time and need help to put their clothes on in the morning but all over the world? It isn't possible, is it?

The Government has already given doctors the legal right to kill old people (by starving them to death, or depriving them of fluids) if they are filling a hospital bed that the administrators want to use for a patient requiring cosmetic surgery or infertility treatment.

So, what's the next step?

Well, the next obvious step is to kill off all sorts of patients with chronic or potentially expensive illnesses such as cancer and heart disease

How on earth could you do that?

How could the politicians possibly get the voters to put up with that?

Well, you could shut down the hospitals – on the excuse that they are needed for the eight million patients expected to fall ill with the coronavirus. It would be like introducing the death penalty by the back door but we won't be killing the possibly guilty; we will be killing the definitely innocent.

You couldn't do that though, could you?

Of course you could.

And they have.

In the UK, there will soon be 10 million people awaiting hospital appointments and treatment. Nearly two and a half million are currently waiting for treatment for cancer.

Many hospital departments are still shut because of social distancing though there is absolutely no reason at all for it. We don't shut hospitals when there is a flu epidemic. And let me remind you – this is not as bad as a flu epidemic.

What if it were all part of a plan to get rid of people who need treatment?

What would you call it when a government decides to kill millions of patients who might need care and cost money?

Genocide, perhaps?

Is it part of the complete reset of our world – as talked about and enthused over by Prince Charles and company at the World Economic Forum?

Why have things changed so much?

It's partly money.

And it's partly eugenics.

It's all part of a wider plan which I will deal with in future videos.

Of course, getting rid of the elderly will remove a big part of the drug company's profits. The elderly take a lot of drugs.

But the new leaders of our new world have solved that – they are making mass vaccination a must for billions.

And, unbelievable as it may sound, things seem destined to get even worse.

Governments around the world are deciding that because of the difficulty involved in dealing with what is now proven to be nothing more than a mild case of the flu they can no longer treat the elderly at all.

Many of the young may shrug at this with indifference but they should remember two things.

First, they may one day be old themselves.

And second, the age regarded as 'old' is likely to be subjected to the standard creep phenomenon.

Those who don't much care about the elderly being killed, will themselves be old sooner than they think. After all young people, if they are lucky, eventually become old people.

And they should remember that the definition of 'old' is getting younger by the year.

Governments have decided that the over 70s cannot be treated. But in some countries the cut off age is 65. And in five years they may reduce the cut off age to 60. And by the end of the decade, the 55-year-olds will be lucky to receive a bottle of aspirin tablets if they have a heart attack or break a leg.

This is a form of euthanasia. Or maybe eugenics would be a better word. Or population control.

It was something the Nazis thought they were good at.

But they were mere amateurs.

You think I'm exaggerating?

The BBC's junior fact checkers will doubtless say I am.

Perhaps I should remind you that, since February, I have been absolutely accurate with all my predictions for the coronavirus.

Check my track record for the last half a century – it's on my website.

Remember too that the BBC receives huge amounts of money from Bill Gates and his pals. And much of the rest of the mainstream media has also been bought.

And then decide if you think I am exaggerating.

Oh and one more thing. As far as I know I am in pretty decent health. I am not suicidal. And I'm careful to avoid accidents…

If anything curious happens and I suddenly disappear please ask questions.

June 28th 2020

Lies, Deceits and Consequences

The world is changing faster than I ever dreamt imaginable, and every day the changes and the discoveries and the threats are of huge proportions. Governments and the mainstream media produce lies with startling ease, and like magicians they distract us by fiddling around with their left hand so that you don't see what they are doing with the right hand. They keep us bewildered and confused, and it is impossible to believe that the disastrous changes and the damage being done could be anything other than deliberate.

The biggest, most outrageous lie is of course the seemingly permanent suggestion that the coronavirus is an unprecedented threat to our health.

Recently, the BBC website's main headline screamed the news that the global number of people infected with the coronavirus had reached ten million.

This, we were presumably supposed to believe, meant that the coronavirus was a major threat to our health, our world, our future, our everything.

But what I didn't see the BBC tell us, and the mainstream media never tells us, is that according to the World Health Organisation, the number of people who caught the flu last year was one billion.

And one billion is exactly 100 times as much as ten million.

The significance of this, of course, is that the death rate from covid-19, the disease caused by the coronavirus which has destroyed the world as we used to know it, is pretty much the same as the death rate from the flu.

Back in March of this year, Dr Anthony Fauci, who is a lead member of Donald Trump's White House Coronavirus Team, wrote: 'the overall clinical consequences of covid-19 may ultimately be more akin to those of a severe seasonal influenza'.

Numerous other doctors have confirmed that the death rate with both diseases is much the same – 0.1%.

And, of course, the statistics show that the vast majority of the people who die of both diseases are over 80-years-old and have a number of serious underlying diseases.

So, it is absolutely clear to anyone capable of rational thinking that the current coronavirus outbreak is approximately one hundredth as serious as last year's flu outbreak. Remember that the total number of coronavirus deaths is widely believed to have been manipulated.

Why didn't governments close down hospitals and the economy last year when the risk to us all was one hundred times bigger than it is this year? The answer, of course, is that it is convenient to do so this year. It fits the plan.

And from that we must conclude, yet again, that there is dirty work afoot. What is happening is very, very sinister.

I know I have said this before but I think it is wise, occasionally, to remind ourselves that everything that comes out of an official spokesman's mouth is part of a massive deception.

And just about everything published in the mass media is a lie.

Distrust the Government, Avoid Mass Media, Fight the Lies.

Some of the lies being told are now becoming a little grey and wrinkled.

For example, those who do not believe in the lockdowns are accused of putting the economy before lives.

This is a pathetic lie but it is repeated endlessly by the half-witted and those without any wits at all.

The fact is, of course, that the lockdowns will result in vastly more deaths than the coronavirus. As soon as hospitals were shut down so that they could cope with the alleged flood of people allegedly dying from the coronavirus, it was obvious that the number of deaths caused by the Government's 'treatment' was going to be vastly greater than the number dying from covid-19.

And so it has proved.

Millions are going to die because of the way governments have reacted to a minor threat.

Moreover, as I warned months ago, the lockdowns have massively reduced our immunity to all other diseases.

We were told the other day that 500,000 people were breaking social distancing rules by crowding together on the beaches. Matt Hancock, the UK's health minister and perpetual nanny, threatened to close the beaches, and some police officers were reported to be threatening arrests.

All this is very confusing because no one seems to me to know whether social distancing rules are rules, requirements, suggestions, advice or laws. And does Hancock have the power to close beaches all around the country? Are there enough policemen? Is he going to arrest the next 500,000 people who totter onto the beaches on a warm day?

Anyway, it is all a load of nonsense because the photos which showed people crammed onto beaches seem to me to have been taken using telephoto lenses – which make people look much closer together than they really were. If you look at the overhead photographs, it seems to me that social distancing rules were being well observed. And even if they weren't observing social distancing rules, who the hell cares? They were topping up their vitamin D levels after months of unhealthy lockdowns.

Bournemouth apparently decided that it was a state of emergency because people were flooding to their beaches. I thought that was what seaside towns rather liked. And I don't remember anyone talking about emergency powers when demonstrators caused mayhem in London and started tearing down statues and damaging public property elsewhere. Mind you it was Bournemouth which wanted to take down a statue of Lord Robert Baden-Powell, the inventor of the boy scouts and a man who doubtless did more for the world than any current citizen of Bournemouth and whose only possible sin was wearing silly looking shorts. Critics of Baden Powell claimed that he was a Nazi sympathiser and had based the boy scouts on the Hitler Youth movement. The snag is that Baden Powell founded the boy scouts in 1907 when Hitler was a boy and adopted the swastika on an early scouting badge nine years before the Nazis used it. Critics don't worry much about history these days.

Some of the papers showed pictures of lots of rubbish left on the beaches. That looked pretty posed to me. I wouldn't put it past our leaders to have deliberately tipped a pile of rubbish on a small stretch of beach just to make us all feel ashamed of ourselves for daring to go out and have a little fun. I visited a number of beaches to check, and none of them had any rubbish left behind. The people running the world today are evil and manipulative and there are no rules and no boundaries. Would you believe they wouldn't do that – after everything else they have done? It would be easy to organise.

It just seems that we aren't allowed to enjoy ourselves at all. The new rules about pubs will make going for a pint about as much fun as taking a driving test. No more darts, bar billiards or pool. No quiz nights, no dancing, no singing, no standing at the bar, no loud music, no laughing, no jokes, no live music. Drinks must be ordered by the aid of a special App, and everyone attending must give their name, address and all contact details to the gestapo agent at the door. Publicans will have to put up with far less income and will have to hire three special employees to do work for the State. There will be one to stand at the door collecting names and phone numbers and addresses. There will be one to stand on guard at the loos, and to clean them between customers. And there will be one to make sure that everyone is sitting quietly and neatly at their designated table and not moving about or making too much noise. I jest not, this is the new world order they want us to accept. It is part of the process of extinguishing all fun and pushing us all towards depression and suicide and an ever growing sense of fear. They know, because the psychologists have told them this, that when we are depressed and fearful we will be more obedient. Have you ever watched the animals in a zoo? After a while they become stuck in their routines. They lose their personality and their sense of adventure. They become like robots pretending to be animals. And the rules about getting married were devised by someone who got the word 'wedding' mixed up with the word 'funeral'.

We are being told that councils all over the country are going broke because of the coronavirus. It has, it seems, in some way caused them huge financial losses.

Really?

Does anyone expect us to believe that?

In what way has the coronavirus damaged their income?

It didn't help, of course, that the malevolent idiots running the councils closed all the car parks to stop people going for a walk in the park or on a beach. But they've been making tons of money from parking fines to make up for that.

Services have been reduced not enhanced.

So precisely how has the coronavirus reduced their income?

Is it possible that the councils were already going broke – largely because of the huge salaries and pensions they pay themselves?

And is it possible that they are just using the coronavirus as a handy excuse to cover up their own greed and incompetence? Is that remotely possible? I have long felt that councils are run by people with a collective IQ lower than their average shoe size and nothing that has happened recently has dissuaded me from that notion.

Whatever the truth, they will doubtless use the coronavirus as an excuse to increase their charges and reduce their services.

Here's another lie which has been doing the rounds.

It has been said that anyone who questions the Government's rules about the coronavirus is a psychopath. And it's being said that this is based on research. One headline I saw was 'Psychopathic traits linked to non-compliance with social distancing guidelines'.

Well I looked at the original lengthy paper upon which this smear campaign was based, and here is what the author actually concluded: 'The results do not (and these words were underlined) mean that it is mostly irresponsible and inconsiderate people who spread viruses. The results do not (and again these words were underlined) mean that people who contract a disease like covid-19, have maladaptive traits.' So, that was more fake news.

Everywhere we look there are lies.

And the lies are all coming from governments and their agents.

Why would they want to lie so much, to terrify people unnecessarily, unless they were planning to take over society, oppress us and remove the last vestiges of our freedom? There are bad things happening here. All of them have been planned for a long time. And those of us who can see what is happening must unravel the lies and identify the people behind them (and it isn't just Bill Gates though if I were making a list of the world's most evil people he would be very high on my list).

The apocalypse to fear is nothing to do with covid-19.

It's the plan that preceded covid-19 that we need to worry about.

Was the coronavirus deliberately engineered and released to trigger all this?

Or was it just a serendipitous occurrence – the rather modest event that the evil deep state dwellers had been waiting for and could use as an excuse. Almost every year there is a nasty new bug around. It was to be expected that there would be one this year as usual.

I don't know the answer and at the moment I don't think it matters.

We have more urgent things to worry about.

The purpose of the coronavirus crime is now clear: it's a takeover of our world and our lives and the destruction of our freedom, our rights and our culture.

If we don't continue to spread the truth far and wide, and persuade the mass of people to understand what is happening, and that our governments and the mass media are lying about everything, then the future is bleak. Indeed, I don't think it is any exaggeration to say there is no future.

But the bastards haven't won.

And we're not going to let them.

July 1st 2020

They're Going to Starve Us and Freeze Us to Death

Have you noticed how the unelected intellectual terrorists leading the way in the coronavirus hoax are keen on phrases to describe what they're doing to us, and what they want to do next, when they've got us all neatly tied up and terrified?

I should explain, by the way, that I am perfectly serious in describing the proponents of the coronavirus hoax as terrorists.

Terrorism can be defined as using intimidation and violence in the pursuit of political aims.

Well, governments everywhere have been certainly using intimidation to pressurise us into being scared of their fashionable version of the flu bug. And if someone threatens to send uniformed men round to arrest me if I don't obey their stupid rules then as far as I am concerned that is violence.

To get back to the phrases they have adopted to describe the world they want us to live in. First, there's the new normal, of course, which should be the new abnormal because it bears absolutely no resemblance to anything I am inclined to accept as normal. I have nothing but contempt for people who are so supine that they willingly wear masks when popping to the shops or who would rather step off the pavement and be run over by a number 29 bus than risk sharing space with another citizen. I've been retired from medical practice for years, and I took my name off the medical register a long time ago but I am thinking of putting it back on so that I can certify as insane anyone who wears a mask or does the social distancing dance on the pavement or in a shop. Masks dehumanise us and take away our human qualities. One of the saddest sights I've seen recently was that of two Ferrari racing drivers standing side by side, proudly wearing their masks. Oh, please. I can't see Fangio, Stirling Moss, Mike Hawthorn or Gilles Villeneuve wearing silly masks.

'Excuse me,' I will say, standing outside one of the new vaccination centres that they will soon be building on every street corner, 'why are you wearing a mask?'

'Gtrjsghe kehek mumble mumble,' they will reply through the requisite number of layers of material, too stupid to know that all masks have pores big enough to let through any imaginable virus.

And then I'll pull out a mental health act form and sign them up for a long, paid holiday in the loony bin. Another one bites the dust.

Then there is the green recovery which sounds far less fun than the pink recovery which I intend to promote when I have a spare minute or two, and no more meaningful than the purple with yellow spots recovery. I have never had much faith in green recoveries since a racing car team painted its car green and claimed it had done so in order to make clear its green credentials. How a car driven round and round in circles and using up a gallon every three miles can ever be green is beyond me. Still, racing car people live in a world of their own. I see that the Mercedes formula one team is painting its cars black this year in some sort of show of solidarity with black people though it seems to me to be more akin with virtue signalling via a paint job guaranteed to gain some publicity. I'm not sure what good a new paint job will do to improve people's lives in Africa, though I suspect it may all be something to do with the fact a young fellow called Lewis Hamilton who drives one of these things is very outspoken about black issues and what needs to be done. I'd have more respect for Hamilton's views if he hadn't buggered off to Monaco or Switzerland as soon as he started earning enough money to pay decent amounts of income tax and make a real contribution to the world. You can't expect to have a voice in social affairs if you don't contribute meaningful amounts of tax. Mind you Hamilton also claims to be keen on environmental issues and yet spends his life flying around the planet in order to drive cars round and round in circles. But then all celebrities live on a different planet to the rest of us. Hamilton would gain a little admiration and respect if he gave half his annual salary to poor people in Africa – in lieu of paying British income tax. Maybe he does; but is keeping it secret.

And, of course, there is the global reset which basically means allowing a bunch of bossy fascists to decide what is good for us, what we should eat, what we should do with our lives and, in due course, what we should think and what we should believe in.

There is a war going on for control of the world, our lives, our minds, our souls and our destiny.

Talking of souls, I am very suspicious, by the way, of the various religious leaders who seemed surprisingly keen to shut down their churches, cathedrals, mosques and synagogues when the flu first arrived a few months ago. Why did they not feel that their congregations might need a little solace at a time like this? Most congregations have been happily practising social distancing for years so even if there had ever been any theoretical risk there had never been any practical risk. Was it just simple cowardice and irreligious self-preservation which led to the betrayal of millions in their time of need, or were they helping to soften us up for a new world in which traditional religion is considered inappropriate and possibly even illegal.

We aren't going to be allowed to have any choice in these matters because these unelected folk (most of whom none of us have ever heard of) know better than we do what we want. There was a time when the people used to vote and choose politicians according to their promised policies. Of course, it was understood that the politicians would lie and that very few of their promises would be kept; but there was a semblance of democracy in the whole business, and politicians knew that if they lied too much they would not be given power at the next elections. But the unelected ones who seem to have given themselves the power to decide our future for us, seem to want to take control with no mandate from the people. Prince Charles, Bill Gates, George Soros and a variety of characters at something called the World Economic Forum have taken upon themselves the authority to decide what is good for us. In my view, these people are morally empty; corruption is burnt into their empty souls. A bunch of people who probably think they are all doing the right thing for the right reasons but who are all doing the wrong thing for the wrong reasons.

The World Economic Forum used to be famous only for its daft Davos conferences at which we all smiled indulgently. But now this and other organisations have shown us their true colours and we are clearly in a fight to the death. It's them or us. The truth, to them, is what they say it is and what they want it to be. How many are using covid-19 to promote their own financial interests at our expense? We are living in Lewis Carroll's worst nightmare.

It is difficult not to feel impressed at the way they are managing to keep us oppressed through the constant application of fear. It's a simple recipe and it works well with the simple minded.

And then there is the oil.

This, like the deliberately engineered coming food shortage is a big part of the future problem we face.

The coronavirus crime has now turned into a global warming crime. The two have become inextricably linked. We are told that the coronavirus appeared because of climate change and that we must therefore put all our effort into tackling climate change – although, as I explained in my video entitled, 'Climate Change is a Lot of Hot Air' this whole argument is childish gibberish unsupported by science and largely promoted by publicity seeking celebrities, the ill-informed and the uneducated. Politicians, business leaders and environmentalists are all fighting one another for the high moral ground as they demand that as the economy is reset it puts climate change top of the list of requirements. The vast majority of the people around the world realise that the climate change nonsense is just that – nonsense. It's propaganda with a sinister purpose.

The manipulators who are trying to take over the world (and doing very well so far it has to be admitted) are using people like Prince Charles, that Swedish kid and untold ignorant celebrities to give them an excuse to take control.

And so we are constantly being told that we must stop using oil and other fossil fuels and rely on alternative sources of energy. As I pointed out in my video, this means relying on biomass – which is wood – because wind and solar don't provide enough energy to power the laptops and mobile phones so beloved by the climate change nutters. And in the UK, the wood we burn comes from trees chopped down in America, cut up into tiny bits and then brought across the Atlantic in diesel powered ships.

What the nutters don't seem to realise is that the oil really is running out. Russia and former USSR countries provide 40% of the EU's supplies – and they are running out. African supplies are also falling. The oil currently being formed deep down in the earth will be ready in 50 million years but I'm not sure I can wait that long.

The shortages are exacerbated by the fact that the big oil companies have been bullied into cutting exploration by 25% – so they obviously aren't finding much new oil.

One of two things is going to happen.

Either the price of oil will soar again over the next few years.

Or millions of people are going to starve or freeze to death as energy systems collapse.

Well, maybe that is what they want.

Certainly, a lot of the unelected people who have started talking about overpopulation and the need for a global depopulation programme, would presumably welcome that.

I know that our world has been pretty well destroyed by a bug which causes a small part of the real health problems caused by flu. I know that we are being lied to constantly.

I know that our food supplies are being deliberately damaged – and if you want to know more about what is happening to our food supplies, just read the transcript of my video on food which YouTube banned because it was full of facts and truths. The video is entitled 'Why You Should Stockpile Food – Now!'. They kept Part II but banned Part I. The video is, I think, still around on places like Bitchute. But the transcript is on this website.

As I have already said, our energy supplies are desperately under threat too and that without oil there will be hundreds of millions of deaths around the world. That's no exaggeration. Without oil, and other fossil fuels, there will be virtually no electricity for farming or cooking. And transport will grind to a halt. That may sound all very nice to the nutters who dream of living in tents in idyllic rural parts, relying on government hand-outs and stealing turnips, but it's a fact of life that they and the frail, the elderly, the very young and most of the rest of us will freeze to death or starve without oil.

Oh, and those who are selfish and greedy enough to be still in love with their electric cars – quite rightly claiming that subsidies mean they are cheap to run – might like to think a little more about how electric cars are made and the fact that they have been shown to make global warming worse.

Fans of electric cars tend to forget that the huge quantities of rare earth metals such as lithium, rhodium and cobalt required for the batteries have to be dug out of the ground – using machinery which is powered with diesel or petrol. An electric car can require 10 kg of cobalt and 60 kg of lithium. And huge amounts of copper are needed too.

The car industry is already struggling to find enough cobalt, lithium to make batteries for electric cars. The planet's supply of these goodies is very limited. Oh, and there is, of course, a massive demand for copper for all the wiring. The mining required to dig up these elements requires lots of huge fuel guzzling equipment.

As an aside, half of all the cobalt needed is mined in the Democratic Republic of Congo. I suggest that electric car fans do a little research into the Democratic Republic of Congo. Many of the rare earths used in the manufacture of electric car batteries are dug out of the ground by children as young as seven. Sanctimonious green electric car buyers will doubtless be delighted to know that they are providing work for so many under 12s.

The price of the materials required for electric car batteries is going to soar and the mines mean much despoliation. The fans of electric cars never seem worried about this. Nor do they campaign to leave the cobalt and the lithium in the ground as they do with oil.

To get back to the electricity supplies: whatever happens I believe there are going to be major electricity outages in the next year or two. Make plans if you can. There are generators and long-term storage batteries available. And at the very least get a kettle that will run off the cigar lighter in a car – then you can at least make a cup of tea or hot soup. Or have a hot toddy when the weather gets chilly.

July 2^{*nd*} *2020*

We're At War

I read an article the other day in which a journalist complained that writing about the coronavirus in Tanzania was dangerous because the Government there is silencing the media.

'When the international media try to report on the pandemic,' moaned the writer, 'they are accused of scaremongering, their attempts described by the Government as a form of warfare.'

This was reported in the British mainstream media as though it were a terrible example of censorship and the oppression of the truth.

Most of my remaining laughs have withered a little in recent months but I managed one for this and I think those who appeared to be shocked by this story need to look a little closer to home, and open their eyes.

There is no freedom of speech anywhere in the world now.

In Britain, for example, the Government owns the mainstream media lock, stock and printing press.

Anyone who questions the 'official' line, which appears to be that the coronavirus which causes covid-19 is a deadly killer which threatens the very existence of the human race, is ignored while every incident or even suggestion which might be used as ammunition to scare people is promoted with hysterical enthusiasm.

If I dare to include too many facts in a video for YouTube the censors will take it down. I've never said anything contentious or illegal or even against the YouTube rules but so far they've taken down five of my videos. After I complained, they did put back two – including one called 'Coronavirus: Why did YouTube ban my video?' I think even they were embarrassed to have taken that down. I've realised, by the way, that if I avoid using words such as 'coronavirus' in the titles of videos then they are less likely to be taken down.

To those of us who care about facts, the BBC is a real nightmare.

It has long seemed to me that the BBC, which receives money from many sources, including some given directly from the Government, the EU and, inevitably, the Gates Foundation, has always been racist and sexist.

There is a Woman's Hour programme on the wireless but the State broadcaster would have a collective fit if anyone suggested a programme entitled Man's Hour. There is a Radio Scotland, a Radio Wales and two stations in Northern Ireland but no Radio England. I suspect that is because Scotland, Wales and Northern Ireland are recognised as regions by the European Union but the EU demanded that England be divided into a number of smaller regions.

Despite its charter and national responsibility, the BBC has always been biased and corrupt but it has travelled further along that road than I ever thought possible. Not content with gouging huge licence fees from the British public, the BBC seems to be happy to accept money from anyone who wants to buy its favours. I have reported before on the massive multi-million payments which have been paid to the BBC by the European Union but many will have been shocked to hear that the BBC also happily pockets huge sums from a wide variety of donors including the Bill and Melinda Gates Foundation. (It is, of course, a coincidence that Bill Gates appears to be revered by the BBC which always seems to describe anything slightly critical of Gates as 'fake news' or 'false claims'.)

We shouldn't forget that the BBC has been using news as a weapon of war for a long time. Goebbels said in 1944 that the British 'know that news can be a weapon and are experts in its strategy'. And it was the BBC which the Government used as the gun.

George Orwell is said to have learned about Newspeak and Doublespeak while working for the BBC and some suspect that his Ministry of Truth in the book '1984' was modelled on the BBC building in Portland Place.

In 1953, the BBC was used to spearhead the British propaganda campaign in Iran which led to the elected government being toppled. And the BBC has a long tradition of blacklisting and denouncing critics. They have perhaps just lost a little of the subtlety in recent years.

Orwell knew, as do all proper writers, that it is a writer's job to stand up for victims, to protect the vulnerable and to oppose oppression. I am appalled that the mass market media has betrayed the people and that just about all the columnists active at the moment seem content to follow the party line. I feel able to offer criticism since I resigned from my last Fleet Street column some years ago when the editor of the newspaper I was working for refused to print a column criticising the Iraq War and Tony Blair's lies about the weapons of mass destruction. As a writer I am disgusted by the way journalists have taken the knee to their editors and proprietors in order to please the Government. It is a journalist's job to behave like dogs and to treat politicians like lampposts.

And as a former GP, I am appalled at the way the science has been distorted and rearranged to suit dishonest motives.

The nonsense about the R number is meaningless because what really matters with an infectious disease is not the number of people who get it but the number who die of it. And we all know that this disease (I daren't say the name too often or this video will be banned because I am considered dangerous) is no more deadly than the flu.

Incidentally, governments are now going to find it harder to push up the death totals. They have already murdered all the vulnerable old people in care homes, and solved the ageing population problem by killing thousands of the over 65s. And many doctors are surely now going to be wary about putting the covid-19 down on every death certificate they write.

And consider the antibody tests, for example.

These have turned out to be appalling unreliable, particularly in the first two weeks of having covid-19 symptoms, but governments are still using the tests as proof that lockdown needs to be reinstated. When you think about what they are doing, it is quite brilliantly wicked in an evil sort of way. At the beginning of this nonsense, months ago, I urged the Government to do more testing – to find out how many people had, or had had, the bug. It seemed sensible. But they steadfastly refused to do this – finding new reasons or excuses on an almost daily basis. 'The dog ate the test results' was my favourite of these. The result is that they can now do more testing, find more people with the disease and, therefore, introduce more lockdowns. They don't need more deaths. They have established that having the disease makes you a menace to society, a sort of Typhoid Mary of our times, and so if there are enough people in one area testing positive they can shut down everyone and everything as a punishment and, mainly, as a message to everyone else.

And the tests are being used to shut down farms and places where foods are prepared. They don't care about the fact that there are many false positives. Part of the plot for our future, and a smaller global population, is to make food scarce and push up the prices.

I feel odd when I say things like that.

I am not a natural conspiracy theorist though I am doubtless now labelled as one. Actually, the odd thing is that I believe that so many people now disbelieve governments and their absurdly, obscenely motivated rhetoric that they are conspiracy theorists – not us. Matt Hancock and Boris Johnson are conspiracy theorists – not you and me.

Everywhere you look they are finding ways to oppress us and make life more difficult. We are told that cash is too dangerous to use, and their yearning for a cashless society is becoming more blatant by the day. Shops and pubs are being told not to take cash – as though it were deadly to do so. It would make more sense to outlaw doorknobs and handles. And those bug ridden plastic recycling bins we are told we must use so that we can pretend we are saving the planet even though our nicely washed old yoghurt cartons are taken off to be burned when they have been collected.

In March alone, 1,250 free to use cash machines were converted to charge a fee when people take their own money out of the bank. And you have to use a machine because banks are too terrified of the plague to deal with mundane activities such as providing their customers with some of their own money over the counter.

No one seems to care that one in five Britons, and the figures are much the same everywhere, cannot cope without cash because they don't have or don't trust plastic, have poor broadband or mobile phone coverage or are frightened of debt. People don't get into uncontrollable debt using cash. But they do get into uncontrollable debt using credit cards.

Of course cash carries bugs. It always has. So just wash your hands after using it.

I feel deeply sorry for anyone under 60 and particularly for those who have small children or grandchildren. If we cannot stop this savage attempt to drive us into the New Abnormal, or the Global Reset promoted by the unelected and self-appointed rulers who have decided that the world is theirs and who are determined to control our lives, there will be little future for any of us.

Everywhere we look there is manipulation of one sort or another. Newspapers and television cannot do anything without sponsorship of one kind or another. I'm proud that these videos and my website are free of advertising and sponsorship but everywhere I find myself raising an eyebrow or two in surprise.

For example, I looked at an interview with Bill Gates the other day that was published by *The Guardian*, the newspaper founded on slave money. The interview was described as being part of their 'Now Generation' articles.

Incidentally, has anyone without a new film or album to promote ever done as many interviews as Bill Gates? The man's hubris, vanity and self-regard are staggering.

The interview was entitled, 'The African youth boom: what's worrying Bill Gates' and the writer was a journalist called Polly Toynbee who met the apparently wonderful Mr Gates at what was rather breathlessly described as his foundation's spacious campus in the heart of his hometown, Seattle.

The blurb said: 'The philanthropist warns that stability in Africa makes a huge difference to the world, and that investing in the health and education of its young people is vital.'

There is lovely picture of Gates looking thoughtful and rather worried about something. Maybe he too has trouble with his damned software. Gates is reported as telling us that Africa is not one country but many, which is kind of him because the rest of us hadn't noticed, and though there isn't much talk of vaccination there is much hagiography here. I saw no mention of all the controversies that have surrounded Gates in recent years. It all seemed rather nauseatingly sycophantic to me. Ms Toynbee didn't ask Gates why he didn't just distribute money directly to individuals and let the recipients use it as best they wanted. She didn't ask why he didn't just build roads and farms so that the poor Africans could better their own lives. She didn't ask him what the devil gave him the right to decide what other people wanted.

'He is reaching for what works best to revive the west's faltering conscience in the face of America first nationalism and rising pull up the drawbridge populism in Europe. The spirit of generosity is under assault as government aid budgets come under constant sniper fire from right wing politicians and their media,' wrote *The Guardian's* Toynbee.

But the best bit of this is at the bottom where a two line note tells us that 'The Now generation' is a series produced in collaboration with the Bill and Melinda Gates Foundation'.

A click on a link tells me that: 'The journalism is editorially independent, commissioned and produced by our *Guardian* journalists.'

Oh dear.

Surely, if you want to maintain the appearance of editorial independence, it is surely wiser to avoid writing puff type articles about your sponsor.

Or maybe that's just me being old-fashioned.

Incidentally, Mrs Melinda Gates has apparently said that black people deserve priority access to the covid-19 vaccine when it arrives.

I don't think this was in response to the recent demonstrations. Perhaps it was more in response to the fact, belatedly recognised, that black people seem more likely to die of the coronavirus.

And why did it take them so long to spot that? I even put it in my book about the coronavirus which was published in April.

But were black people more likely to die, because of poverty, overcrowding and co-morbidities rather than racial differences? Has anyone done any research? I don't think so.

Or are black people deliberately being given the coronavirus bug because some of our new unelected leaders want to give them the vaccine?

If I were representing black people I would want to look closely at this. I would want to look at the Gates' words about the size of the world population and at all the strange stories about the vaccination programmes associated with the Gates foundation. I would want to know how well the vaccine had been tested, who had made it and what the death rate was likely to be.

And I wonder why the wife of a billionaire software maker felt able to decide who should and who should not be vaccinated.

I've noticed too that it is being claimed that some of the regions that have seen the highest incidences of covid-19 infection have high levels of pollution.

Gosh.

Of course people who breathe polluted air are more likely to suffer from respiratory illness. And when the air pollution is high it is usually because there are lots of people living closely together. And infectious diseases tend to spread more in crowded areas than in places where folk live 100 miles from their nearest neighbour.

This all comes under the heading of what I would call 'completely crappy and pointless research'.

More relevantly, right from the start of this crime, I have been wondering whether the covid-19 deaths could be more common in patients who have been given a recent flu jab.

A number of doctors have asked this.

But as far as I know, no one has attempted to answer the question – though it wouldn't be difficult to do so.

Indeed, doctors are being actively discouraged from looking at ways to treat or prevent covid-19. In a previous video, I discussed the way that hydrochloroquine was mis-investigated.

I have previously reported that at least one doctor in the UK has, to my certain knowledge, been struck off the medical register for daring to question the coronavirus crime. And I heard the other day about a small group of GPs in France who had used antihistamine drugs to modulate the severe symptoms of covid-19 and who have been trying to get a controlled study done for the last three months. Instead of being encouraged, the doctors have been threatened with sanctions or being struck off. Their crime? They contacted the media.

Make no mistake, these are dark and difficult times, as Victorian novelists probably liked to say.

You won't find the truth in the mass media.

But you will find it here.

No advertising, no sponsors and definitely no money from Mr Gates's ungodly Foundation.

July 2nd 2020

Just a Little Prick – The Bill Gates Story (Part One)

Bill Gates is often described as a philanthropist.
Interviewers generally seem to treat him as a cross between a saint and a prophet. In a way this isn't difficult to explain. After all, the Bill and Melinda Gates Foundation is a partner with many media companies, tossing money around with remarkable generosity. In the UK, the BBC and *The Guardian* are just two of the recipients of Gates largesse.
It would, of course, have been possible for Gates to have used his vast wealth to change poor countries in a very straightforward and positive way by, for example, using his billions to help with road building programmes or to help poor farmers to improve their land and their farms by digging wells. Using $10 billion to set up water supplies would have doubtless saved many lives in a simple, honest way. But you can't control the world quite as easily simply by doing practical, honest things which save lives. And Gates seems to me keen to take control of every aspect of our lives. To me he seems to be a strange hybrid of those mad fictional characters Dr Strangelove and Ernst Stavro Blofeld – the James Bond baddie.
I'm afraid I don't believe any of Gates' projects have anything much to do with philanthropy. There is too much intermixing of donations and business. What do the Gates family really want? I cannot help thinking it's more about power and unspoken plans.
Gates got rich through the Microsoft software company, allegedly because his mum knew the chairman of IBM and got Gates his big break. There are accusations that Gates stole some of the ideas for his business. Personally, I feel that Gates has made himself obscenely rich by making the world a far more stressful and annoying place than it was before Microsoft appeared. In my experience, there were other much easier to use word processing programmes but Gates steamrollered the opposition out of the way with ruthless efficiency. Gates original partner, Paul Allen, claimed that Gates tried to screw him and charged his partner, with mercenary opportunism. Before Gates arrived on the scene, people who wrote software often gave it away free. Gates took over the world of personal computing, acquired a monopoly position and took full advantage of it to make himself very rich. Additionally, there have for some time been doubts in my mind about how close Microsoft is to the National Security Agency in the USA.

The Microsoft billionaire seems to have learned his hometown boy act from veteran investor Warren Buffett who didn't get to be rich by being a hometown boy but has a good line in simple charm. Gates has described himself as a health expert. He frequently offers advice and predictions about health matters though personally I'd have thought his only area of expertise with viruses involved those usually found in computers. He has stated that the world will not return to normal after the coronavirus until all or most of the world's population has been vaccinated. Because he has a lot of money, and tends to distribute it widely, politicians and bureaucrats and scientists listen to his advice and accept what he tells them – parroting his line about vaccination with great loyalty.

It would, I think, normally be unusual for a bloke with no formal medical training to give health advice to the world but Gates has managed to buy himself a seat at the table by giving huge sums of money to organisations such as the United Nations and the World Health Organisation – in my own view now two of the most evil organisations in the world. The Bill and Melinda Gates Foundation is said to be the second largest contributor to the WHO and If the United States really does stop its donations, then Gates will be the biggest contributor. That sort of money buys a lot of access and, I think, an unhealthy amount of influence – especially when you also spend a good deal of money on publicity designed to show the world what a good egg you are. Gates is also linked to the World Economic Forum, which reckons that the coronavirus is a great excuse to change the world and which has a plan called The Great Reset which, like most of these plans which have emerged since the coronavirus, seems to me to have been prepared some time before the arrival of covid-19.

Gates, of course, also gives a good deal of money to Imperial College in London – the place where Neil Ferguson works. It was, of course, Ferguson whose rubbishy forecasts about the coronavirus resulted in the lockdowns, the social distancing, the ruin of the British and American economies, untold deaths in care homes and so on. Gates has also funded work done by Dr Chris Whitty, the UK's current Chief Medical Officer. And the Gates Foundation has even given money to Public Health England – a UK Government organisation, sponsored by the Department of Health, which allegedly exists to protect and improve the nation's health. Public Health England appears to be desperately keen on vaccinations which is a big surprise, of course.

One of their documents carries the slogan Keep Calm and Carry on Vaccinating – which seems a little cheesy to say the least.

Before I go any further it is important to point out, and bear in mind, that Gates believes the planet is overpopulated. He thinks this is a real problem. Is it still a secret passion? Who knows? Interviewers, who often seem to come from organisations with financial links to the Bill and Melinda Gates Foundation, rarely ask searching questions about difficult issues.

The Bill and Melinda Gates Foundation is an odd organisation in that as well as having philanthropic aims, it also invests in a good many companies designed to make a profit. Indeed, the Foundation seems to be doing very well and seems to me to operate as much like a family investment trust as a charity.

The Gates Foundation has a mass of interlinked projects and commercial holdings. And it seems to an outsider as though he is more interested in controlling the world than in helping people.

Here are just a few of the things Gates is currently doing with his money.

First, of course, there are the vaccines. I have already dealt with some of the controversies associated with the Gates's obsession with vaccines in previous videos.

Gates seems obsessed with vaccines and now seems to favour ones using very new technology. He is terrifyingly keen on giving his experimental vaccine to billions of people – ideally to the whole population of the planet. It doesn't seem to occur to him that even relatively safe vaccines have been known to cause many thousands of deaths, might enhance susceptibility to disease or indeed cause and spread infections. If it has occurred to him it doesn't seem to be something that worries him unduly.

On the surface, Gates seems to see vaccination as the answer to most of the planet's health problems and sees them only doing good and incapable of doing very much harm. 'We're not going to return to normal until most people have been vaccinated,' he has said, after warning that the coronavirus would otherwise result in millions of deaths. 'You will never be free until we have a vaccine,' seems to be the mantra. Naturally, the politicians and the scientists agree with the man with the money even though experts seem to agree that a vaccine may never be found. If no vaccine is found then much of the world will remain in a state of terror and social distancing and masks and occasional lockdowns will become a normal part of life. Is that what

Gates wants? The politicians and the big business people with a yearning for control will be delighted.

Moreover, Gates seems to have decided that we won't have a vaccine for 18 months – and, naturally, the world's politicians and scientists (many of whom are on the Gates payroll) agree with the world's least qualified but most powerful 'doctor'. So it seems that the artificial lockdowns and the unnecessary social distancing and masks will remain in place.

Incidentally, I usually avoid the words vaccine and vaccination because they tend to result in censorship. On this occasion, however, it seems impossible to do so.

Since Gates is convinced that the planet is overpopulated, it seems odd that he would be keen on vaccinating huge swathes of Africa. You might think that vaccinating children would mean that there would be fewer deaths and that the population would go up. But Gates argues that if you vaccinate children and they don't die then mothers will have fewer babies and instead of having eight babies in the hope that two will live they will just have three, believing that the vaccines will keep them alive. I am not at all sure how this means that vaccination will result in a fall in the population but Gates says it will and the politicians and the scientists and the journalists all nod wisely, pat their wallets and agree with him. I haven't been able to find any real, solid evidence for this claim, which seems to me to be a combination of the bizarre, and the unbelievable, laced with wishful thinking, apart from the evidence from Gates himself. I don't like to point this out but religion seems to play a part in the number of children a woman has. In the UK, for example, the figures show that Muslims tend to have an average of three children per family whereas Christians usually have only two.

There are, of course, those who are concerned that Gates's mass vaccination programme is part of his plan to reduce the world's population to 500 million or so – a figure that many who are keen on population control regard as acceptable. Personally I cannot see the difference between an untested vaccine, used globally, and genocide. But then I'm perhaps a little old-fashioned in liking to see drugs and vaccines properly tested before being rolled out to large populations. And although interviewers rarely seem to mention it, there are some very worrying stories circulating about some of the vaccination programmes promoted by Gates and/or the WHO. These are not, however, worries that get aired in those parts of the media supported by grants and partnerships from the Gates Foundation. I allow absolutely no advertising or sponsorship on my videos or website. But great chunks of the media, popular and specialist, seem to enjoy close, financial links with the Bill and Melinda Gates Foundation and it is important to remember this. I have no doubt that many websites are also given money or support by the Foundation.

I will deal with Bill Gates's obsession with vaccines in the second part of this two part series entitled Just a Little Prick.

But there are many other topics which must first be mentioned.

First, the Bill and Melinda Gates Foundation has invested in a company called Monsanto.

I have always regarded Monsanto as the most evil company on the planet and I've thought of it this way for several reasons...

First, Monsanto has long been a leader in the development of genetically modified plants. These terrify me because as far as I have been able to find out, they have never been properly tested to see what long-term consequences there might be. What damage could there be to crops in a few years' time? Could they become more susceptible to disease? And are there any risks to the people who eat genetically modified food? For some years now, Monsanto has taken to patenting its seeds and, as a result, small farmers who have traditionally grown their crops from their own seeds have found that they have been unable to do so. There are said to have been many thousands of suicides as a result of this – as farmers found that they weren't allowed to grow the seed they had saved from their own crops but had to buy seed they couldn't afford to buy. I have reported on this many times in the past. And, of course, Monsanto is the manufacturer of Roundup – a doubtless effective but equally doubtless nasty weed killer.

Unfortunately, there have been a number of claims that Roundup causes cancer and there were 125,000 lawsuits as a result. The German company Bayer bought Monsanto a little while ago. Bayer is alleged to have paid $63 billion for Monsanto and to have paid $10.9 billion to settle the claims relating to Roundup.

Bayer, now the new owner of Monsanto, has an interesting history which is worth a short detour while we're here. Think of this as our equivalent of a side trip to Barnard Castle.

In 1925, a group of important German companies, which included Bayer, formed a cartel called IG Farben. Their aim was to obtain control of global markets in key industrial sectors – specifically: chemicals, pharmaceuticals and petrochemicals. History shows quite clearly that it was the formation of this cartel, and the creation of IG Farben, which led directly to the Second World War (and all its associated atrocities) and ultimately the European Union. IG Farben's need for cheap labour was so great that the company built a huge factory at Auschwitz where there was a large reservoir of slave labour. Bayer, the company's pharmaceutical division tested its drugs on prisoners. IG Farben also made huge amounts of money by providing the gas for the killing of prisoners in concentration camps throughout Germany.

At the end of the Second World War, IG Farben was broken up into four new companies, one of which was Bayer, and all of Farben's assets (including the profits from manufacturing the gas used in the infamous gas chambers) were transferred to the new companies – all of which were managed and run by the people who had run IG Farben. So, the bottom line was that although IG Farben had been run by war criminals, no one was really punished and things carried on much as they had done during the war. The only thing that changed was that a good deal of company notepaper had to be redesigned and freshly printed.

The new companies denied any responsibilities for the actions of IG Farben on the basis that they were new and had not existed during the war. This disgraceful self-serving legal move was accepted without a murmur of protest. Bayer, which had been a part of IG Farben, had used concentration camp victims for its experiments and for testing new drugs but the company was allowed to keep all the profits from these experiments.

By the mid-1960s, Bayer had become ever richer and more powerful. And there seemed to be no shame about the past. Bayer actually set up a foundation to honour a Nazi called Fritz ter Meer on his 80th birthday, and started the foundation off with a donation of two million deutschmarks. (It was not until 20 years later that Bayer changed the name of the foundation.) It did not seem to bother anyone that Herr ter Meer had overseen the building of IG Auschwitz and had been found guilty of war crimes (including genocide) and sentenced to just seven years imprisonment in 1948. Naturally, he did not serve the full sentence. Fritz ter Meer, one of the most evil Nazis, was released in 1950 and immediately re-joined the board of Bayer.

That's the end of the detour.

Will Bayer be making a coronavirus vaccine or treatment? Who knows. Would you want it if they did?

The bottom line is that I cannot imagine why anyone who really cares for people and the planet would put any money into Monsanto or Bayer.

Many investors try to avoid what they think of as 'dirty' companies who do or have done bad things to people or the environment but this doesn't seem to bother Gates.

Oddly enough I haven't been able to find any evidence that interviewers from *The Guardian* or the BBC have asked Gates whether he is comfortable with his investment in a company widely regarded as rather worse than wicked. Have I mentioned, by the way, that both the BBC and *The Guardian* are partners with the Bill and Melinda Gates Foundation – by that I mean that they have received money from the Foundation? That is, of course, the sanctimonious *Guardian* newspaper which was founded with the aid of money from slavery.

Next, Gates has been funding scientists at Harvard who are trying to block out the sun's rays in an attempt to stop global warming.

If you haven't heard of this before just stop and think for a moment. The scientists want to spray millions of tons of dust into the stratosphere to stop the sun's rays reaching the earth.

One plan is that every day, more than 800 large aircraft would lift millions of tons of chalk dust to a height of 12 miles above the Earth and then sprinkle the dust to stop the sun's rays getting through.

Another plan is to send up hot air balloons to release powder into the atmosphere.

There are, you won't be surprised to hear, a couple of problems with this.

Obviously, the first is that no one has yet proved that global warming is taking place and is anything more than a natural phenomenon.

Moreover, there are a lot of scientists who believe that we are heading into a phase where the planet is actually cooling.

And there are those who think that Gates's money and the scientists throwing dust into the sky could help create droughts, hurricanes and mass deaths. It seems fairly well agreed that altering the atmosphere to cool the planet could have unpredictable effects. In 1815, a volcanic eruption created crop shortages and disease outbreaks.

Some might say, of course, that all this could be considered a bonus by a man who wants to reduce the world population.

No one seems to have told him, by the way, that 800 large aircraft taking off every day and flying to 12 miles up, would require a good deal of aviation fuel. And what sort of dust are they planning to have sprayed? Well, some say calcium. But I have also heard talk that barium, alumina and strontium might be used. Whatever it is won't improve the quality of the air we breathe. Bottom line is that this seems to me to be a way to reduce the world's population rather than protect it – all in the guise of dealing with the climate change hoax.

Next, Gates is funding scientists at a company called Oxitec who are genetically modifying mosquitoes. This project has received authority in the US, and the genetically modified mosquitoes will be released in 2022. What could go wrong? I have no idea. I don't think anyone else does either. But I can think of a number of good reasons why this is breathtakingly dangerous. There is even talk of research into mosquito delivered vaccines.

Gates is also helping to pay for researchers who are making breast milk from cultured mammary cells. This seems to me to be the ultimate in hubris. Why does Gates always want to interfere with nature? The female body produces the perfect breast milk. There is no need for substitutes. I remember that when attempts were made to introduce powdered milk into developing countries, it was a disaster. Women were told to stop natural breast feeding and to follow the example set by Western women – and to use artificial milk. One problem was that the water used to rehydrate the milk was often badly polluted. And many babies died. If Gates wants to help women and babies, he would surely do better to encourage natural breast feeding.

You will by now see a pattern developing. Gates seems to me to be a mad scientist manqué. He seems to have massive faith in the idea that scientists can solve everything by interfering with nature – often using global warming as an excuse for his plans. His attitude seems to be that he knows much better than God how things should work, and so he is going to use his money to pay for the improvements he thinks we need.

Next, Gates is funding the developing of fake meat. This will be very handy when his other projects such as blocking the sunshine destroys traditional farming. The Bill and Melinda Gates Foundation funds the Cornell Alliance for Science which supports the agrichemical industry. All this takes the power from small farmers and gives it to big chemical companies, in my opinion. If Gates's projects damage natural farming then his foundation's investments in laboratory food and artificial breast milk will doubtless prove to be extremely profitable. Gates, through his Foundation, has also invested in microchipped biomedical, track and trace and payment transaction systems such as cryptocurrencies. He seems to prefer digital payment systems to old-fashioned cash and appears to be enthusiastic about ID systems and health passports, which he describes as being good for keeping an eye on people, making sure that they pay their taxes and have their Gates-approved vaccinations.

And I think it is fair to say that he is probably rather more enthusiastic about trans-humanism than I am.

And then there is the organisation known as ID2020, which is believed by some to show more than modest enthusiasm for mandatory vaccination programmes and mandatory track and tracing programmes. Since 2016, ID 2020 has promoted digital ID. The promoters or partners are Microsoft, the company which made Gates rich and GAVI, the alliance which links drug companies and the Bill and Melinda Gates Foundation – among others. One of the Gates Foundation's aims is, of course, investing in vaccine development and surveillance.

'It's exciting,' they say, 'to imagine a world where safe and secure digital identities are possible, providing everyone with an essential building block to every right and opportunity they deserve.'

If I trusted Bill Gates, I might be a trifle more enthusiastic. But I'd rather ask Donald Trump to hold my wallet than ask Bill Gates to hold my identity.

Gates and or his Foundation or Microsoft have also invested in Onfido which is preparing technology to develop a phone app to scan faces so that people can work or travel.

And I doubt if Gates would object to the suggestion that we all have medical certificates vaccinated into our bodies to prove that we have had the covid-19 vaccination.

What else is there?

Well, there is the Pirbright Institute, where they study infectious diseases affecting farm animals. The Pirbright Institute is one of those curious hybrid organisations which is government funded but also a charity and, as you have probably guessed, its major stake holders include the Bill and Melinda Gates Foundation. I was a little surprised to find Gates supporting an institute researching farm animals until I discovered that the Pirbright Institute had taken out a patent on a coronavirus with the European Patent Office. Big companies do that a lot these days and it seems institutes do, too. I wonder why anyone would want a patent on the coronavirus – though, of course, the patent might be useful for a vaccine.

And there is something called CEPI – which is the Coalition for Epidemic Preparedness Innovations. This was launched in Davos in 2017 by the governments of Norway and India, the Wellcome Trust, the World Economic Forum and the Bill and Melinda Gates Foundation. It has been given large chunks of taxpayers' money from Germany, Australia and the UK.

One of CEPI's goals is the development of platforms which can be used for rapid vaccine development against unknown pathogens. One of the board voting members is someone from the vaccine business unit at Takeda Pharmaceutical Company and the scientific advisory committee includes someone from Pfizer, of course. And CEPI and GlaxoSmithKline have announced a collaboration, which is nice. And CEPI works in partnership with Imperial College, which is where Ferguson works and where work is being done on vaccines. You will remember Ferguson. It was his outrageously wrong prediction which led to the lockdowns and the social distancing and the desperate call for a vaccine to end all our misery. Oh and CEPI also works with GAVI which we will come to in part two of 'Just a Little Prick'. GAVI has announced its enthusiasm for identifying and registering children around the world.

Just how Gates, the world's leading expert on health, keeps up with all these organisations is beyond me. I wouldn't know whether I was at a CEPI meeting or a GAVI meeting or simply in the counting house counting out my money. But I expect our wonderful billionaire has lots of help. And there is always Mrs Gates, of course.

Gates, through his Foundation, has bought support and influence everywhere but he has, in my view, left a trail of damage and concern. And all that brings us back to the vaccines, of course. No story about Gates would be complete without details of the vaccines – past and future.

I will deal further with Mr and Mrs Gates' obsession with vaccines in the next part of this two part series. It's an obsession which seems to me to be distinctly unhealthy though perhaps not for Bill and Melinda. I don't think it is too healthy for people in developing countries and it is probably not going to be healthy for those of us in developed countries either.

When asked when we would get back to normal after the coronavirus hoax, Gates said 'when almost every person on the planet has been vaccinated against coronavirus'. He has colourfully described the vaccine for covid-19 as the final solution. Inconveniently, many experts say that it may not be possible to make a vaccine. Some point out that making a vaccine often takes many years. And I am not the only doctor to worry that if a vaccine is made very quickly, with inadequate testing, then the global consequences could be absolutely catastrophic. Injecting 7 billion people with an experimental vaccine sounds to me like a potential recipe for a disaster previously unknown on the planet. In his less bombastic moments, Gates realises this and has, therefore, insisted that there be legal indemnification for those making and distributing vaccines. In other words: if the vaccine kills you or destroys your brain then you're on your own. Don't expect any compensation. In the US, manufacturers and distributors have had immunity from February 2020. I'm not sure whether the immunity will cover doctors and nurses so that's something they might like to worry about. Patients should see my video entitled, 'Advice for anyone not wanting to be stuffed'. Or read the transcript on this website.

Part Two of this series gets even more extraordinary. And watch it soon just in case it gets removed and mysteriously disappears.

YouTube has announced that it will remove any video deemed to be in contravention of advice being given by the WHO (that must be tricky, given the WHO's ability to change its mind but there you go).

And one of the biggest providers of money for the WHO is, of course, what's its name, oh yes, the Bill and Melinda Gates Foundation.

Still, if that happens you can always read the transcript on my website www.vernoncoleman.com – as long as that remains in place.

July 3rd 2020

Just a Little Prick (Part Two)

Welcome to part two of 'Just a Little Prick', the unauthorised Bill Gates story. Obviously, the term 'little prick' refers to what happens when you have an injection and is naturally in no way meant in a pejorative way. Heaven forbid. If I were to be rude about Mr Gates his subsidised friends at *The Guardian* and the BBC would doubtless need to be revived with smelling salts.

In the first episode of 'Just a Little Prick', I dealt with a few of Mr Gates's connections, aspirations and investments. But I made it clear that he and his wife seem to have one first love: vaccines.

Some people love cats, mountain climbing or horse racing. But Bill and Melinda Gates love vaccines. They yearn to inject everyone, and to them vaccines appear to be the eighth wonder of the world. I wouldn't be surprised if they spent their honeymoon watching vaccines being made or watching vaccinations being given to tiny African children. I bet they spend their evenings drooling over vials of vaccines. And at Christmas they probably give each other unusual vaccines they've found.

Unravelling the Bill and Melinda Gates Foundation and its links with the world of vaccines and vaccinations has taken weeks and given me a headache. Thank heavens there isn't yet a vaccine for headaches.

Among the many partnerships and so on which the Bill and Melinda Gates Foundation has developed in recent years, there is one with an organisation called GAVI.

Now GAVI is rather odd in that it is a partnership between the Bill and Melinda Gates Foundation, the World Health Organisation (which itself is very well financed by the Bill and Melinda Gates Foundation) the World Bank and a variety of other bodies.

So, for example, GAVI also has close and loving partnerships with what I think are some of the world's biggest, dirtiest, most disreputable multinational drug companies including GlaxoSmithKline and Pfizer. Perhaps not surprisingly, the organisation 'Doctors Without Borders' has I think alleged to have said uncomplimentary things about GAVI, alleging that large multinational drug companies working with the Bill and Melinda Gates Foundation put high mark ups on their prices and that GAVI spends oodles of money subsidising large companies. One of GAVI's stated aims seems to be to create a healthy market for vaccines.

You will probably not be surprised to hear that Gates has close links with a number of multinational drug companies but you may, or may not, be surprised to hear that he doesn't seem to me to be terribly fussy about the company he keeps. On the other hand it would I suppose be quite difficult to find a drug company partner that didn't have a reputation that would make Al Capone blush with shame. If you get into bed with a drug company you have to be prepared to wake up in the morning with a bit of scratching and itching and so on.

In a previous video entitled, 'Would You Trust These People with Your Life?' I detailed some of the bad things that GSK has done over recent years and I pointed out that if it were a human being, GSK would be described as a recidivist. It would probably have regular appointments with a parole officer.

GSK is one of the world's biggest pharmaceutical companies and, in my view, if it made teaspoons, you'd need to be a special sort of person to buy a teaspoon from them.

In 2014, for example, GSK was fined $490 million dollars by China after a Chinese court found it guilty of bribery. The court gave GSK's former head of Chinese operations a suspended prison sentence, and they gave suspended prison sentences to other executives too.

Sadly, that misadventure in China wasn't GSK's only little 'Oh dear, whoops, how did that happen?' mistake. Here are some others.

In 2009, in Canada, a five-year-old girl died five days after an H1N1 flu shot and her parents sued GSK for $4.2 million. The parents' lawyer alleged that the drug was brought out quickly and without proper testing as the federal government exerted intense pressure on Canadians to get immunised.

In 2010, GSK paid out $1.14 billion because of claims over a drug called Paxil. And they settled lawsuits over a drug called Avandia for $500 million.

In 2011, GSK paid $250 million to settle 5,500 death and injury claims and set aside $6.4 billion for future lawsuits and settlements in respect of the drug Avandia.

And then there are the accusations of fraud, misbranding and failure to report safety data.

In 2012, GSK pleaded guilty to federal criminal offences including misbranding of two antidepressants and failure to report safety data about a drug for diabetes to the FDA in America. The company admitted to illegally promoting Paxil for the treatment of depression in children and agreed to pay a fine of $3 billion. GSK also reached a related civil settlement with the US Justice Department. The $3 billion fine also included the civil penalties for improper marketing of half a dozen other drugs.

There's more interesting stuff about GSK on my video entitled, 'Would you trust these people with your life?'

Oh, and there are a couple of other things you should know about GSK.

First, GSK is one of the top earning vaccine companies in the world. And in 2010, there were reports of narcolepsy occurring in Sweden and Finland among children who had the H1N1 swine flu vaccine. It is reported that not all the safety problems were made public.

In Ireland, the Irish Government kept inviting people to get vaccinated even when it was clear that the pandemic was on the wane and it was nowhere near the catastrophe portrayed by influenza researchers, governments, industry and the media. One member of the Irish parliament, told the Irish Prime Minister. 'The Health Service Executive decided to purchase Pandemrix and continued to distribute it even after they knew it was dangerous and untested.'

It is perhaps worth noting that Professor Neil Ferguson, the Eddie the Eagle of mathematical modelling though perhaps without the innocent and patriotic charm, had predicted that the swine flu could lead to 65,000 deaths in the UK alone. In the end, the swine flu killed 457 people and had a death rate of just 0.026 per cent of those infected. Just another of Ferguson's cock ups. Cock ups seem to be a speciality of his in more ways than one.

Second, Sir Patrick Vallance, is the Chief Scientific Adviser in the United Kingdom and, I suspect, a key figure in dealing with the coronavirus in the UK and the plans for a vaccine. Vallance worked for GSK between 2006 and 2018. By the time he left GSK he was a member of the board and the corporate executive team. Fines and so on which I have listed took place while Vallance was working as a senior figure at GSK.

As I say, you can find out lots more exciting stuff about GSK and about Astra Zeneca in my video entitled, 'Would You Trust These People with Your Life?' If the video disappears, you can, as always find the transcript on my website www.vernoncoleman.com

Oh, and there's one more thing I nearly forgot to mention. GlaxoSmithKline was fined £37.6 million for cheating the National Health Service. I wonder what Vallance thought about that.

The Bill and Melinda Gates Foundation also has a relationship with Pfizer and to be honest with you, Pfizer's record isn't anything you would want to boast about. If you worked there you'd keep quiet about it I think and say you worked for the tax people or robbed banks for living.

So, for example, in the UK, Pfizer was fined £84.2 million for overcharging the NHS by 2,600% and in the US, Pfizer was hit with a $2.3 billion fine for mis-promoting medicines and paying kickbacks to doctors.

You might think that a foundation wanting to have a clean reputation might avoid relationships with companies like those.

But Bill Gates doesn't seem to mind about all these little peccadillos; the cheating and the deceiving and so on. And in a way why should he? He has a team of PR people willing and able to make sure that his halo is constantly being repaired and polished, and I doubt if any of his many press and broadcasting partners will want to damage their financially advantageous relationship by mentioning anything which might caught embarrassment. After all, we must not forget that the Foundation he shares with Melinda, Mrs Gates, seems to me to have investments with bought much of the world's media; doling out fairly huge chunks of cash to no doubt grateful partners. Did I remember to mention that those two sanctimonious organisations the BBC and *The Guardian* are partners with the Gates Foundation?

It cannot be that Gates isn't aware of the problems associated with vaccination because his own foundation has allegedly had its own little peccadilloes to think about. I've described some of those controversies in other videos.

In India there was trouble over a Gates-funded vaccine programme. A government investigation claimed the programme, an observational study, violated the human rights of those being injected and failed to report properly adverse effects. That, as we have seen, is not entirely unusual drug company practice. A parliamentary investigation concluded that the Gates funded Program for Appropriate Technology in Health had been engaged in a scheme to help ensure 'healthy markets' for GlaxoSmithKline and Merck (another drug company). An eminent Indian editor said, 'it is shocking to see how an American organisation used surreptitious methods to establish itself in India. Another complaint was that Indians were used as guinea pigs.

In Africa, a meningitis vaccine project, funded by Gates, led to reports of up to 500 children allegedly suffering seizures and convulsions and becoming paralysed.

And back in India, it was reported that over 490,000 people allegedly developed paralysis as a result of the polio vaccine that was given. Remarkably and horrifyingly it was claimed that 80% of polio cases were derived from the vaccine.

There are complaints that the Gates Foundation has taken over public health for the benefit of big drug companies. The links between the Gates Foundation and other organisations and the pharmaceutical giants seem never ending. There seem to me to be a good many unanswered questions.

Gates has long argued that the world is overpopulated, and to help further this end the Gates Foundation is said to have funded Marie Stopes, an organisation, which performs over three million abortions a year and has also worked with a charity called Gynuity which is experimenting with a second trimester abortion trial in Africa.

But it is vaccines which seem to interest Gates most, and despite all the known hazards the enthusiastic Gates remains gung-ho about them. He must know that there are very real dangers with vaccines but curiously it doesn't seem to worry him. I wonder if he really has any idea what he is talking about when he discusses vaccines. There seems to me to be little awareness of the risk-benefit ratio.

For example, I have seen an interview in which he agrees that if 7 billion people are vaccinated against the coronavirus there could be 700,000 people damaged by the virus. There could, of course, be many deaths but I don't think Mr Gates likes to talk about that scenario. He says that there could be 700,000 people with side effects, and he dismisses this as though he is talking about a bit of soreness or a slight rash.

Not necessarily so, Mr Gates. I've been studying and writing about vaccines for over 50 years and the side effects from vaccination are often life changing. It is perfectly possible, for example, that there could be 700,000 people with severe brain damage after the first tranche of the vaccination programme has been completed.

I wonder if Gates has any idea what a brain damaged person looks like; how devastating it is not just for them but for their relatives.

And of course the covid-19 disease, the subject of the Gates's determination for a global vaccine, has, as I keep reminding everyone, killed far, far less than the ordinary flu can kill in the same sort of time period.

What is all this about? Who is doing what for why and who is profiting and how?

Well, the drug companies are making money. Loads of it. The Bill and Melinda Gates Foundation is getting more control over global healthcare. And Bill and Melinda are becoming ever more powerful and ever more able to pursue whatever other goals and agendas may be dear to them. And wherever they go they are treated like royalty. And Bill Gates himself is said to be richer now than he was a decade ago. Indeed, during the decade of vaccines promoted by Gates, his personal worth is said to have doubled to over $100 billion.

The bottom line, however, is that I can't help suspecting that if Gates hadn't made so much money and hadn't doled so much of it out to buy influence, everyone would laugh at him, ignore him or dismiss him as a nutter. Is there a hidden agenda? How much does Gates' fear about overpopulation influence what he does? And how much does that family interest in eugenics affect the aims of the Gates Foundation? Many rich people do wonderful things with their money – but they do it without trying to change the world and without wanting to alter the way people live.

Although Gates is a university drop-out with no more medical degrees than your fridge, he is regarded as a saviour and his views on vaccination are treated as though they had been carved in stone and handed down from on high. What Gates wants is what we get. It seems to me that Gates is ignorant, deluded, arrogant and enormously dangerous. In my view, he is doing, and will do, infinitely more harm than good.

And the other half of this strange joke is that whereas I am medically trained and have studied vaccines and vaccination for half a century my questioning, cautious view, asking only for more medical or scientific evidence to be produced in support of the claims which are made, is regarded as unacceptable and I am the one libelled, demonised and dismissed as a nutter, targeted by trolls, demonised as too questioning and regarded as too dangerous to be allowed onto Facebook lest I terrify the 'community' with too many truths.

Putting aside my scepticism and doubts about vaccination (and my conviction, after much research, that vaccines are neither as safe nor as effective, as we are assured by their ignorant supporters) I am deeply concerned about the safety of any coronavirus vaccine. I feel that anyone who accepts a coronavirus vaccine as proposed or supported by Bill Gates or his Foundation, should perhaps be placed in protective care for their own protection. I pray that no parents will allow their children to be given a vaccine that has been hastily produced. Those who believe in vaccination should demand that any vaccines are thoroughly tested for safety and efficacy – and that all test results be made public. Still, there is a bright side to all this. When the inevitable biopic of Gates' life is made, I hope they will use my title 'Just a little prick'. It seems so suitable for a man who appears to be dedicated to vaccinating the world.

July 4th 2020

Who Is Pulling the Strings?

Japan didn't have proper lockdowns because the Government there was hoping that they could still go ahead with the 2020 Olympics. I gather there was also a problem with the constitution which doesn't really give the Government in Japan the authority to shut down the country.

They didn't do much in the way of testing. They focused on quarantining the people who appeared to have the coronavirus. That's the usual textbook way of dealing with an infection. You keep the patients with the infection isolated. You don't isolate all the healthy people.

Since the Japanese didn't quite follow other countries, you might expect that the death total from covid-19 in Japan would be terrifyingly high.

It wasn't.

The Japanese death total from covid-19 to date is 977.

Less than a thousand.

And to save you looking it up, the population of Japan is 126 million – just about twice the population of the UK.

The UK death total is now alleged to be 44,000 – and though we all know what we think of the way the numbers have been added up in the UK, there is no doubt that the care home deaths alone will far, far exceed the total in Japan.

What more proof does anyone need that the lockdown and all the other legal paraphernalia was unnecessary, brutal and politically motivated rather being scientifically or medically based?

The statistics show that the death rate is falling everywhere. And since most of the deaths occurred in care homes where the people who died were already suffering from numerous serious disorders, it doesn't seem likely that covid-19 is going to make much of a return. Around the world, the vast majority of the deaths occurred among already sick over 80-year-olds. And many of the over 80-year-olds with many diseases are now dead so they can't die again.

If the coronavirus does return, if there is a truly deadly second wave, then I won't believe it isn't planned. Indeed, if there is a second wave I will have great difficulty in believing it's the same infection.

Meanwhile, our world gets crazier by the day.

If this were merely a pandemic of a flu-like illness, we could all be getting back to normal. We could be wondering what idiots mismanaged things so badly. We would demand that there should be a proper enquiry – and we might expect that a number of people were charged with fraud. If someone steals your money by pretending that something is what it is not then that's fraud. You might think that there are a number of people who deserve to be questioned and doing some explaining. Why, for example, were the predictions of one mathematical modeller with such a terrible track record given so much importance? And what was the role of the 77th brigade of the British army during all this?

If we ever manage to get back to democracy those are questions which will need answering.

But it's not going to be that easy, is it?

Because this isn't about a simple virus infection; there is much more going on.

Governments will now do more testing so that they can find more hotspots so that they can close down areas or towns. And smart phones will be used to track and trace people just as though we were all living in a 21st century version of Nazi Germany.

And, incidentally, here is a good reason to use cash.

If you buy something with a credit card just five minutes after another customer and the other customer turns out to have been in contact with someone else exhibiting symptoms of the new political flu, then you will be a target of the contact tracers. And, since you used a credit card, you will be easy to trace.

The demand that we wear masks is growing rapidly. In parts of America, you can't go into a food store if you aren't wearing a mask. In Texas, the governor has issued a state-wide executive order requiring most individuals to wear a face mask both indoors and outdoors. Wearing masks in Scotland is going to be compulsory from 10th July so presumably something is going to happen at midnight on 9th July that will make the coronavirus change its habits. The wearing of masks will be mandatory except for a few exceptions and for children under five years of age.

And yet, as I showed in my analysis of the research evidence, we know that wearing masks reduces blood oxygen and can cause all sorts of health problems.

Figures published by the United States Center for Disease Control, show that as the number of deaths from pneumonia, influenza or covid-

19 went up, so the total number of deaths went down. The total number of deaths actually went down. The only explanation I can think of is that many of the people who were put down as having died of covid-19 or the flu would, in other years, have been put down as dying of their heart disease, lung problems, cancer or whatever.

Moreover, although we obviously won't be able to compare the figures until the end of the year, the statistics appear to be showing that the total number of people dying in 2020 is not going to be very different from the total number dying in 2019. Actually, I am being generous and bending over backwards to be fair to those claiming that we are living through a crisis.

Look at these figures.

In week 10 of the year the number of deaths in 2019 was 58,490 but in 2020 the death total in the same week was 54,157. In week 15 in the US the total number of deaths in 2019 was 55,477 whereas in 2020, the total number of deaths was 47,574.

I took those weeks at random but the pattern is clear – fewer people have died in America in 2020 than died in the same period in America in 2019.

And this in the middle of a pandemic which has closed down hospitals and the economy.

In the UK, the rules are impossible to understand. Well, I can't understand them anyway. Hairdressers and pubs can open but some hospital departments are still shut. Indeed, some hospitals are still shut – despite what the official spokespersons might be saying. You can go into an amusement arcade where people are usually all crowded together but you can't go into a bowling alley where people are usually well separated from other players.

I can no longer remember whether or when social distancing must be measured at six feet six inches and when it can be three feet three inches. Not content with wasting most of our money, the Government is now introducing endless new rules, regulations and guidance to tell us how we are to use that tiny portion of freedom which we are allowed to keep. Although, as I have said before, a rule, a regulation or a piece of guidance which is enforced by the police and which can result in my being fined or imprisoned is a law.

The zombies are still desperate to obey the rules. They are like enabling victims, conscientiously doing as they are told and shouting abuse or threats at those who have woken up and can see the truth. They are not very bright but they are slavishly obedient. They telephone the police if they see someone they think might be breaking the regulations. They would have made good concentration camp guards. And, talking of concentration camp guards, in big shops the members of staff who are designated to ensure that customers follow the rules have that vacant look, that air of superiority, that comes so naturally to those enjoying power they have borrowed and which they can enjoy without having to temper it with any sense of personal responsibility.

I am consumed by questions. How many people know what is going on? How many people are in on the secrets that will define our future? Why do the authorities feel the need to suppress anything and everything which might produce a smile or two? Going to the beaches or a pub becomes a sort of state crime – threatening the lives of us all. If I hear again about 'civic duty' I think I shall scream.

Who persuaded the unions into deciding that we couldn't or shouldn't open schools? Why is it that 31% of private schools are delivering four or more hours a day of live online lessons whereas among state schools the figure is just 6%?

What is Boris Johnson's advisor, Dominic Cummings planning to do when he leaves government employment at the end of 2020? Does he have plans? Is he going to have a wonderful job with the Bill and Melinda Gates Foundation? Or where else?

Why did Britain import $10 billion worth of human and animal blood? Why so much and what for? Just two years ago, the Government said that the UK was self-sufficient in blood. Where is the blood all coming from? And where is it going? And why?

How many of the services which were temporarily suspended or reduced will return to normal when all this is over?

No, sorry, that's a silly question. I already know the answer to that.

Why is the Government in the UK apparently determined and desperate to destroy small investors and pensioners who don't have a civil service pension? Without dividends being paid, pension funds are going to have to pay pensioners out of capital. And we all know what that means in the long run.

When was all this planned? The coronavirus bill which was passed back in March was over 350 pages long. They didn't write that in twenty minutes. We never saw what was coming but it has clearly been coming for years. All this planning took a long time. Who planned it? And why?

We are told that there will soon be a vaccine. The usual 15 year time period to prepare a new vaccine will be cut to months, presumably by cutting out some of the testing. The vaccine will then be made available for everyone on the planet.

How mandatory is this vaccine going to be? Will those who have the vaccine proudly wear a tattoo? Will those who refuse the vaccine have to wear a badge marking them as unclean? A yellow star sewed onto their clothing, perhaps?

Why is the coronavirus not transmitted among those who attend Black Lives Matter demonstrations but dangerous among people having a day on the beach or in a pub? Why is it legal to attend a mass demonstration for Black Lives Matter but illegal to watch a football match or a cricket match? Are we supposed to believe that the virus doesn't work at demonstrations but does at sports grounds? What lunacy is this? Why is it illegal for a man to open his shop but perfectly legal for demonstrations to trash it and loot it?

The world seems to have turned upside down. And the police have exchanged their slogan 'protect and serve' for a new one 'punish and enslave'.

Why are thousands of privileged, self-righteous, elitists and Philistines demanding that we trash our history when they should really be worried about the future we don't have.

Who is pulling the strings to make us dance like puppets to whatever tune they play?

And where is all this going to end?

Just a couple of days ago, in America, in Los Angeles, the city of angels, a court removed a child when a parent tested positive for covid-19.

The parent had made alternative arrangements for the child to be cared for by someone else but the court simply took the child away from the parents.

How long before other parents avoid having the test done in order to protect their children? How many people will just flee into the wilderness and live off grid? This insane, obscene madness has gone far enough. No, actually, it's gone too far.

It is no longer a case of the maddest lunatics having taken over the asylum. We now have a situation where the most dangerous prisoners have taken over the prison.

July 5th 2020

What Did You Do In The War?

There is no doubt that the world is full of a good many bizarre and unsupportable claims and notions. Trying to pick your way through the quagmire of claims, counter-claims and general nonsense is harder than it has ever been.

The basic problem, of course, is that governments and official sounding organisations have been lying, deceiving and manipulating since the coronavirus first emerged from hiding and yelled 'boo'.

All honesty has gone out of the window. Governments have lied, distorted truths and threatened us with the full authority of the law if we question their orders.

I've been writing about medical matters for a long, long time and I am pretty well accustomed to the fact that governments and official bodies hide truths, suppress facts and spout a lot of nonsense to keep us all looking in the wrong direction so that they can carry on deceiving us. But I have never known anything like this.

These days the world's governments and the major global organisations have taken things one stage further by employing people to take down information they don't like, whether it is true or not, to spread confusion and bewilderment along with the fears, and to put up false information to mislead and to guide us into deadly traps. The British Government even has a part of the British Army, the 77th Brigade, spying on its citizens and protecting the Government line. Exactly what are they doing, I wonder. Are they taking down material that doesn't fit the official line, even if it's true, or sneering at those trying to provide solid, honest information? Are they using our taxes to plant misinformation and fake news? I don't have the foggiest. Is this really what the soldiers of the 77th Brigade joined the army to do? Don't they realise that by suppressing the truth and suppressing debate they are endangering their own lives and their families' lives?

YouTube apparently now has a policy to censor doctors or scientists who disagree with the view of the World Health Organisation. Putting aside the difficulty I find in knowing exactly what the view of the WHO might be at any one time this blanket endorsement of an organisation which I find rather iffy to say the least seems to me to be terrifying. The WHO recommended wholesale quarantine and lockdowns which resulted in the civil rights of billions of citizens being removed. Moreover, the WHO policy will result in more deaths than covid-19.

The BBC seems to have become addicted to spreading what is now called 'fear porn' – using government propaganda to terrify people into submitting to whatever lunatic ideas are currently in vogue. Since government advice changes regularly, so the advice given by the media changes too. The result is confusion and more bewilderment. Should face masks be worn, for example? And if so by whom and when and where? Ofcom, the UK's broadcasting watchdog has advised broadcasters that they must exercise extreme caution when broadcasting statements that seek to question or undermine the advice of public health bodies on the coronavirus or otherwise undermine people's trust in the advice of mainstream sources of information.' Since the public health bodies and mainstream sources of information have all been provably wrong about the coronavirus – right from the start and in almost every respect – the public have been officially prevented from hearing the truth!

I don't consider myself as being involved in social media at all – I'm just a retired doctor and a book author – so I can say this: I've worked extensively for national newspapers and TV stations round the world and I can tell you that the best researchers, writers and broadcasters are currently working online – and not in mainstream media. The mainstream media is a disgrace.

The whole question of the virus is of vital interest to us all – including those employed by the Government.

The mainstream media, both print and broadcasting, has been bought – either by governments or by private individuals or organisations – and so any attempts to provide an alternative view, to question the official, party line or to discuss contentious issues will be banned. There is no longer any freedom of speech.

And things are getting worse by the day.

Numerous private pressure groups, charities and so on are constantly demanding that material which offers a point of view which they consider unacceptable be removed from the internet – as well as from the mainstream media.

And so there are pressure groups demanding that anyone who dares to question the claims of those who believe that our climate is changing should be silenced. Mainstream media has already been silenced but now these pressure groups want the internet prefects to remove any videos or articles which offer a point of view which does not agree with their own.

They probably don't see it as censorship – they just see it as getting their own way and silencing the opposition.

But it's the sort of thing that fascists have favoured even since Mussolini woke up one morning, had breakfast couldn't think of anything better to do, and invented fascism.

Amazingly, big commercial advertisers have got in on the act. They too want information to be suppressed if it doesn't agree with their corporate policies. And so recently we had the bizarre sight of Volkswagen, fresh from being caught cheating on its emission tests, and endangering the lives of millions, withdrawing its advertising in an attempt to police the internet. If they don't stop doing that I shall be tempted to remind the world that the Volkswagen beetle was designed by Adolf Hitler.

The game has changed.

And the problem is that suppressing free speech and silencing debate simply leads to more conspiracy theories, more false information and more confusion.

Some of the stuff I have read in the last day or two has been startling – to say the least. And yet untangling the truth from the fiction is extraordinarily difficult. For example, weeks ago I found a site called deagel.com which contains a forecast for 2025. The site suggests that by 2025, the population of the USA will have fallen from 326 million to 99 million and that by 2025, the population of the UK will have fallen from 65 million to 14 million. The site tells us that the population of China and Russia will be much the same as they are but that Germany will have fallen from 80 million to 28 million and that Australia will, in just five years, have gone from 23 million to 15 million.

These figures are both startling and terrifying.

A note at the bottom of the page informs readers that the information was obtained from a variety of institutions including the CIA and the United Nations and the International Monetary Fund.

What the devil is going on? Can this really be true?

I have no idea.

It's just one of many mysteries.

How accurate are the figures for 2025?

Your guess is as good as mine.

But if the CIA and the UN and the IMF really are providing these figures then they clearly know something we don't know.

Albert Camus, the Nobel Prize winning author of *The Plague* wrote that the only means to fight the plague is honesty – and although he was writing about a different plague, and a fictional one, his words ring loud and clear today.

The problem, of course, is that when you suppress truths you create a vacuum in which mysteries and conspiracies can thrive. We are being told to do as we are told by the State and not to trust anyone who disagrees. We are being told not to trust our neighbours but that we must trust people who are proven liars. We have lost all our civil rights and our natural, God given freedoms and we have lost our freedom of speech.

I can't help wondering if the powers that be, the authorities who are both hiding the truth and suppressing debate, are not deliberately creating a climate in which conspiracies can grow.

Maybe they just want to confuse us.

Maybe they want to be able to feed us misinformation to build up our sense of fear.

Maybe they want to use misinformation to help them discredit those who are struggling to tell the truth – so that they can dismiss everything not on official, government press release as fictional.

How long will it be before all of those who question the official line are silenced?

I have no idea.

All I can tell you is that I will continue to try to find a way through the dense woods of information out there in order to provide honest, accurate appraisals of what is true.

And if I discover information which means that I change my mind – then I will tell you and explain why.

Meanwhile we live in a world where those who are in charge of the policing process are constantly trying to fill our minds with their propaganda.

Perhaps they want to encourage people to put up bizarre claims so that they can suppress everything – claiming that they are doing so to protect us.

And this, of course, is exactly what happens in a war.

Truth, as has always been said, is the first casualty of war.

And truth was certainly an early casualty of this war.

The Government and the mainstream media made sure of that.

I've said it before and I will say it again.

We're fighting a war.

But, sadly, tragically, we are fighting a war against our own government and against most other governments in the world.

World War III has started – and it will be over before many people, the zombies, know it has even started.

Who would have ever thought it could come to this.

We all have to be prepared to answer the question: 'What did you do in the war?'

July 7th 2020

The Madness is Everywhere

Everywhere I look there is madness.

The posh papers and magazines are full of articles by journalists writing about their experiences under house arrest. Oh, how brave they have all been. Having their stupid dinner parties by video, doing their silly dances and listing all the books they've read, the films they've seen and the foreign languages they have learned.

They write about the coronavirus crime as though it's been an adventure. A weekend's camping expedition or a sleepover with chums.

They look at everything through their privileged and slightly stupid eyes. They seem to think that everything will soon be tickety boo and they can all go back to evenings out to a nice restaurant and an evening at the theatre.

It doesn't seem that way to us here.

I wake up thinking I must have imagined what has been happening. And then when I realise that I haven't I feel as though I am living in a bad science fiction movie.

Yesterday, someone close to us, who has cancer, told me that she constantly worries that her cancer has gone to her brain and that no one will tell her the truth. The nightmare in which we are living cannot possibly be true. Sometimes she thinks she may have had a fatal car accident and must be living in purgatory.

I understand totally. I sometimes wonder how many million people are contemplating suicide as the only way out of this obscene piece of global manipulation.

The reporting of this massive take-over of the world has been a disgrace. The mass media has been bought and simply does its best to ramp up the fear and drive the yearning for a vaccine as the only way out of the chaos. The BBC has always been a propaganda machine but I am surprised at how cheaply the rest have been bought. And now those of us fighting for freedom and truth have to battle our own army too

Don't the members of the 77th Brigade, with the proud golden Burmese lion, realise that what is happening to us is happening to them too. Their health service and schools have been destroyed. Their parents and grandparents are being killed. They too will almost certainly be forced to accept an untested vaccination against a disease that is no worse than the flu.

The mass media announced with great excitement that retail sales rebounded since the end of the lockdown. Imagine that! Shops are open and people can leave their homes and the chattering classes are surprised, amazed and delighted that retail sales have gone up.

Pubs and hotels are about to open but the rules are so absurd that if I owned a pub or a hotel, I'd give up and do something else. The social distancing rules will have to be reduced to three feet and a bit if the entire leisure industry isn't to be destroyed but even that won't be enough. Pubs will be patrolled by traffic warden types so that the social distancing laws will be properly observed. What sort of person would take such a job?

Anyone wanting to visit a pub will be told to order their drink on a phone app so that the Government will know what you order. Presumably, those of us who wouldn't know an App if it stood up and barked will have to do without.

In restaurants there will have to be disposable menus, fewer items available and no buffet food and the waiters will have to wash their hands so often that there will be a global water shortage by October.

In hotels, guests will be advised to have meals delivered by room service – with the food left outside their room door so that isn't too warm when they eat it. Oh what a lot of fun holidays and weekend breaks will be. I feel for all those folk who love putting on posh clothes for dinner. Getting all spruced up to sit on the bed to eat your dinner just won't be the same.

How are trains going to manage social distancing in the future? According to the Department for Transport, the busiest train in the UK used to be the 17.11 service from Sutton to Luton which, in pre-lockdown days, carried an average of 1,579 passengers. If all the passengers now have to keep two metres apart then the train will need to be a mile long and will require 80 carriages.

Banks may only be open from 10 a.m. to 2 p.m. (the coronavirus apparently isn't active during those hours) but they're doing their best to make life miserable. I've heard several reports of Barclays Bank refusing to accept coins from customers paying in money. Since cash is legal currency, this is doubtless illegal and anyone who is faced with a snotty teller refusing a bag of coins should take the teller's name and the manager's name and make a report to the Bank of England, their MP, the police and anyone else they can think of.

The madness is everywhere. The City of London Corporation has banned bathing in Highgate Ponds in case its lifeguards are asked to resuscitate bathers who have the coronavirus. What danger could there possibly be to young healthy lifeguards?

There are calls from demonstrators for the police to be disbanded or defunded, as has happened in some parts of America. Don't those demanding this realise that to do so would lead us straight into martial law? Do they not have the sense to realise what martial law looks like? Or is that what they want?

In India, over 122 million people lost their jobs in the month of April alone. In Qatar, there is a penalty of three years in prison for not wearing a face mask in public. And in Panama, where the lockdown allows men and women to leave their homes on alternate days, transgender citizens are complaining that they can't go out on either day.

If I put this stuff in a novel I'd be stoned to death by the readers.

For three months the local hospital physiotherapy department has been shut. The local hairdresser will be open in a couple of weeks but the physiotherapist department has no idea when it will open. What is wrong with these people?

And now that journalists have noticed that the loos are mostly shut, there are articles about how to pee in public without getting arrested. The key to the law is, apparently, not alarming members of the public – though personally I think peeing on people wearing masks is perfectly OK because they are zombies and not members of the public.

Seaside towns are going to be totally destroyed by what is happening. Empty hotels and boarding houses mean that the shops and cafes and ice cream parlours have no customers. Just about every British seaside town will be a ghost town by Christmas. Even the charity shops are closing.

Everywhere you look politicians, civil servants and the mass media are busy doing everything they can to spread fear.

In one of my brainwashing videos I mentioned that in the guidance given to the British Government, it was pointed out that 'a substantial number of people still did not feel sufficiently personally threatened'. Wow.

That's us they're talking about. We are not sufficiently personally threatened. Why would they want us to be so threatened? What ulterior motive could there possibly be? Could I have been right back in March when I suggested that one of the reasons for the hoax was to get us ready for mandatory you-know-what?

Their effective, clinical winding up of the fear process has been designed to cause the greatest harm.

When we are under, stress our bodies produce a hormone called cortisol. Lots of stress equals lots of cortisol in our bodies.

And guess what: patients who have lots of cortisol in their bodies are more likely to die from covid-19 than people who are calm and relaxed. And, of course, since elderly, frail people with illnesses are more likely to die anyway, they are the ones who are going to be most affected by stress.

So there we are: one of the reasons why the Government has been deliberately terrifying us is because they know that we will have more cortisol in our bodies and they know that the extra cortisol will push those who have co-morbidities over the edge.

It's yet another type of mass murder.

No one seems to care about mass murder any more.

There was a huge fuss about a killing in a park the other day. The papers splashed the terrible story over their front pages.

But there has been very little fuss about the tens of thousands of old people who have been abandoned and killed during the last few months.

When I think about it I realise that they've been planning this takeover for years.

When I was young and didn't know anything very much, I was frequently invited to lecture to doctors, nurses and medical students. I presented a number of TV and radio series for the BBC and ITV and for stations abroad.

But as I acquired a little more experience, a little more knowledge and a reputation for questioning the establishment and saying professionally unsayable things that turned out to be right, so the invitations dried up.

Don't misunderstand me.

I don't want to appear on TV or radio and I don't want to give lectures to doctors any more. But it does worry me a little that a combination of original thinking and experience scares the establishment quite as much as it obviously does. And I find it a bit sad that younger doctors who are involved in the media seem to decide that the easy way to be successful is to support the establishment and toe the official line.

What surprises me most, and saddens me enormously, is the way that members of the medical and nursing professions have accepted this takeover of our lives.

Even if they don't think there is anything sinister behind what is happening, they must by now realise that the whole response to the coronavirus has been wrong. The politicians and their advisors all got it wrong. The most generous way of looking at things is that they mistook a fairly ordinary flu virus for a version of the plague.

As a result, hospitals have been closed. Patients with cancer and other serious disorders have been denied essential treatment. Thousands of patients in care homes have been murdered as a result of inept policies and management. Schools have been closed and the lives of millions of children have been ruined. They know that is no exaggeration. The Government has been employing brain washing techniques to control us and to create a fake affection for the health service.

Doctors and nurses all know this is true. They know that the clever three word, three phrase slogans, the encouragement to take part in weekly clapping sessions and the advertising were all designed to build up the fear and to create a sense of national obedience.

Even if there were no ulterior motive, this is still the biggest cock up in medical history.

Medical doctors and nurses know that the spin doctors have been doing everything they can to exaggerate the number of deaths. Patients with the coronavirus were listed as having died of it.

If the truth about what has happened ever emerges then the medical and nursing professions are going to be embarrassed and humiliated to put it kindly. People in both professions are going to go to jail.

It is time to insist that hospitals and clinics are opened immediately without any of the social distancing which every thinking person knows was never necessary.

The media has found many curious heroes in the last three months, mostly as part of the propaganda process I'm afraid. Now is the time for the professions to earn their plaudits. The nation needs to have its health service back.

It would be a big step forward on the road back to real normality. And together we can do it.

A few years ago, there were a lot of threats about ID cards and iris scans being introduced. I wrote about them and helped campaign against them.

The public thought about it, considered the evidence and said a very loud, 'no thank you'.

We need some of that good sense and determination again.

All the round people are fighting their own governments. It happens from time to time in history.

In the UK Johnson, Hancock and company have made themselves our enemies just as Hitler and company were our enemies in 1939 and the 1940s. Johnson is a gullible simple minded buffoon who is dancing on the end of a piece of string being jiggled by Cummings. Hancock is just a pompous, half-witted prefect who would be out of his depth if he were a small town mayor.

They want to destroy freedom and democracy.

Well the bastards aren't going to win.

July 7th 2020

Old Lives Matter

This is not a fashionable thing to say but black people are not the most ignored, oppressed, misused and discriminated against group of people in the world.

The most ignored, oppressed, misused and discriminated against are the elderly.

And it isn't difficult to find the evidence.

For example, UK broadcasters run a non-profit organisation called the Creative Diversity Network which exists to measure diversity in the UK's broadcasters. They study 30 channels in the UK.

Their latest report showed that BAME people make up 12.9% of the population but 22.7% of onscreen contributions. Disabled people and transgender people are also over represented on TV screens.

But there is one group which is under represented – the over 50s.

Curiously, inexplicably and rather offensively these broadcasters seem to regard 50 as elderly. To me it seems very young.

The over 50s make up 36% of the UK population but are under-represented at 24.6%.

So the evidence clearly shows that black people are over-represented and the elderly are much under-represented.

Why then is the BBC spending £100 million of taxpayers' money to produce yet more diverse content?

Sadly, this is nothing new, of course.

In 1967, Barbara Robb put together a book about the abuse of the elderly. It was entitled, *Sans Everything – a Case to Answer*. (The title is, of course, taken from Shakespeare's 'As You Like It' and the full phrase is 'sans teeth, sans eyes, sans taste, sans everything').

The book developed because on 10th November 1965 a letter appeared in *The Times* protesting about the plight of old people in hospital. The writers of the letter complained about the evil practice then all too common of the staff in general and geriatric hospitals of taking spectacles, dentures and hearing aids away from the elderly and leaving them 'to vegetate in loneliness and idleness'.

That was 1965.

C.H.Rolph pointed out that we needed 'to protect the defenceless invalid against physical discomfort, emotional exploitation and deprivation, indifference, exasperation and neglect'. He went on to say that practices in one British hospital were 'a catalogue of cruelty, callousness, filth and depersonalisation such as I have not read since I was reviewing the reports of the Nuremberg trials'.

The truly alarming thing is that the treatment of elderly patients is now worse than it was in the 1960s.

It is hard to believe but true that doctors and nurses have been given official authority to deprive the elderly of food and water so that they die as quickly as possible.

The elderly used to be respected and admired, and consulted for their wisdom and experience.

Today, I'm afraid that the elderly are too often ignored, abused, despised and taken advantage of; dismissed as nuisances, invisible in fifty shades of beige.

Politicians seem to do everything they can to belittle and demean the elderly. Newspaper commentators have weighed in with their heavy boots too and several have claimed that the elderly should not be allowed to vote. Why? Most pensioners have spent their lives working and paying tax so why should they be deprived of a voice just because they've passed a certain birthday. A good number of older folk have far more get up and go than most youngsters and their knowledge of current affairs is surely helped not hindered by their experience and accumulated wisdom.

I am convinced that when utility companies put the elderly onto special lists, it is not so that they can provide them with extra services but so that they can charge them extra and treat them appallingly. All that patronising stuff about wrapping up when the weather is cold and drinking plenty when it's hot. Really. Oh and don't forget to breathe.

It is hardly surprising that so many older folk are now so desperate to deny their age that they spend a fortune on cosmetic surgery in an attempt to preserve the youth they have lost. (Oddly enough, however, it is customary for such individuals to take pride in telling those they meet their real age. There is something charmingly contradictory in having plastic surgery to disguise your age and then telling everyone you meet precisely how old you are.)

Worse still, of course, the elderly are now being officially slaughtered in just about every country in the world. Governments know that because of the absurd levels of expenditure on the coronavirus hoax they will not be able to provide a decent health care service. They will expect younger citizens to look after themselves (by losing excess weight and controlling bad habits such as drinking and smoking) and they will deny health care completely to those who disobey. The elderly will merely be denied treatment.

I find it impossible to believe that administrators around the world all made the same terrible mistake in sending hospital patients into care homes.

No, there has been a coordinated, massive extermination programme. The only logical conclusion is that thousands of old people around the world have been murdered. As a result, governments around the world have saved themselves billions in long-term health costs. And those same governments will also save themselves billions of pounds a year because of the pensions they won't have to pay.

It has been a holocaust.

Incidentally, the dictionary defines a holocaust as slaughter on a mass scale.

And I cannot think of a more appropriate word because that is what this has been.

We have to remember the obvious: that the residents in care homes are there because they are ill and need care. Most have several serious disorders. They may have heart problems, respiratory problems, neurological problems, cancer or any number of other serious health disorders. And because they probably don't eat well, and don't take any exercise, their immune systems are pretty well shot.

It is inconceivable that health care administrators didn't know that. And yet they sent untested hospital patients who were thought to have the coronavirus, and some of whom might have had it, into those care homes where the vulnerable patients caught the infection and died.

Were those patients sent in as Trojan horse killers?

The result would have been the same if the patients being sent from hospital had the flu.

You wouldn't put a patient with the flu into a care home, would you? It would be criminal.

But they did that with suspected coronavirus patients.

And things were made worse because the staff in the care homes had no idea about barrier nursing and they had no equipment.

And, worst of all, they were terrified that the coronavirus was going to kill everyone who caught it because evil governments, and evil journalists had spread lie after lie after lie about the disease. Care home staff were told to keep out relatives and friends – for absolutely no sane reason – and some care home staff simply ran away, with about 40% of staff simply disappearing in France for example.

In the North East of England half of care homes had a coronavirus outbreak. In Scotland nearly half of all coronavirus deaths occurred in care homes. Nearly half of all coronavirus deaths in Sweden occurred in care homes. In Spain, two thirds of the coronavirus deaths occurred in care homes. In Italy, no one seems to have any idea how many old people died in care homes – alone, without staff or family. Many of the elderly didn't actually die of the coronavirus – though that was put on the death certificates – they died of thirst.

In England and Wales in the 11 weeks until 22nd May, there were 50,000 care home deaths. That's double the expected number.

Is anyone going to try to convince us this was all an unfortunate accident?

How many were killed by this wicked plan?

I have no idea. And nor does anyone else. But the exaggerated figure for the total number of coronavirus deaths includes a very high percentage of elderly patients who need not have died.

If I had to make an educated estimate, I would suggest that the number of elderly patients murdered globally between the beginning of March and the end of May 2020 was somewhere between 100,000 and 150,000. That's a fairly conservative estimate.

If any other group of people had been slaughtered so deliberately and so ruthlessly, there would be unbelievable outpourings of anger visible on our streets.

Imagine if 100,000 teenagers had been deliberately murdered in three months – because they were teenagers.

Imagine if 100,000 women had been deliberately murdered in three months – because they were women.

Imagine if 100,000 black people had been deliberately murdered in three months – because they were black.

Why have there been no demonstrations about the old people who were killed?

How many celebrities have you seen or heard shouting out about the murder of old people?

No, nor me.

The real tragedy here is that although this is the worst mass slaughter of the elderly in modern history, it isn't actually anything new.

Old people have been murdered for years without anyone taking any notice. My video on the subject was taken down by YouTube. There is only one serious –ism in most developed countries today – ageism. It is deeply offensive that this is not taken seriously. We all know that black lives matter but don't old lives matter too?

Euthanasia (sometimes admitted and sometimes not) is now commonly practised in so-called civilised societies around the world, and the elderly are invariably the victims.

For many years in the UK, doctors and nurses were encouraged to follow something called the Liverpool Care Pathway.

This was a murderers' charter, which allowed doctors and nurses to withhold food, water and essential treatment from patients who were over 65 and who were, therefore, regarded as an expensive and entirely disposable nuisance.

Then the Liverpool Care Pathway was replaced by something called Sustainable Development Goals (which originated with the United Nations and which is, therefore, global).

Sustainable Development Goals allows the doctors and hospitals to discriminate against anyone over the age of 70 on the grounds that people who die when they are over 70 cannot be said to have died 'prematurely' and so will not count when the nation's healthcare is being assessed.

Governments everywhere love this new rule because it gives the State permission to get rid of citizens who are of pensionable age and, therefore, regarded by society's accountants as a 'burden'.

In Holland, one eminent doctor has claimed that the elderly are not admitted to hospitals – and certainly not to intensive care units. 'The Netherlands does not hospitalise the weak and the elderly in order to make room for young people.'

Don't believe me? A survey of 6,600 patients in the Netherlands found that treatment – including drugs, food and water, were most likely to be withheld from the over 65s. And in 56% of cases, doctors didn't bother to discuss their failure to provide treatment with their patients or patients' relatives.

I have also seen claims that the elderly are routinely killed in Germany, France, Italy and Spain. Age has become a criterion for triage.

Genocide is coming to a town near you – if it isn't already there.

Back in 2015, when doctors in America were reported to be withholding treatment from elderly patients, doctors said it wasn't ageism. They didn't say what it was though. It certainly wasn't stamp collecting. And it wasn't kindness or proper, decent medical practice.

Michael Bloomberg, the billionaire who nearly became the Democrat Presidential candidate in 2020, said America should deny healthcare to the elderly. There was no suggestion that the morality of it be discussed.

In Canada, patients have been buried without post-mortems and, as elsewhere, they were said to have died of the coronavirus if they were thought to have the bug. If a patient with a knife sticking out of their chest had sneezed within 14 days of their death then they died of coronavirus.

This isn't entirely new, of course.

In the UK, it was way back in February 2005 that it was revealed that the British Government had advised that hospital patients with little hope of recovery should be allowed to die because of the cost of keeping them alive.

The key words were 'little hope of recovery'.

Those words that don't mean anything.

Any doctor worthy of the name will tell you that they've seen patients get better despite there having been 'little hope of recovery'.

But Tony Blair's Labour Government suggested that 'old people' be denied the right to food and water if they fell into a coma or couldn't speak for themselves.

So, patients should be killed if they couldn't speak for themselves.

So much for any hope for stroke victims.

Blair's Government suggested that the need to cut costs came before the need to preserve the lives of patients, and decided it had the right to overturn a right-to-life ruling which had been made when a judge ordered that artificial nutrition and hydration should not be withdrawn unless the life of a patient could be described as 'intolerable'. The judge had added that when there was any doubt, preservation of life should take precedence.

Depriving the elderly of food and water is done all the time. Drinks or food are put on a tray and, if the patient is too ill or weak to reach them then they are taken away untouched. In most hospitals, no one bothers to feed patients who cannot feed themselves.

Meanwhile, the Government pours money into vanity projects and wastes money on foreign aid programmes which result in crooked politicians putting billions into Swiss bank accounts.

But the elderly are classified as the 'Unwanted Generation'.

Anyone of pensionable age is a political embarrassment and to be ignored or dumped or killed.

Elderly individuals facing blindness from age-related macular disease are denied drugs that might have prevented their blindness because they are considered expensive, useless and expendable. The theory is that they don't contribute and rarely vote and can, therefore, be disregarded.

How have we managed to forget that in the 1930s the Nazis deliberately starved and dehydrated elderly and vulnerable patients because they were regarded as a useless burden on society?

That is exactly what we are doing today.

We're killing people off if they are old and can't complete an Iron Man Triathlon.

Governments around the world are deciding that because of the difficulty involved in dealing with what is now proven to be nothing more than a mild case of the flu they can no longer treat the elderly at all.

Many of the young may shrug at this with indifference but they should remember two things.

First, they may one day be old themselves.

And second, the age regarded as 'old' is likely to be subjected to the standard creep phenomenon.

Those who don't much care about the elderly being killed will themselves be old sooner than they think. After all young people, if they are lucky, eventually become old people.

And they should remember that the definition of 'old' is getting younger by the year.

Governments have decided that the over 70s cannot be treated. But in some countries the cut off age is 65. And in five years they may reduce the cut off age to 60. And by the end of the decade the 55 year olds will be lucky to receive a bottle of aspirin tablets if they have a heart attack or break a leg.

This is a form of euthanasia. Or maybe eugenics would be a better word. Or population control.

It was something the Nazis thought they were good at.

But they were mere amateurs.

July 8th 2020

Hand Sanitisers Can Kill You

I tottered to the shops today.

And what a sad, depressing experience it was.

The ambitious new world leaders, led by the Bill and Melinda Gate Foundation (which I think of as the Myra Hindley and Ian Brady Foundation, Josef Stalin's Academy for the Weak Spirited and the Mao tse Tung school of obedience) have destroyed the High Street.

Small shops were already suffering – destroyed by a combination of the internet, charity shops and obscenely high local taxes – but now the shops are on the ward where everyone walks on tip toes and whispers. The sort of ward where, in the old days, you'd be as likely to see a priest, a vicar, a rabbi or an imam as you would to see a doctor or a nurse. These days, of course, the men and women of religion are all hiding in the cupboard under their stairs, shivering with fright.

There weren't many people buying anything. Shopping has become a miserable experience. The charity shops were all shut so I took a pile of DVDs to an establishment which would have been called a junk shop in the old days but which is probably a curio specialist or an antique dealer now. The woman behind the counter seemed pleased enough.

Not many people were wearing masks and I was pleased to see that most people seemed to be happily ignoring the rules about social distancing.

But there were some terrified souls about. There were a couple of young families, all masked up, with even tiny tots wearing masks, and one or two older folk were wearing masks too. Half of them were, I noticed, wearing their masks over their mouths but not their noses which made the effort pretty pointless, of course. One middle aged couple were wearing masks, yellow rubber washing up gloves and hats to which they'd sewn material so that their necks were covered. I wish I were making this up. Honestly, I wish I were making it up. I bet they'd blocked their back door keyhole so that the bug couldn't get in that way.

They looked so truly pathetic that I felt sorry for them and I was filled with anger for the people who have been busy promoting the fear.

Tom Hanks, who appears to have completed a medical degree since his last film, has been telling us all that he won't respect us in the morning if we don't wear our masks like good little children.

Well, screw you Tom. Your arrogance in thinking that I give a toss about your respect is matched only by your arrogance in thinking that you know what you are talking about.

It is reported that a scientist from the Royal Society has said much the same thing, though as far as I know he didn't have a film to promote. He didn't seem to have a medical degree either.

A professor of chemical engineering also said we should wear masks. I wonder if any of them know that two Chinese boys died wearing masks. I wonder if any of them have watched the video I made about the research that has been done into mask wearing.

These, and people like them, reminded me that when I was younger and we were allowed out more, I used to go and watch cricket and if there was a Test Match on there would invariably be a call for a doctor to go to the pavilion because one of the players needed medical attention.

I would go along and find myself at the back of a queue of blokes all anxious to help. And none of them would be medical doctors. One would have a doctorate in philosophy, another would have a doctorate in music and the third would be a bishop with a doctorate in theological studies. They all turned up wanting to get into the dressing room and rub shoulders with the cricketers, and they all seemed surprised that they weren't needed.

'Oh, I didn't know you needed a medical doctor,' they would say, apparently astonished, as they backed out of the dressing room when their inappropriate skills had been rejected.

Dr Tom thingy and the bloke from the Royal Society reminded me of those idiots.

And now, of course, a pile of 239 assorted scientists have decided that the bug can hang around long after someone has sneezed. And the World Health Organisation has leapt on the idea as enthusiastically as a 7-year-old leaping on the sticky bun plate at a children's party. The quickest way to become important and famous is to say something that fits in with the WHO's current lunacies and pro-vaccine propaganda. Gosh and golly what a surprise that was. The bug can hang around. Who would have thought it? I bet they want us to have more social distancing. A hundred yards perhaps, or maybe two hundred yards out of doors and a slightly longer distance indoors. I don't know if any of them were doctors but what does any of this matter other than as a means to terrify the ignorant and the susceptible? If 239 market gardeners had said we all needed to smear ourselves with custard, the

WHO would have been thrilled. As long as Mr Gates approved, of course. I can't wait for the Manchester United supporters club to make a statement on the use of masks.

Meanwhile, I wonder what you call 200 moronic scientists.

A diarrhoea of scientists, perhaps?

None of these buffoons seems to have noticed that it isn't how many people get an infection that matters – it's how many die of it. And you have to look at the risk benefit ratio. You have to look at how many are harmed by wearing masks. You have to look at the way people's quality of life is affected adversely.

If we need to wear masks because of the coronavirus then we need to wear masks all the time to protect us against the flu. Is that really what people want?

Back to my shopping expedition.

In one establishment I was asked to take a photograph of one of those funny squiggly black and white things on my phone and to download an app so that they could make a record of all my details. I showed them the old phone which I carry with me. It was built in the 1990s and it doesn't have a camera. It'll only just about make and receive calls.

'Oh, that's alright, sir,' said the bloke at the door, looking rather sorry for me. 'Just write your name, address and phone number on a piece of paper and leave it with us.' He pointed to some scraps of paper and a cheap pen.

I thought that was fine. I don't mind anyone knowing that my name is B. Johnson, that I live at 10 Acacia Avenue in Milton Keynes and that I happen to have the same telephone number as Buckingham Palace.

Three days ago, I was D. Crockett of The Alamo, Texas. Sometimes I'm Dr John Holliday of the OK Corral. If my very good lady and I go out together, we are Bonnie Parker and Clyde Barrow and we are moving about a good deal so can't give a permanent address.

'Are you any relation to Davy Crockett?' asked a youth, the last time I was D. Crockett. I said he was my great grandfather and that I'd still got his coonskin cap in a drawer at home.

You mustn't do this, of course. It might be naughty. I'm in so much trouble it no longer makes any difference.

Oh, and before you think I might get found out by my credit card - I always pay cash. If they won't take cash I don't buy.

As I wandered around the shops, I couldn't help noticing that there was a lot of sanitiser around. Every time I went into a shop I was invited to try their sanitiser. It was like passing the perfume counter in a department store. Would you like to try this after shave? A squirt here and a little squirt there. Visit six shops and you'd have had six squirts of sanitiser. Well, some folk might have. I said no thanks and marched past them and no one ran after me. The few customers who were around couldn't buy anything because they were all constantly trying to wipe the goo off their hands. When you've used six lots of sanitiser, the layers of stickiness must take hours to remove. The ones doing social distancing looked very strange as they rubbed their hands and dodged first to the left and then to the right and then back again. My level of social distancing is to try to avoid bumping into people.

What none of these shoppers knew is that there is evidence that it isn't just masks which can kill people. Sanitisers can be deadly too.

In America, the FDA has warned of a sharp increase in the number of hand sanitiser products that are labelled to contain ethanol but which actually contain methanol – which can be toxic when absorbed through the skin and can be life threatening if swallowed. So some hand sanitisers can cause nausea, vomiting, headache, blurred vision, permanent blindness, seizures, coma, permanent damage to the nervous system or the ultimate side effect – death. That's the type of death that you only get once. If repeatedly used as a hand rub, skin absorption can cause chronic toxicity and sight damage.

A paper I have seen in 'Infectious Diseases Consultant' confirms the danger. And there is a two year old paper in the International Journal of Environmental Research and Public Health entitled, 'Methanol as an unlisted ingredient in supposedly alcohol based hand rubs can pose serious health risk'.

It's nigh on impossible to know which sanitisers are deadly because some of them are mislabelled. And besides, when a shop insists that you use their hand sanitiser are you really going to try to read the label? Even if it's got a label. They probably got the stuff from a bloke who usually does their drains and bought a supply from a mate on the market who knows someone in China. You could use some sanitising gels to strip paint.

If a shop assistant ever does run after me demanding that I use their store sanitiser, I shall simply say that I have a skin allergy and that I'll develop a serious rash and possibly go into anaphylactic shock if I succumb to their blandishments.

'I have two lawsuits outstanding against retail establishments,' I'll point out regretfully. 'But if you insist on taking the risk, could I have your name first?'

I'll lay decent odds they'll suddenly decide I don't need to use the goo after all.

July 9th 2020

It's Going to Get Worse

Everywhere I look I see the mainstream media warning us that a second wave is coming.

They have, I think, realised that the coronavirus hoax is running thin. Too many people realise that it is a con.

And there are too many problems.

In America, some doctors are using budesonide steroid spray to treat coronavirus patients. Indeed steroids and simple hay-fever remedies are being used everywhere. And more and more doctors say there is no need for a vaccine.

The plan is in trouble.

So the enemy needs a replacement; a stand-in; an understudy.

And so they're threatening us with a new disease. They need something new and even nastier than the coronavirus. There is serious talk of the bubonic plague coming back, though to be honest it never went away. And the BBC website, where they specialise in scare stories and coronavirus nonsense, ran a headline the other day which read, or rather shouted, 'Flu virus with pandemic potential found in China'. The story went on to warn that researchers were concerned that it could mutate and trigger a global outbreak.

And maybe it will be that one. Or something else.

The only certainty is that the publicity will tell us it will be nasty and worse than the coronavirus. Covid-19 was just a prelude. The practice infection to build up our fear and turn us into terrified slaves to the state.

They aren't finished with us yet. Not by a long chalk. In fact they're having fun with us and just getting started. Since February, they have been testing us and training us for their new world order, the green revolution, the global reset. They want to see how far we will go, what we will put up with, how much they can humiliate us. They want to break our spirit and turn us all into zombies. And so the zombies are everywhere. They're the ones who wear those deadly masks and scowl at those not wearing them. They're the idiots who insist on social distancing.

It has for more than a month been obvious that they will need a second wave, of course. The fear levels are drifting down a little and more and more people now realise that the whole coronavirus scam is part of a plot to take over the world and control us with digital surveillance,

CCTVs, the internet of things, track and trace systems, driverless cars, crypto-currencies, education via the internet and a health care system which keeps patients well away from doctors.

I feel crazy saying all this. But it's palpably true. I did a video a month ago warning that the second wave was coming.

And it is all happening above government levels, of course.

No government in the world would happily exchange its own currency for a share in a global cryptocurrency. The politicians don't know what is going on. This is happening way above the heads of Johnson, Trump, Macron or Merkel. In the UK, I suspect that Cummings probably knows what is going on. But in the UK I doubt if Hancock or anyone in the cabinet knows any more than you or me. Probably less. You can tell who isn't part of the plan by checking to see what they think will happen next. The Bank of England seems to think that the UK economy will recover quickly. So they are out of the loop. So are most financial commentators.

The global warming nonsense is all part of it, of course. There's no science behind it but they picked three spokespersons who seemed beyond criticism. A little Swedish girl, a slightly potty Prince and an old TV presenter. And then they got school children everywhere believing that the world would end before Christmas if we didn't all stop using oil and gas.

And the Black Lives Matter protests are part of the plan. In the UK, every bit of our history is being demonised. Americans are told that George Washington and Abraham Lincoln were bad, bad people. The police, presumably acting under orders, arrest people having picnics but allow masses of demonstrators to break the lockdown laws and to destroy statues and public property with impunity. We are being told we must forget our history completely. Forget the old world. Forget our pride. Why? They need us to forget about nationality so that we accept the idea of becoming global citizens. The celebrities who promote all this hysteria have absolutely no idea what they are doing. They want to keep track of us and so before we go into a pub or a restaurant we have to give all our personal details. This is happening globally. What a coincidence. Privacy is a thing of the past.

And now, belatedly they are doing tests. They are using antibody tests which are so useless that they ping positive if you have had the common cold in the last ten years. And every time someone has a positive result, they lock them in. And lock in all their friends. And lock down the factory where they work – especially if it's a place where food is prepared. In March, when I suggested that more testing would be a good idea, I innocently assumed that they would devise a reliable test.

And so what is the overall plan?

Well the final plan is to reduce the size of the global population, to take away all our freedoms and rights and turn us into slaves of a new, all powerful world government run by a bunch of psychopathic billionaires without souls. We will all be in the clutches of The Myra Hindley and Ian Brady Foundation.

Globalists and multinational companies want to control everything. They want a global recession and massive unemployment so that they can 'reset' the economy. They want robots and a global digital currency. And they want us all vaccinated and implanted and tattooed. I promise you I feel mad saying all this. I don't believe I am saying it. But I do believe what I'm saying. And, as Sherlock Holmes said: once you eliminate the impossible, whatever remains, however improbable, must be the truth.

It's all based on big lies. But as Hitler said, if you tell a big enough lie then you'll get away with it because people won't possibly believe that you'd lie that much.

The plan is to eliminate all small businesses because they are messy and a nuisance and difficult to control and they allow people to be independent of the state.

They're getting rid of religion. That's just old-fashioned and a nuisance. And they need to deprive us of spiritual comfort. So church services are banned and no one can sing hymns anymore. And religious leaders around the world bow to all the nonsense either because they are brain dead or because they have been bought. You can demonstrate against statues but you can't sing a hymn.

And, of course, to do with away traditional medicine as we know it. So, for example, the Royal College of General Practitioners said the other day that the pandemic had resulted in positive changes to general practice. What they mean is that fewer patients are being seen in the surgery. 'New research is needed,' they said, 'to determine if the new system (whereby GPs treat most patients online or by telephone) diminished or increased the burden on GPs'.

That was it.

Whether the new way of working is better or worse for doctors. Not patients.

I've got a slogan which I will offer free to the medical establishment and which fits nicely in with the current fashion for brainwashing everyone:

Bugger the patients. Stuff good care. Think of yourself.

GPs are excited about the plan to vaccinate everyone. You know why? Because GPs earn tens of thousands of pounds a year for giving vaccinations. Actually, they don't even have to give the jabs themselves. A nurse or health care assistant or possibly a cleaner passing by does the actual injecting.

And the doctors and politicians who do recognise that the whole coronavirus thing is a hoax are so embarrassed and ashamed that they're frightened to admit the truth. They're frightened of being sued for all the mistakes they've made. So they keep quiet. It's the same as it has always been with vaccines. Anyone with two neurones to rub together knows that vaccines are neither safe nor effective. But they maintain the myth, and demonise people like me, because it would cost trillions in damages to tell the truth.

The healthcare scandals are horrendous. We know someone who has breast cancer and who has been waiting over five months for radiotherapy. That's not incompetence – it's criminal.

A friend was recently refused antibiotics because he is over 65. That was the only reason. His age. It's outrageous, medically indefensible ageism. But it's the new way. Doctors don't seem to see anything wrong with it. Dr Mengele would feel comfortable working in health care these days.

And they haven't finished with us, yet.

They've hardly started.

Now they know that most people are stupid, and so the globalists are getting confident. They've got us cornered.

And so the second wave is coming. It'll be here by the autumn unless we convince enough zombies to recognise the truth.

Meanwhile, just in case, we all need a survival plan. We have to become survivalists.

I'm working on a plan.

And in a future video I'll tell you what we're planning to do.

July 10th 2020

That's Not Science: It's Propaganda

Doctors like to give the impression that they have conquered sickness with science but that's just promotional baloney. There are, at a conservative estimate, something in the region of 18,000 known diseases for which there are still no effective treatments – let alone cures. Even when treatments do exist their efficacy is often in question. It's not surprising that the treatments for the coronavirus are completely confusing and it's not surprising that many people, me included, suspect that effective treatments are being ignored or suppressed because they might interfere with the need for a nice expensive vaccine that would make billions for drug companies and establish a greater need for compulsory annual vaccinations for everyone.

Modern clinicians may use scientific techniques but in the way that they treat their patients they are often still more like quacks and charlatans, loyal to existing and unproven ideas which are profitable, and resistant to new techniques and technologies which may be proven and effective.

One report a few years ago concluded that 85% of medical and surgical treatments have never been properly tested.

The fact that a doctor may use a scientific instrument in his work does not make him a scientist – any more than a typist who uses a word processor is a computer scientist. The scientific technology available to doctors may be magnificent but the problem is, and don't tell anyone I told you this, that the application of the scientific technology is too often crude, untested and unscientific.

Drugs which are commonly prescribed have often never been properly tested. And there are scores of simple questions which go unanswered. Why, for example, do doctors prescribe the same dose of an antibiotic for a 7 stone woman as they prescribe for a 27 stone man? I've been asking that question for decades and no one has ever got an answer. Or the other way round. Most drugs are given in similar doses to patients who are 16-years-old as to patients who are 86-years-old – even though their bodies will be very different.

Modern doctors, whether practising as physicians or surgeons, do not see the human mind and the human body as a single entity (which is why the medical profession has been slow to embrace the principles of holistic medicine and doubly incompetent in its attempts to deal with stress-related disorders) and they rely more on hopes and assumptions than on evidence and objective clinical experience. I'm afraid that too many modern doctors are as narrow-minded, and as influenced by their personal experiences and interpretations as their predecessors were 2,000 years ago.

Most patients probably assume that when a doctor proposes to use an established treatment to conquer a disease, he will be using a treatment which has been tested, examined and proven.

But I'm afraid that is often not true.

The first problem is that there are tens of thousands of medical journals in the world and it is difficult for anyone to keep up with new papers – even in a small speciality and even with the aid of computer search engines.

Amazingly, only about 15% of medical interventions are supported by solid scientific evidence' and 'only 1% of the articles in medical journals are scientifically sound.

What sort of science is that? How can doctors possibly regard themselves as practising a science when six out of seven treatment regimes are unsupported by scientific evidence and when 99% of the articles upon which clinical decisions are based are scientifically unsound?

How can doctors regard themselves as scientists when it is known that a kind, compassionate doctor can have a healing rate 50% better than his or her crueller colleagues – simply because patients respond better to his or her remedies?

How can doctors regard medicine as a science when it has been proven many times that at least a third of patients will get better if given a placebo – a medicine that contains no active ingredients?

How can doctors regard medicine as a science when it is known that a large proportion of patients expecting to have heart surgery will get better if they are merely given a scar on their chests and told that they have had an operation?

Medicine is no science. It's an art. Mysticism.

But these days it is polluted by business. And money.

The savage truth is that most medical research is organised, paid for, commissioned or subsidised by the drug industry. This type of research is designed, quite simply, to find evidence showing a new product is of commercial value. The companies which commission such research are not terribly bothered about evidence; what they are looking for are conclusions which will enable them to sell their product. Drug company sponsored research is done more to get good reviews than to find out the truth.

A study published in one major journal found that one in five researchers in the life sciences had delayed publication of their results, or had not published them at all, because of their relations with business firms.

Whenever I have accused scientists of being prejudiced and 'bought' because of their allegiance to their corporate paymasters, the answer has invariably been the same: 'Everyone does it. There isn't a scientist in the world who hasn't taken corporate money.'

Sadly, this is probably true – and is one explanation for the fact that many allegedly independent Government bodies are almost always packed with men and women who work for (or have taken fees from) the large corporations their Government body is supposed to be policing.

It is also a fact that most of the doctors and scientists writing articles, papers and reviews for medical and scientific journals have received money, grants and freebies from drug, chemical or food companies.

And it is also worth remembering that many allegedly and apparently independent journals accept corporate advertising and some accept payment in return for running articles.

With a very few exceptions there are no certainties in medicine. The treatment a patient gets will depend more on chance and the doctor's personal prejudices than on science. The unexpected seems to happen so often that it really ought to be expected and the likelihood of a doctor accurately predicting the outcome of a disease is often no more than 50:50.

Even in these days of apparently high technology medicine, there are almost endless variations in the treatments preferred by differing doctors. Doctors offer different prescriptions for exactly the same symptoms; they keep patients in hospital for vastly different lengths of time, and they perform different operations on patients with apparently identical problems.

There is, indeed, ample evidence now available to show that the type of treatment a patient gets when he visits a doctor will depend not so much on the symptoms he describes but on the doctor he consults – and where that doctor practises. And yet most doctors in practice seem to be convinced that their treatment methods are beyond question. Many GPs and hospital doctors announce their decisions as though they are carved in stone.

But for me the big worry is that today's research is largely controlled by and for the pharmaceutical industry. Doctors are unquestioning. Most don't read original papers (and couldn't read between the lines or assess papers accurately even if they did). The majority obtain 99% of their information from two biased and thoroughly unreliable sources: drug companies and the Government.

No one bothers to look for evidence that vaccinations actually work or are safe or don't cause problems when several different vaccines are injected into the same body. I wrote a book called, *Anyone who tells you vaccines are safe and effective is lying.* And no one in the medical establishment has ever tried to dispute that statement.

Young doctors are told that what they are taught are facts. And they are taught (and then believe) that medicine is a science. But the fact is that outside the anatomy room and, possibly, the physiology laboratory, there are no facts in medicine. The gaps in our knowledge about the body are far greater than the extent of our knowledge.

Medicine is not a science. It is an art and a craft. With a smidgen of science stuck on the side. Economics, psychiatry and psychology are all pseudosciences with no more relation to real science than astrology or iridology. Medicine is somewhere in between real science and economics. But it isn't a science.

Doctors like to be thought of as scientists because it contributes to their aura of infallibility. Drug companies like to think that doctors are scientists because it encourages patients to have faith in the remedies they produce. And research doctors like to pretend that they are scientists because it makes it easier for them to obtain grants and to tell convincing stories to the media. Too often, I'm afraid, modern medical scientists decide on a commercially acceptable solution and then select the facts which support the solution they have selected.

That's not science: it's propaganda.

And it's not surprising that the whole coronavirus hoax has been allowed to meander along unhindered by proper debate.

July 11ᵗʰ 2020

Doctors and Nurses Betrayed Patients – and Themselves

A growing number of doctors and nurses appear to be waking up and questioning the absence of any science behind the coronavirus hoax. That's very nice, and I congratulate them.

But what the devil took them so long?

Why did they wait so long to speak out?

Their silence betrayed their patients, their profession and themselves.

Only a complete moron could have thought that this manufactured 'crisis' necessitated the closure of hospitals and GP surgeries.

How could doctors stand by seeing cancer patients deprived of essential treatment? The NHS should have been stoned not clapped.

There was never any greater risk than there is with the flu every year. Indeed, the figures show that the ordinary flu bug has always posed a much bigger risk than the coronavirus.

So far this year the coronavirus has affected 10 million people.

The flu can affect 1 billion people in the same period.

And the mortality rates for the two are almost identical.

We don't close down hospitals and clinics whenever the flu appears.

So, obviously, this was a politically motivated closure of hospitals, shops, businesses and so on. And doctors should have seen that.

And just as the closure of hospitals will result in far more deaths than covid-19, so the wearing of masks will result in far more deaths than could possibly be saved. Wearing a mask reduces blood oxygen levels. I have seen car drivers with masks on. I've even seen bus drivers wearing masks. These things reduce blood oxygen. There will, before long, be a disaster with a bus crashing because the driver was wearing a mask and became hypoxic.

Why else do you think governments everywhere admit that people with respiratory or heart problems don't have to wear a mask?

And the stupid rules about social distancing were never justified. There was never any science to support them.

Anyone who believes in the twin heresies of social distancing and masks is, by definition, either certifiably insane, a cretin or on the dark side of the human race. Most are left wing, pro EU fascists and believers in the climate change nonsense.

Doctors and nurses who are now waking up to the fact that they've been tricked are claiming that they were told that if they spoke out they would be punished.

Well, it's true that the authorities are punishing doctors who dare to question the official line. I know of a doctor in the UK who was struck off the medical register for questioning the coronavirus story. And in the USA, Dr Scott Jensen, a doctor who is also a state senator, is being investigated for making statements about the similarity of the coronavirus to the flu and about the way death certificates were being signed.

And it is also true that simple and effective remedies have been banned or demonised simply so that we could all be prepared for the vaccine. But if most of the doctors in a big hospital spoke out, no bureaucrat would dare to strike them all off the register. If 500 doctors stood up for the truth, it would be impossible to take away all their licences.

'I work in a hospital,' wrote one brave NHS employee. 'So far none of the nurses, doctors or domestics has been off sick. And patients with the coronavirus are transported all around the hospital, to X-ray, to CT scan and to the ward and yet mysteriously no one gets infected.'

What sort of spineless people are working in health care these days? That's the sort of excuse popular with lesser war criminals.

Still, looking on the slightly bright side, some of them are waking up and now realise that the coronavirus hoax was exactly that – a piece of political trickery, conceived and executed by people with hidden agendas. The damage done by the hospital closures will be massive. And the mental issues caused by the fear will be long lasting – even permanent. Millions are suffering from severe depression as a result of the lies that have been told. Suicide rates are going to rocket.

Any doctors who are still social distancing and wearing masks outside the operating theatre should be ashamed of themselves. They, like much of the rest of the population, have been made fools of and if they had any professional pride left they would be red-faced, embarrassed by their own gullibility and ashamed of how easily they've been made part of a wicked conspiracy and made to look like fools.

Now is the time for the medical and nursing professions to stand up and to demand some answers and explanations from the leaders of their professions and from the administrators who gave the orders which have led to tens of thousands of unnecessary deaths.

They should also insist that hospitals are now opened fully and that patients are told that there is nothing to fear.

For although a growing number of doctors now realise that the coronavirus scare is a hoax, there are still hospitals and administrators who are behaving as though we were in the middle of an outbreak of the bubonic plague.

The latest piece of lunacy in the NHS is for the people in charge to suggest that patients who want treatment at an Accident and Emergency department should telephone and make an appointment. NHS England's national medical director has reportedly told the House of Commons health and social care committee that the health service wanted patients to telephone first and be given a timed slot to attend the A&E department.

I've heard everything now.

Patients who are desperate for help, bleeding, in pain, with bones sticking out at funny angles will be expected to telephone and make an appointment to be seen in the accident and emergency department. Triage will, it seems, now be done by teenagers on the telephone. What qualifications will they have? GCSE in woodwork, perhaps?

Distraught relatives will have to telephone and fix an appointment before going to the hospital. Is the plan simply to kill more patients? Did the hospital closures not kill enough?

I will tell you what is going to happen.

Everyone is going to ring for an ambulance. And who can blame them? As for hospitals, well even the Royal College of Physicians admits that many NHS services will not get back to full capacity for more than a year.

Millions of patients will wait too long. Patients in pain will have to wait for more than a year for treatment. Waiting times will be obscenely long. Tens of thousands will not be seen until it is too late. Tens of thousands of people who could have lived will die.

Around the world, the death toll from the hoax will be measured in millions.

Comparatively few will have died of the coronavirus.

The vast majority will have died because they were shut out, abandoned or too frightened to seek help.

And the medical and nursing professions have to take responsibility for all that pain, that sorrow and those deaths.

Doctors should not have accepted the unscientific gibberish behind the coronavirus hoax. Before allowing hospitals to be shut down they should have asked questions. It was never difficult to see that mistakes were being made.

Doctors and nurses betrayed their patients and their professions but they also betrayed themselves.

Too many were happy to accept the weekly applause and the praise when they knew that they deserved neither.

It is time now for the healing professions to make amends.

They should make it clear to the administrators and the politicians that they are no longer prepared to accept the coronavirus nonsense.

They should demand their government's medical advisors be sacked. They should demand that all members of the elite, medical establishment be sacked too.

They should demand that social distancing be abandoned and that masks should be burned.

They should tell the public that there is nothing to fear.

And they should be prepared to work long hours to clear the backlog of patients as quickly as possible.

There really is no choice.

If doctors and nurses do not stand up then they will be truly unworthy. I hope this video stays up for a day or two so that one or two people can see it. YouTube is taking down almost anything these days and what appears to me to be political censorship appears to have become arbitrary.

July 12th 2020

Is There Anything They Won't Do?

So now the Gestapo are calling themselves Public Health officials. The name is the only discernible difference. They can come to your home and, if they see a child playing in the garden or riding a bicycle up and down your road, they can take the child away to be tested, assessed and isolated.

The parents don't need to be there. Their permission is not required. Their child can be legally kidnapped and removed if the Public Health official thinks they might, note the word 'might', be infected.

It's the same for all of us, of course. We are living in a totalitarian world. Boris Johnson, who has been playing a pantomime buffoon for years, has led a coup that should eventually land him and his war criminal colleagues in prison. We have a truly evil government. They aren't removing the last vestiges of our freedom for our benefit. The disease against which this is directed is becoming less of a problem as each day goes by. As I seem to have been saying forever, it was never more than the flu.

Johnson and co aren't actually lining us up to be shot if we fail their stupid test. But maybe that will be next. Nothing is now impossible. And all this, remember, is happening as the infection becomes ever less of a threat. In many countries, deaths from all causes are now lower than average for this time of the year. And as more and more doctors are finding the courage to speak out and tell the truth. One doctor has even offered $5,000 to anyone who can produce evidence that the damned virus actually exists.

I don't know how much Johnson and his cabinet know about the plan to take over the world but I suspect they don't know all that much. I wonder if there is anyone in the UK cabinet important enough to be allowed into the cabal with which the United Nations is planning a world takeover.

Still, that doesn't alter the fact that this latest piece of trickery is pure, unadulterated evil. And the rest of the House of Commons might not exist. I haven't heard many MPs protesting about human rights, freedom and democracy. As long as they get their fat salaries and their expenses they don't give a damn about us. You wouldn't think they worked for us, would you?

Have you noticed how so few of our so-called leaders have any statesman like qualities. They all look as though they were put together in the dark and in a hurry by someone who couldn't understand the instructions because they were written in Japanese.

Having us kidnapped and dragged off to secret locations for no good reason isn't Comrade Boris's only new innovation.

It seems that bonking Boris has now gone completely barking for he is apparently going to insist that we all wear masks whenever he tells us to.

I suspect that Comrade Sturgeon is as potty as a damp kilt but Boris is now thinking of following her mad example and making face masks compulsory in Scotland in shops, pubs, offices, restaurants and lunatic asylums.

Boris, like Sturgeon, appears to be following the revised advice given by the WHO – now seemingly majority owned by the Myra Hindley and Ian Brady Foundation. Sorry, I naturally meant the Bill and Melinda Gates Foundation.

There is, let me remind you, no unequivocal evidence that masks help prevent the spread of anything other than bits of food from messy eaters. But there is evidence that they kill. And there is evidence that if you wear one for a while your blood oxygen levels are likely to fall to a dangerously low level.

The only other explanation for this piece of official lunacy is that our government, like many governments around the world, wants us dead. The people who give in and wear masks are not only a bit simple-minded but they are also clearly suicidal since the hypoxia masks can cause can be deadly.

Everything is getting madder by the day.

If this were not a plot to deprive of us every morsel of our independence and our freedom, the government in the UK would by now be arresting the idiots who produced and promoted the lunatic predictions which led to the lockdowns and the social distancing.

Ferguson, like bats and seagulls, appears to be a member of a protected species. Why hasn't he been arrested for producing the most egregiously incorrect forecast in the history of forecasts? And why haven't all the Government's advisors been sacked and thrown into the Tower of London?

Everywhere I look there is more madness.

Not content with attempting to do away with cash, there is now talk that they want to get rid of credit cards and debit cards so that everything we purchase goes through an App on our phone. I know the red fascists will applaud this, and I'm sure the entire staff of the BBC will applaud the idea, but they don't count as human beings.

The Government has generously opened the pubs (though there was never any reason to shut them) but they made it impossible for owners to make a profit or for punters to have any fun, so the pubs will slowly close and politicians can claim it's not their fault because they tried.

And then there is the social distancing. Instead of playing Simon Says, we are all playing Boris says. But this is no party game.

It is now clear that social distancing was developed by the CIA as a form of torture. And it is known that it causes depression, poor sleep, impaired brain function, reduced immunity to infection, poor heart function and so on and on. Following social distancing rules is said to double the risk of death. It is, indeed, equivalent to being obese, smoking 15 cigarettes a day and being an alcoholic.

Children who are forced to follow social distancing rules will grow up severely damaged. They will never recover. And yet children are far more at risk of injury or death by travelling to school than because of the coronavirus. The CDC in America reckons that the covid-19 risk to those under 19 is as near as damnit to zero. No child has passed the coronavirus to an adult. Asymptomatic individuals don't seem to pass on the infection even if they have it. There was never any need to close schools or to introduce any social distancing nonsenses. Why the hell are teachers demanding daft and destructive rules for children? In my view, any teacher who refuses to go to work unless social distancing is introduced should be fired.

When social distancing was first widely introduced about 70 years ago, it was regarded as the ideal way to break down prisoners. It caused more damage than beating them or starving them. Prisoners of War have said that they felt that social distancing and isolation were as bad as any physical abuse. There is no doubt that social distancing is a cruel and inhuman thing to do. Indeed, it is a war crime.

And where did they get the six feet distancing from?

Out of someone's head apparently.

Allegedly, mad scientists felt that the British people wouldn't know what a metre was and so they doubled it just for fun.

And the sick joke is that social distancing actually increases the spread of illness. And social distancing in schools is a form of child abuse. Because of masks and social distancing, we will never acquire immunity to disease, our immune systems will deteriorate and we will never acquire herd immunity.

Forget what I said about teachers being sacked. That's not enough. They should be arrested and tried for child abuse if they insist on social distancing in schools.

The Government's advisors in the UK keep saying that we cannot halt social distancing. They don't say why. But my fear is that they are just keeping people terrified until the damned vaccine is ready. The UK Government has already ordered 65 million syringes and needles. And one drug company is already making a vaccine that has not yet been properly tested.

Remember that Vallance, the Chief Scientific Advisor to the UK Government, used to work for GlaxoSmithKline, a big vaccine manufacturer. And that Dr Whitty, the Chief Medical Officer in the UK, did research funded by the Bill and Melinda Gates Foundation. In my view, both of them should be fired for having a potential conflict of interest.

Incidentally, I see that Mr Gates, the self-appointed doctor to the world, has allegedly said that singing, laughing and talking can all spread covid-19. I hesitate to suggest this but maybe, if Mr Gates were to stop talking for a few years we might all be safer.

Meanwhile, we are now living in an occupied country. Everyone not already a member needs to join the Resistance Movement.

If the Public Health Officials come for you, do not resist with violence but I suggest that you film everything – or ask someone to film everything. Then send the film to as many people as you know. And write down details – including names and times. And tell the official that you will sue them personally for kidnapping you. When they tell you that they are immune because they are acting for the State remind them that at the end of World War II that was not considered an acceptable defence at the War Crimes Tribunals.

July 13th 2020

The Screw is Tightening

The number of people dying from the coronavirus is falling fast and yet the screw is tightening everywhere. In many countries, death totals are lower than they usually are at this time of year. You would have had to have had your skull scooped out and filled with concrete not to realise that there is something really sinister and evil going on.

The fear being promoted with such enthusiasm is clearly nothing to do with a fairly ordinary virus and everything to do with the ambitions of those who want a world government and total control over every aspect of our lives.

Everywhere I look I see evidence that attempts are still being made to push the fear and to terrify people.

The testing programme shows that more and more people have or have had the virus. Indeed, almost everyone who is tested seems to have a positive result. Actually, that isn't so surprising because it seems that some tests ping positive if you've had a cold or flu vaccination in the last decade. It probably shows positive if you've ever sneezed.

Apparently, one test showed positive when tested on a goat. The test was even positive when tried on a papaya fruit.

Still, the test is proving very useful to those who want to destroy the country so that the UN can rebuild it the way they want it to be according to Agenda 21.

And so, around the world, towns are being closed down and the citizens punished for absolutely no good reason at all. If anyone in government were interested in the science they would know that lockdowns don't work. They were never going to work. They were always a terrible idea. They came out of Ferguson, of course. The lockdowns and the hospital closures merely made things worse. They resulted in all the care home deaths. They stopped people developing immunity. They made people depressed and unhealthy. They will result in millions of entirely unnecessary deaths around the world. And they are wrecking the economy.

We are constantly being promised the vaccine – as though it were the Holy Grail.

My position on vaccination is very simple: I am pro truth. And I expect, or rather demand, that if I am going to be given a vaccine or drug then it will have been properly tested beforehand. And that the risk-benefit ratio will have been properly investigated. Sadly, the evidence shows clearly that the risks far outweigh the benefits.

After years of observation, I am convinced that there is one big difference between the people who are devoted to vaccination at all costs and those who are concerned about its safety and effectiveness. Most of those in the first group have never done any research at all whereas most of those in the second group, the cautious doubters, have done a good deal of research, are alarmed by what they have seen, and know what they are talking about.

Sadly, many doctors know very little about vaccines and vaccination except that it is an extremely profitable activity. The average GP can make many thousands of pounds a year by giving injections. In practice, of course, she or he doesn't have to give the injections – a nurse or assistant does that. And nurses, health visitors and so on, know only the propaganda I fear.

How many know that the UK Government has to pay out so much money to the parents of children damaged by some vaccines that they have a fixed fee of £120,000 per severely damaged child. In the United States, the Government has paid out over $4 billion for vaccine injuries. That money has been paid on behalf 18,000 individuals.

That's a lot of money for governments to pay out for treatments that are supposed to be perfectly safe.

I bet you won't read that in the *Daily Mail* or *The Guardian* or see it on the BBC.

They have destroyed our education system with the lockdowns and the social distancing and a whole generation of children has been indoctrinated into fear. I predict huge mental health problems for two whole generations – at the very least.

And they have, as they planned to do, destroyed untold small businesses – leaving the way clear for the multinationals to control all our purchasing.

There are still some innocent souls who believe that the economy will bounce back in a few months. Financial commentators blithely tell us that everything will be fine long before Christmas.

Those dunderheads probably still believe in the tooth fairy because they clearly have no idea how much damage has already been done. They have no idea how much damage is continuing to be done by social distancing and so on. I suspect they have no idea how businesses are run. And they appear to have no idea that they are being manipulated just as we are.

Or maybe they are part of the plan to deceive and to manipulate, to oppress and to misinform.

But I doubt that.

I think many of those who seem to be in charge are acting blind. They are panicking and have no idea what is going on. Some are continuing with stale and stupid arguments because they are frightened to admit that they got it all wrong – that the whole coronavirus story has been wildly exaggerated.

I am convinced that many of the politicians in government have absolutely no idea what is going on.

And I am equally convinced that there are some advisors who know exactly what is going on.

I also suspect that a former Prime Minister whom I won't name other than to say that his first name is Tony, his second name begins with a B and he is widely known as Britain's most famous war criminal, knows a good many of the people who know exactly what is happening – and the role of the United Nations.

If there is anyone in the world who trusts Blair, they should be locked up for their safety and for ours.

Our strings are being pulled by the people behind the United Nations, the World Health Organisation, the Global Economic Forum and so on. And it is becoming clear that their agendas are no longer quite so hidden. They plan to take over the world; to control our bodies and our minds in every conceivable way.

I am convinced that a small chunk of rich and powerful people planned this disaster and are still organising things so as to make our current lives as difficult as possible so that they can break us. They are using old psychological tricks to wear us down. If you haven't watched it then do please either watch my video on brainwashing or read the transcript on my website.

The same people who were pulling the strings of the global warming nutters, and hiding in the background, are now controlling the demonstrations and the riots, the interracial conflict and the attempts to eradicate our national histories.

They are doing everything to destroy the world we know so that they can recreate things to their advantage.

You would have to be extremely naïve not to realise that our world is being manipulated by some very evil people indeed.

I am fully aware that saying this will ensure that the trolls will have a field day. Well, if they had the brains and the courage I would happily debate with them. Unfortunately, they don't have the brains or the courage. And I'm banned from all mainstream media anyway, largely because of my views on vaccination and drug companies.

And while mentioning a debate let me just repeat my challenge to Dr Whitty, the British Government's Chief Medical Officer. I will happily debate vaccination with Dr Whitty, live on national television or radio. This would give the establishment a chance to destroy publicly the fears that I have, and that many share, about the safety and effectiveness of vaccination.

But Dr Whitty won't debate, of course.

And you can read into that whatever you like.

There are, of course, many people who say there never was a virus and that all we are seeing is the usual standard flu. Certainly, the infection rate and the death rates are similar to those of a fairly ordinary flu. Indeed, remove the care home deaths and this is a very mild flu attack. But I don't think any of that really matters very much in practical terms.

The only thing that matters at the moment is that a mild problem has been wilfully exaggerated, fear has been created and our lives have been totally disrupted.

When we finally extricate ourselves from this mess, which we will, there will have to be a good many questions about who did what and why. I'd like to see Ferguson in court. His model was clearly as much a load of rubbish as others he's produced over the years. And I would like to see in court the people who accepted Ferguson's predictions without submitting them to any sort of peer review.

And I would like to know how many people who have been giving advice have past or present links with the vaccine industry and its advocates. But our immediate need is to understand the tactics and strategies of the people behind the United Nations, the World Health Organisation and the other bad organisations. We need to know who they are, what they are trying to do – and precisely what they want. Let us not forget: we are fighting a war.

And in a war, information is the most vital commodity. This is a time to re-read, among others, Machiavelli's The Prince, Sun Tzu's the Art of War and the Emperor's Napoleon's thoughts on strategy and tactics. I've dug out my copies of all three.

July 14th 2020

Your Body and Mind Aren't Enough – They Want Your Soul

It is abundantly clear that the whole coronavirus hoax is being organised and scripted by psychologists who specialise in brainwashing and what are known in military circles as psychological warfare.

The statistics show clearly that the coronavirus is no longer an epidemic. Doctors everywhere admit that there are now very few deaths from the disease. Indeed, many doctors are admitting that there never was an epidemic. The whole thing was a sleight of hand trick; a massive manipulation.

Doctors and nurses have been told that they will be fired, and probably never work again, if they speak to the media at all. A few have spoken out anonymously and have admitted that hospitals have not been busy. There have been very few cases of covid-19. I've been told that the few patients who were found were tested many times – and on each occasion the test was submitted as though it related to a new patient. So each patient who tested positive became 10 or 12 cases of coronavirus. The whole story has been created, and we have been tricked, conned and manipulated. In some hospitals, doctors and nurses apparently wore masks only when members of the public were around. Social distancing rules were never obeyed unless there were cameras around recording doctors and nurses dancing and clapping themselves. In the UK, GPs surgeries have been effectively closed – with patients forced to telephone if they wanted to speak to a doctor. Now accident and emergency departments are going to be open only to patients who have telephoned and made an appointment.

'I shall be breaking my leg next Wednesday afternoon, so could I have an appointment, please? Around 3.30 p.m. should be the right time. '

'I think I will be having a stroke on Thursday evening. Could I have an appointment for 10.45 p.m. please?'

GPs surgeries and hospitals will soon be accessed via the internet only. Face to face medicine will be a thing of the past. Artificial intelligence is taking over. Telemedicine will replace traditional medicine.

Operations, when they are essential, will eventually be performed by robots. Doctors and nurses haven't understood it yet but they will be redundant.

It is no accident that shops are struggling.

Forcing everyone to wear masks and forcing shops to put social distancing tapes on the floor is designed to make shopping such an unpleasant experience that everyone will do their shopping online. Telling shops not to take cash is utter nonsense – it seems designed to put small shops out of business by making the whole experience unbearable for many. The current system seems designed to destroy High Street shops.

Similarly, pubs and restaurants are being destroyed by social distancing rules, by forcing us to wear masks and by insisting that everyone leave all their personal details with the pub or restaurant staff. The psychologists know that although one or two people will visit pubs and restaurants for a while most will soon tire of the system that has been put into operation.

Advised by the brainwashing specialists, politicians are teasing us and controlling us by giving a little freedom, and then taking it away. We are told that we can take holidays abroad without having to spend two weeks in quarantine when we return. But the rules may change while we are away, in which case we will have to go into isolation for two weeks. And the list of countries which we can visit without quarantine is changing all the time. You'd have to be mad to fix a holiday abroad not knowing what the rules might be while you are away or when you arrive back.

The plan is to disconcert us, to keep us on edge, depressed and fearful. That is what our governments are doing to us – deliberately.

Governments always lie to us. Remember Vietnam? Cuba? The twin towers? The weapons of mass destruction that didn't exist?

But the lies have been elevated to new levels. They now want to control everything.

We are constantly being told of draconian measures being introduced in other areas. And since the rules change from one area to another we never quite know what punishments to escape. In one part of America you can be sent to prison for a year if you fail to wear a mask. In another part of America you have to pay a 2,000 dollar fine but there is no prison sentence. In Texas, some people have been told that they should wear masks in their own homes. In one shop a guard pulled a gun on a man who was not wearing a mask. In California, people have been telephoning the police if they've heard a neighbour coughing or sneezing. The snitches and sneaks, eager to please the system, are part of the mass surveillance system.

And yet if you buy a boxful of disposable masks you will probably see, printed on the side of the mask, a warning that the mask does not provide protection against viruses such as the one which causes covid-19. Of course it doesn't. The viruses go straight through the mask, like a bluebottle fly through chicken-wire.

If you are beginning to feel as though you are being treated like a prisoner of war then you're beginning to understand the situation. There has been a global coup, led by the United Nations, the World Health Organisation, the Bill and Melinda Gates Foundation, the World Economic Forum and a variety of other billionaires. Their aims are quite straightforward: they want to reorganise the world, they want a world government, they want to destroy everything which we regard as 'normal', they want to destroy our history (they are using the Black Lives Matter campaign to help with that) and they want to force us to use the internet for everything. They want us all vaccinated, regularly, and they want us to carry immunity passports if we want to leave our homes, buy things or obtain medical assistance. They want us tracked and traced every minute of the day. They want us to use self-driving cars because they can be controlled from afar. They want us to have smart meters installed so that they can turn off our electricity supplies if we misbehave. They are creating so-called smart motorways which seem deliberately designed to create more queues. Ever changing speed limits cause more traffic jams and plenty of fines. They want us to use telephone apps for all our purchases and they want us all to be dependent upon the State. They want to eradicate small companies so that large multinationals can satisfy all our needs. And they want to replace people with robots. The future they have planned for us bears very little resemblance to the world to which we are accustomed.

The coronavirus is a key part of the plan. It is the virus which is going to terrify us into obeying their orders without question. And they are using psychological warfare techniques to keep us under control. The only plague around is a plague of corruption. The individuals who are helping with the compulsory testing and tracking are today's concentration camp guards.

There has been a global coup and our lives are being micromanaged by a group of very evil people and organisations which are determined to take control of the world in order to redesign it to suit their own selfish, commercial and political interests. Our political system has failed us all completely.

They want to get rid of the elderly, the middle classes and schools. They want to get rid of anyone who isn't deemed to be an asset to the State.

They want children to be educated via the internet and they aren't terribly interested in how well educated they are at the end of their schooling. Forcing children to follow social distancing rules is completely unnecessary and so cruel it can only be described as evil. It will create emotionally damaged children who are germophobic, suicidal, homicidal, neurotic and psychotic. Many will become psychopathic. And I now believe it has been planned by the numerous teams of psychologists and military mind control specialists in countries everywhere who are helping to mastermind our new global world. I wouldn't be surprised to see children forced to wear masks. At first I thought that the social distancing in schools was being imposed through ignorance but I no longer believe that. This is being done to destroy and it is evil almost beyond comprehension. What sort of people deliberately use CIA torture techniques on children? Psychologists, politicians and teachers all around the world are guilty and should be tried at the war crimes court.

They want to reduce the global population. They know that forcing us into isolation, making pubs unbearable and closing nightclubs will help stop boys meeting girls and vice versa. It is no coincidence that the authorities have for the last few years been encouraging homosexuality, transsexuality and gender reassignment. Fewer babies that way.

This is all a question of power, control and money – but not necessary in that order.

Our food supplies are being controlled. They are planning shortages that will lead to panic and mass starvation – particularly in the underdeveloped parts of the world. All around the world farms and food packing and distribution centres are being closed down because employees (usually asymptomatic) are tested and shown to be positive. (Why, you might ask, does it seem that food workers are being targeted for testing?)

Thanks to the climate change nutters, who have been manipulated very successfully, there are going to be massive shortages of energy. There will be no electricity for long periods of time. Heating and cooking will, for many, be nigh on impossible.

The recent Black Lives Matter demonstrations have been manipulated to call for the defunding of the police. The plan is to replace the police with the military and with drones and robots. It is quite remarkable how easily the Black Lives Matter demonstrators were manipulated into helping the coup that will wreck their lives.

They want to control everything.

They want our bodies, our minds and our souls.

And unless we fight back we will soon be nothing but slaves of the system. We are fighting a war of terror – but our enemies are our governments and international organisations such as the United Nations and the World Health Organisation.

We all have to stand up against the system.

Doctors could help protect us all by making it clear to everyone that the so-called pandemic never existed and that it was a trick designed to prepare us for the takeover, the coup.

Once the covid-19 hoax has been properly exposed for the sham that it is, the whole plan will fall apart. And it will be impossible for the manipulators, the plotters – the enemy – to try the same trick again.

July 15th 2020

Mask Wearers are Collaborators Who Could Destroy Us All – They Should Be Locked Up for Helping the Enemy

So now they're turning up the heat. The evil Gates subsidised monsters who are trying to take over the world and turn us all into slavish zombies must be feeling very cocky. In the UK, the Government decided that we all have to wear masks in shops. On July 24th, the coronavirus is going to mutate, stop being a fairly feeble flu-like bug and become something as deadly and dangerous as one of the Clintons. And so on the 24th July, we have to start dressing up as bank robbers whenever we go shopping. The shop assistants don't have to wear masks but the shoppers do. Apparently, according to Boris the Buffoon, the coronavirus can't jump to or from a shop assistant but can jump to or from a shopper. How clever the coronavirus is to know this. Of course, if a shop assistant pops into a neighbouring shop they have to put on a mask because then they become a customer and when they are a customer they can catch the virus and spread it.

Another oddity is that although the coronavirus can infect shoppers it can't infect people who work in offices. It seems that this very intelligent virus seems to say to itself `I can infect these people because they are just out shopping' but 'I must not infect those people in that office because they are working'.

If all this sounds like totally unscientific gibberish that is because it is totally unscientific gibberish.

How clever too for the authorities to know that people in shops must wear masks but not give their names and addresses whereas people in pubs must give their names and addresses but not wear masks.

If we weren't fighting a war against the most evil cabal ever put together in the history of mankind then it would be laughable.

And look at the history behind this latest change of heart.

Professor Jonathan Van-Tam, Deputy Chief Medical Officer previously announced that there was no need to wear a mask.

And Michael Gove, a weedy little British politician who is about as far removed from being a statesman as Bill Gates is from being a doctor, said that the UK government didn't plan to insist that we all wore masks in shops. I bet he feels an idiot now.

Because within hours Boris Johnson, our Fuhrer, backed up by laws which would have been envied by Stalin, Hitler and Attila the Hun, not to mention Vlad the Impaler and Genghis Khan, suddenly decided, seemingly all by himself, that the entire nation should wear masks whenever they ventured into a shop.

Everyone knows the disease has almost died out. It'll soon be less of a threat than athletes' foot. If the coronavirus were a pop record it would be about to slip out of the Top 100 and slide into oblivion.

So, what had happened to change the pint of rancid pond-water that Boris doubtless refers to as his mind?

Well, the only thing new that I could find was a bit of research performed by a team at Cambridge University. They seem to have concluded that wearing masks was a good thing. And guess what the bloke who did the research does for a living? His name is Richard Stutt and he usually models the spread of crop diseases. Crop diseases! He is another bloody modeller like Ferguson. 'Our analyses support the immediate and universal adoption of facemasks by the public,' Stutt is quoted as saying. And he works on crop diseases and suddenly he knows all about whether or not we should wear face masks. You'd think Boris would be wary of modellers wouldn't you? But then maybe not if they give him the news he wants. My researches suggest that there is going to be a glut of mathematical modellers receiving knighthoods in the New Year's Honours List.

Did Stutt recommend the wearing of masks to stop the flu last year? The mortality risk with the flu is pretty well identical to the risk with covid-19. Has he recommended the wearing of masks to stop the spread of TB? A quarter of the global population is said to be infected with TB, a disease which kills over one and half million a year. If we need one mask for the coronavirus then we need four masks each for TB.

'We have little to lose from the widespread adoption of facemasks,' said a Dr Retkute.

I think the mistake this lot have made has been in focussing on the R number – the number being infected. Bugger the R number. It's of absolutely no real significance. What matters is the D number – the number dying. And the D number has fallen dramatically because they've stopped killing old people in care homes. If Stutt and Retkute were doctors they might understand this better. Why don't they stick to crop diseases?

Nothing to lose by wearing masks?

I know of two people who died because they wore masks and the hypoxia killed them. How's that for nothing to lose?

But then we must remember that it is the Government's plan to help reduce the world population – and thereby win the hearts of Bill and Melinda Gates.

Maybe my scepticism about anything coming out of Cambridge University, where the crop disease bloke works, has been heightened since the University accepted $210 million from the Bill and Melinda Gates Foundation.

Everywhere you look the Gates Foundation has left its dirty fingerprints.

The bottom line is that I am convinced that there is no sound medical reason to wear a mask. Masks are bad for us physically. And they are bad for us mentally. If you look at the risk benefit ratio then the risks are far greater than the benefit.

The only reason for our being forced to wear masks is to oppress us, to frighten us and to turn us into pathetic slaves of the beast. If you wear a mask they own your body, your mind and your soul. That's it. Game over.

And now that they've made mask wearing compulsory, when will they ever reverse the law?

What do you think? In three months' time? Six months? Twelve months?

The correct answer is: probably never.

They've said we'll have to wear masks in shops until the vaccine is ready. And that could be 5, 10 or 15 years. Or Longer. This is going to be part of the new abnormal.

How many people will be killed by masks in the next twelve months alone? Your guess is as good as mine – and almost certainly better than that of any politician.

A friend of mine who suffers from anxiety intends to tell shopkeepers that wearing a mask gives her a panic and fainting attack and would they therefore please have someone trained in first aid to follow her around the shop.

Those with respiratory and heart disorders fear that if they don't conform and wear masks they might be subjected to abuse from mask wearing zombies.

The utterly loathsome Hancock, the UK's Minister of Gibberish, says that shop staff should call the police if a customer isn't wearing a mask. If they don't then another busy body customer will probably do the snitching for them. To me it seems as if it's all part of the plan to smash society and create distrust. And, of course, the mask wearing will help destroy shops so that we all do all our shopping online. Hancock is to me like the appalling Macron in France, living proof of the validity of the Peter Principle – that members of a hierarchy are promoted until they reach the level at which they are no longer competent. Come to think of it that's clearly true of Johnson too. Shame on the Conservative Party. Let's have a general election and dump these evil bastards onto the political scrap heap. Compared to Boris Johnson, the pathetic and utterly woeful Theresa May was a beacon of strength, probity and wisdom. I can't believe I said that but it does show the level of contempt I have for Johnson. It is now clear that the buffoon act wasn't an act. He is a buffoon – clearly as under-endowed in the brain department as you can imagine. Incidentally, the psychologists advising the Government obviously think that the term 'face covering', the new preferred term, is somehow more acceptable than the word 'mask'. Or maybe their contempt for us is so complete that they think we won't notice that there is something of a similarity between an item called a face mask, which covers the lower half of the face, and something quite different called a face covering which covers the lower half of the face.

Boris, you crooked, ignorant, deceitful, two-faced, cheating, betraying bastard, we would know they were masks if the psy-op specialists suggested you call them lemon meringue pies.

Alternatively, is it impossible that masks are part of some satanic ritual – along with the constant hand washing, the social distancing and the house arrests?

When we have got through this war, and won the conflict against our own government, we will never forget Boris Johnson's perfidy – or his government's total betrayal of the voters. Johnson will join Blair as a candidate for the War Crimes Tribunal.

The terrible thing is that many people have already fallen for the nonsense.

The other day I drove to a local supermarket. I spotted just a few wearing masks, from their eyes half of them looked arrogant and very pleased with themselves – as though they had just been given a gold star or appointed milk monitor for the term. The other mask wearers looked terrified as though they were expecting to be dead before they reached the safety of the checkout.

Outside the supermarket I saw several people wearing masks. A young couple with a four or five-year-old – all wearing masks. A pair of teenagers wearing masks. A few middle aged folk masked up and a couple of old ladies in masks they'd obviously made themselves. Oddly enough I didn't see any elderly men wearing masks. Dunno why.

The town looked so sad, by the way. Apart from the supermarket the only shops open were two nail parlours (both empty), an ironmonger (I was the only customer there) and a charity shop. Everything else was closed. Probably permanently.

It is clearly not being unfair to say that the mask wearers are not God's brightest creations.

However, the really sad thing is that the mask wearing zombies are too stupid or too ill- informed to realise that they are playing into the enemy's hands.

Some of the zombies actually think they're helping to save lives. If you try to tell them about the dangers of mask wearing they will point out that surgeons wear masks in the operating theatre. As though this had any relevance. What they don't realise is that surgeons wear masks to stop bits of saliva ending up in the wound. They don't wear them to prevent the flow of disease, they don't usually wear them all day long, they don't wear them outside the operating theatre and they certainly don't wear them while walking about and requiring extra oxygen.

How can there be people who don't realise that in wearing masks they are aiding and abetting the thieving criminals who are stealing our freedom and our future.

Anyone who wears a mask is a spineless and moronic collaborator helping the worst people this world has ever seen.

Independent research by a bunch of florists has shown that mask wearers aren't capable of thinking for themselves; they are not very bright, they are followers, the sort of people who, as children, dreamt of being concentration camp guards. They never do anything or achieve anything; they are saddos, nerds and remainers – invariably devoted to the European Union.

Put on a mask and you are bending a knee before Gates, Soros, the Rothschilds and the Rockefellers, Blair and the Clintons.

What an evil, soulless bunch.

I've recorded two videos about Gates. Please watch them if you haven't. The first video is called Just A Little Prick part one. And, with startling originality that I am very proud of, the second one is called Just A Little Prick part two.

The mass media invariably describe Bill Gates as a philanthropist. The BBC and *The Guardian*, both sharing some of the Gates wealth, probably think he should be known as St Bill.

However, I am going to try to get the Oxford Dictionary to revise its definition of the word philanthropist.

It should read: 'A philanthropist is an evil crook who has absolutely no interest in the welfare of others but who uses large donations of money to buy power and control and to make even more money'.

I'll suggest that synonyms of philanthropist should include: 'slimy, single cell organism usually found at the bottom of filthy ponds'.

Just remember that next time you see anyone describing themselves, or being described as a philanthropist.

The idiots wandering around in their little masks are bending the knee to the toxic Gates; in my view a being so dangerous and diseased that he should be rammed into a test tube and kept in Madam Tussaud's Chamber of Horrors. Mothers could take their children and point him out as the definition of evil.

And they are bending a knee to more candidates for the chamber of horrors: Blair, the hideous Clintons, the foul Obama and the rest of the malignant crew.

Oh and the wretched Boris Johnson too.

The mindless mask wearers are collaborators and when war ends you know what happens to collaborators. Most of them are political innocents who voted Remain because they didn't bother to do enough research to know that the EU had been set up by Nazis to enable post-war Germany to control Europe.

Finally, I'll leave you with my mantra:

No silly mask

No deadly vaccine

No social distancing

Please learn it, recite it and share it with the collaborators who seem determined to drag us down with them – but who will fail because those of you who have seen the light have a monopoly on wisdom, courage and integrity.

And two other small things.

First, the channel is growing so fast that YouTube doesn't always seem to manage to send out notifications about new videos. I'm sure this is just a technical hitch. We try to research, write, edit, record and put out a new one each day at 7.00 p.m. – though this doesn't leave much time for sleeping and eating and virtually none for dealing with emails.

Second, as you know, we don't accept ads or sponsors or any money for the channel or the website and I promise that we never will. However big the channel gets, or the website gets, there will never be any outside money involved. Unlike the BBC, for example, which sold out years ago and cannot be trusted to tell the time, this is a genuine non-commercial public service channel. We specialise in the truth, served with a little spice I hope, and leave bias, prejudice and fake news to the vastly overpaid cretins at the BBC.

July 16th 2020

They Want to Kill Six Billion of Us – Here's How They'll Do It

There are people around who believe that if we all wear masks, obey the social distancing laws and become true slaves to the system, then everything will be back to normal by Christmas at the latest.

In the last 24 hours I have read, and been dismayed by, three articles by writers who believe that if we all behave properly, and do exactly as we are told to do, the coronavirus will slink off and all will be well with everyone back at work, the economy beginning to boom and the world well on its way to a recovery. There are even some who were shocked at the suggestion that taxes will rise dramatically in the next 12 months or so. Where do these people think the money came from – the money that an ex Goldman Sachs, currently the UK Chancellor, was throwing around with such gay abandon.

Of course, they add as a rider, we won't be able to forget about social distancing, and we may have to keep on our masks until the vaccine is ready, but everything will be normal apart from that.

I wonder what these people have inside their skulls. Porridge? Those little white polystyrene balls that are used for packaging? Bubble wrap? They certainly don't have brains.

The people now planning to rule the world, a group of billionaires and would be billionaires who I will, for ease, refer to as the enemy, have decided that there are too many people in the world, and that the earth would be more comfortable for them if the total were reduced to around 500,000,000.

Since the current population is around 7 billion that means that at least 6 billion of us are surplus to requirements, unnecessary, not wanted on voyage. Since their ambition has a convincingly eugenic flavour, they will presumably want to get rid of the weak and the poor and the elderly and the frail.

So how are they going to do that?

Well, the ignorant, scare mongering climate change nutters have done some of their work for those who want us dead. The brainwashed children and idiots who believe in man-made global warming are helping the enemy enormously. Cutting back on our use of oil and gas will kill hundreds of millions who will die of hunger and cold.

And I have no doubt that the enemy will manage another 'plandemic'.

The abominable Gates and his wife have already said that people will pay attention when the next pandemic arrives. And I thought they both smirked very knowingly when Bill made this prediction.

It wouldn't be difficult.

They could just say that the coronavirus which caused covid-19 had mutated. Or they could blame a pig virus or a cuckoo virus or maybe a virus from the Gates family – something unpleasant.

It wouldn't really need to be something too nasty. After all, a really bad virus might kill off some of the billionaires.

I rather suspect that we are going to have more alleged virus health calamities coming up. If it isn't the coronavirus in a pre-ordained second wave it will be something else. If they can make up one crisis then they can, and will, make up many more.

All it needs is good marketing, and organisations like the BBC will provide all the myths and fake news that the enemy will need.

The BBC, *The Guardian* and the *Daily Mail* could turn tapioca into a deadly threat.

Of course, the plan to reduce the global population is already doing well. The enemy has got everyone social distancing. And that is known to cause illness and to kill people. The CIA reckon that social distancing is one of the most powerful weapons there is for controlling large numbers of people.

They managed to murder huge numbers in the care homes and they have killed vast numbers of the sick by closing down hospitals for absolutely no good reason.

They put everyone under house arrest – and isolation damages the immune system. Prisoners of War have confirmed that isolation does more damage than physical torture. Stress and anxiety affect the immune system too.

The masks will kill quite a few people too. It's well known that they reduce blood oxygen levels, and those with respiratory and cardiac disorders will die. It's true that surgeons wear masks but the circumstances are entirely different. Women's movement enthusiasts used to burn their bras. Perhaps, we should burn our masks – in an environmentally acceptable way, of course.

Even the sanitising gel they insist we use a dozen times a day will kill some people. (If you haven't seen it, watch my video on hand sanitisers. Or read the script on this website.)

And then there is the cold in the winter months. They are stopping us using gas and there are going to be electricity outages. Many will freeze to death in the winter months.

But I think their biggest weapon is food.

That's how they are going to bring the population crashing right down. Food shortages are coming and the cost of food is going to rise even faster than it has been doing. And it isn't because of global warming or whatever other lies they tell you – it is, however, a side effect of the coronavirus hoax.

All around the world food is in short supply. The price of the world's most important staple food – rice – has risen by 70%. Food prices in the US have recently seen a historic jump and are, I believe, destined to stay high and go higher. Countries which have good food production are halting their exports. Vietnam, for example, has stopped exporting because they need their food supplies at home. And you cannot blame them. Some authorities condemn it as nationalism but all countries, all villages, all homes would do much the same.

And it is the managed over-reaction to a virus known to be no more dangerous than the flu that is causing the problem – and that will result in millions of deaths to add to the millions who are going to die as a result of the lockdowns.

The global death rate because of the food shortage is going to be measured in hundreds of millions – and eventually in billions. Africa and Asia are going to see the worst levels of starvation ever seen. I fear that those countries which have some grain will flog it to America – despite massive starvation. Black lives matter protestors, who have been manipulated by professionals, would be wise to forget about Cecil Rhodes's statue, and where they'd like to see it placed, and concentrate instead on helping Africans who are going to be subjected to the worst genocide in history.

So, how is the coronavirus scandal responsible for the food shortages that are coming?

That's easy to explain.

Processing plants and distribution centres all around the world have been deliberately severely disrupted by the massive over-reaction to this fairly ordinary virus.

Around the world, more and more testing is being done. And although the tests are about as trustworthy as Gates, Clinton and Soros – your local purveyors of fear and death – they are treated with undeserved reverence. Curiously, it seems to me that farms and food distribution centres are being tested more than, say, civil servants or tax officials. This is odd because the chances of the virus being carried on food are roughly the same as the chance that the moon is made of cheese.

And so if one worker on a farm or in a warehouse falls ill with flu-like symptoms then the authorities will close down that farm or the warehouse. Delivery systems have been massively affected as drivers are sent home for two weeks and all their colleagues sent home for two weeks too.

As a result, huge crops of vegetables and fruit are being ploughed into the ground. Millions of animals are being slaughtered and then buried or burnt because the supply chains have been shut down. America, almost unbelievably, has been importing beef because of the shortages.

The world lockdown, and the mass 'house arrests' that were engineered to keep us all subservient, mean that thousands of farmers cannot get their crops picked. Fruit in particular is likely to rot in the fields and tankers full of milk are being poured away. Controls on transport have meant that it has been difficult to move food from where there is a glut to where there is a dearth. It would have been easy for governments to insist that furloughed workers should help pick the crops but they didn't do so. And why would they? The plan is to eradicate the poor and the weak.

And the unsurprising consequence of all this is that there are going to be massive shortages of fruit and vegetables and prices are going to rocket.

In the UK, the most toxic of the Remainers, the fascist EU loving lunatics, bigoted, soaked in their own prejudices and consumed by ignorance, will blame Brexit for the shortages. But then, if they develop a bald spot or lose their keys they blame Brexit.

In the US, the media will doubtless blame Trump for the food shortages. Sadly for them all, the shortages will be global.

All around the world there will be a shortage of almost all foods.

This isn't the sort of fear-porn favoured by irresponsible mainstream media giants such as the EU-and-Gates-supported BBC.

This is real.

Other factors are going to ensure that the shortage just gets worse.

If and when the economy is allowed to stutter into action again, the price of oil will doubtless eventually rise because the existing supplies are diminishing rapidly and most oil companies have pretty well given up exploration.

The rising price of oil will mean that farming and transportation costs will rise and that will push up the price of food still further.

I tell you this not to scare you but because when you know something is happening you can do something about it.

You may think it is worthwhile building up your stocks of long-dated food staples such as rice and pasta. Dried and tinned foods which have long dates are good. As you eat your stocks, replace them with more. Governments tell us not to store stuff but the military don't buy bullets the day they need them, do they? If you have a garden and can grow your favourite vegetables or fruit that's probably a good idea but watch that no one climbs over your fence and steals them. I don't recommend having an allotment – the chances of you being able to harvest your own crops are too remote because they will be stolen. It might also be a good idea to stock up on vitamin and mineral supplements if you usually take them.

I've always been a bit of contrarian, though I don't suppose anyone would notice, and I'm convinced that the time to panic buy is when there is no panic.

I hope the advice here will help those who watch these videos: do a little quiet food stock piling now so that you and your family will have a better chance to be strong and healthy. Countries look after themselves and we all need to do so. It isn't selfish. It's survival. If you buy food you will eat anyway, and you store it carefully, what have you got to lose? If I'm wrong and there is no enemy and there are no food shortages then you can always eat what you've stored.

If and when your government finally warns you of this problem it will be far too late.

And tell your family and friends to watch this video soon. The last time I warned about the coming food shortages YouTube removed the Part One video within hours. Curiously, they left the second video in the two video series.

Remember: you should stockpile food now – don't wait for the panic

July 17th 2020

Why is YouTube Protecting Government Lies?

YouTube was doubtless a good idea when it started. I expect the originators may have had good intentions – they, perhaps, hoped to provide members of the public with a place for new ideas and for discussion. And I appreciate the fact that most of my videos are still available.

But I fear that the platform has allowed itself to become a tool of the devil-worshipping oppressors who are working hard to destroy mankind.

If you do stupid things on roller skates or leap out of a tree into a vat of blancmange then your videos will be safe. YouTube doesn't censor the puerile or the pathetic.

But it seems that the platform's censors do not approve of free speech, original thought or any sort of public debate.

I have absolutely no idea why they choose to take down videos these days. They've taken down a number of my videos. Indeed they've taken down a good many videos made by doctors or including interviews with doctors doubtful about the official line on the coronavirus. Worse still, they've removed some channels completely. So, for example, David Icke's channel was apparently banned. It was a diabolical example of censorship to remove his channel completely. I discussed YouTube's censorship policy in an earlier video of mine entitled, 'Why did YouTube ban my video?' which is worth hunting for if you haven't seen it. It's still available on my channel.

YouTube seems to ban anything which departs from the WHO's instructions – but those are not the law and they are often debatable. And so videos which deal with social distancing, masks and vaccination may be removed.

It sometimes seems to me that they simply look for videos which contain words of more than six letters and then take them down on the dubious grounds that anything which contains big words must be dangerous. The blancmange and the roller skating gerbils are fine. But anything which includes facts and opinions is likely to find itself on the equivalent of the cutting room floor. I made another video entitled, 'Everything you are allowed to know but I can't tell you what about' which also attacked the YouTube curious policy on health matters.

The pathetic lies and abuse from the feeble-minded trolls are easily ignored – the trolls who so eagerly spread libels are clearly a bunch of ignorant half-wits. Their lies and deceptions are blatant and laughable. Talking of abuse, I have a fine collection of screenshots of libellous remarks made on the pages behind my Wikipedia entry. Excellent and useful evidence.

But in theory the censorship of free speech is threatening the last remaining vestiges of our freedom. And in practice too.

The internet is important because as we have seen the mainstream media have been bought. The BBC was always going to defend the indefensible – it has, after all, taken money from the European Union and Bill Gates – but I am shocked and saddened at the way that other television stations and national newspapers have managed to bend their knees and, at the same time, bend over to facilitate the desires of the remorselessly wicked cabal so clearly determined to rule the world.

I sincerely hope that YouTube will revise its attitude to freedom of speech and debate. If it doesn't then sadly the one certainty in my mind is that when this fiasco is over, and we have reclaimed the world and rediscovered our freedom, there won't be much of a place for an organisation which appears to have sold itself to the public enemy. My experience suggests that YouTube may have taken sides and I don't believe they're going to end up on the winning side.

Meanwhile, I know that we cannot be silenced.

If I have to find a soap box or stand on street corners handing out hand written leaflets then that's what I will do.

We have built this society. It is our responsibility. If we stay silent then the evil will be done with our blessing.

It has always been up to us to shout 'stop' when we have had enough of the wickedness around us. We all have a voice we can use and we all have a duty to make sure that our voice is heard. If we remain silent then we are just a part of the evil which is corrupting and destroying our world.

We have to ignore the sad individuals who scoff or mock – either because they have been bought with a purse of silver or because they are too unintelligent to understand the nature of the war we are fighting. We must not allow ourselves to be put off by scorn, derision, undisguised contempt or a lack of support or encouragement from others.

Look through history and we can all see that imaginative, thoughtful and creative individuals have always had a hard time. Look back and you will find countless examples of citizens who were harassed or persecuted simply because they dared to think for themselves – and tried to share their thoughts with others.

The sad fact is that our world has never welcomed the original, the challenging, the inspirational or the passionate and has always preferred the characterless to the thought provoking.

Those who dare to speak out against the establishment have always been regarded as dangerous heretics. The iconoclast has never been a welcome figure in any age.

Confucius, the Chinese philosopher, was dismissed by his political masters and his books were burned. Those who didn't burn his books within 30 days were branded and condemned to forced labour. Two and a half thousand years later, Confucius's influence was still considered so dangerous that Chairman Mao banned his works.

Described by the Delphic Oracle as the wisest man in the world, Greek teacher Socrates was accused of corrupting the youth of Athens, arrested for being an evildoer and 'a person showing curiosity, searching into things under the earth and above the heaven and teaching all this to others'. Socrates was condemned to death.

Dante, the Italian poet, was banished from Florence and condemned to be burnt at the stake if ever captured.

After they had failed to silence him with threats and bribes, the Jewish authorities excommunicated Spinoza in Amsterdam because he refused to toe the party line, refused to think what other people told him he must think and insisted on maintaining his intellectual independence. He and his work were denounced as 'forged in Hell by a renegade Jew and the devil'.

Galileo, the seventeenth century Italian mathematician, astrologer and scientist got into terrible trouble with the all-powerful Church for daring to support Copernicus, who had the temerity to claim that the planets revolved around the sun.

Aureolus Philippus Theophrastus Bombastus von Hohenheim (known to his chums as Paracelsus) made himself enemies all over Europe because he tried to revolutionise medicine in the sixteenth century. Paracelsus was the greatest influence on medical thinking since Hippocrates but the establishment regarded him as a trouble-maker.

Ignaz Semmelweiss, the Austrian obstetrician who recognised that puerperal fever was caused by doctors' dirty habits was ostracised by the medical profession for daring to criticise practical procedures.

Dr John Snow fought two huge battles. He introduced anaesthesia for women in confinement and by removing the handle from the Broad

Street pump in Soho he helped prevent the spread of cholera in London. Both battles brought him enemies.

Henry David Thoreau, surely the kindest, wisest philosopher who has ever lived, was imprisoned for sticking to his ideals.

These are all my personal heroes. They show that original thinkers and people who do not fit neatly into the scheme of things have never gone down well. You and I are in good company. (I'm not speaking to the trolls, by the way. They pressed the thumb down button within a second of the video starting and they've been back in their cells for some time now.)

And nothing has changed over history.

Today, incompetence and mediocrity thrive and are subsidised, supported and encouraged by our increasingly bureaucratic and intrusive society. Among bureaucrats and administrators, incompetence and mediocrity are esteemed virtues; these be-suited morons revere the banal and worship the bland.

The unusual or the eccentric attract scorn and ridicule. Politicians are frightened of anything new or challenging. They reject the innovative, the creative and the imaginative in favour of the accustomed, the comfortable and the ordinary. It is hardly surprising that the sensitive, the thoughtful, the imaginative and the caring find twenty first century life almost too painful to bear.

But this isn't simply a battle for the right to say new or unthinkable things.

We are fighting a war for our right to say anything; we are fighting for the right to question our rulers.

Whenever we feel that something is wrong, it is our duty as human beings to stand up for our principles, to shout and make our voices heard.

There is a chance that some people will regard us as lunatics. Many small-minded people will sneer and tell you that in trying to change the world and root out dishonesty, corruption and injustice we are tilting at windmills. But there is also a chance that our voice will be heard; that others will respond and that we will win our battle.

But we really don't have a choice.

If we fail to fight then we will lose the world we know.

On this occasion, the benefits of victory far outweigh the insults of the insignificant. And, after all, only when you've found something you are prepared to die for will you really know what life is all about.

The battle you and I are fighting against the coronavirus hoax is the most important battle any of us will fight. It's crucial to our lives, our world, our beliefs, our humanity, our mental and physical health, our spirituality and our future. It's crucial too to future generations and to the world God gave us.

It's just a pity that YouTube appears to have chosen to side with the forces of evil and to censor and remove what I believe were perfectly sensible and well-researched videos – apparently because they used facts to question official policy.

But that won't stop us and I predict they will find themselves on the losing side.

I fear that YouTube will probably remove this video, and they will doubtless remove this channel. Why would they do that?

It has been widely reported that doctors and nurses have been forbidden to question the official line – even when it is patently wrong. They have been banned from speaking to the media.

Have the bosses at YouTube been told to suppress those who dare to question the lies – even if they are medically qualified?

That, I think, is the difference between them and us.

You and I prefer to think for ourselves, and to do the right thing whatever the cost, and we cannot be bought or pressured to do the wrong thing.

This channel has never been monetised – there are no ads and no sponsors. And there never will be.

July 18th 2020

How the Greens Will Destroy Our World

The mad Greens and other proponents of the myth of climate change (nee global warming) say that the oil in the ground (or under the sea) will have to stay there. They want to stop us using oil, gas, coal and uranium. They want us to get all our energy from renewables such as solar and wind power and through their power in the EU they are forcing through policies which fit with these aims.

Presumably, the mad Greens want to fly to their regular climate change conferences by solar powered jet and to use solar power to charge their websites and their laptops.

They want the big oil companies to go bust, and because of the political pressure they've exerted, numerous investment and pension companies are refusing to invest in oil companies.

This is lunacy and if I had a pension with a company which bowed to these loony activists, I would withdraw my money immediately.

The plan is clearly to destroy oil and coal companies, and their shareholders. It obviously has not yet occurred to the Greens around the world that without coal and oil there won't be enough electricity for their little diesel powered electric cars as well as their coal fired laptops.

(I discovered, by the way, that people in electric or low emission cars are far less likely to stop at zebra crossings than are people driving petrol or diesel engine cars. The drivers of electric cars are, it seems, so bloody pleased with themselves that they feel they can treat everyone else with disdain and contempt.)

The nutters are wrong for a number of reasons – which also make them dangerous.

First, the climate change silliness has been developing for well over a century. The campaigners like to think they invented it but pseudo-scientists have been putting forward the theory that greenhouse gases could change the climate since the 19th century. Only the converts (the pseudoscientists who see the whole business as a way to become rich and famous) think the evidence is convincing. Independent scientists admit that there is no genuine evidence that the earth is heating up. (I was taken in during the 1970s and 1980s but I no longer accept the dubious evidence as honest.) Moreover, even if the earth were getting hotter, there is no way to know if this could be caused by burning fossil fuels. (There is actually more evidence that it is getting cooler.)

Second, the alternatives to fossil fuels are frighteningly inefficient. For example, it takes more energy to make a windmill than the windmill will ever produce. So, the more windmills we produce the more energy we waste. Wind farms and solar farms are examples of entirely pointless rural vandalism; tributes to the self-serving sanctimoniousness and rank hypocrisy of an ignorant generation.

Third, the clever alternatives to oil and the internal combustion engine are silly. Using food to make fuel (the biofuels nonsense) exacerbated the starvation problem and the Greens have condemned hundreds of thousands, probably millions, to death by campaigning for yet more food to be turned into fuel for rich people.

Fourth, electricity, though very nice and useful stuff, only provides about 20% of our energy needs. The other 80% comes from nasty old gas, oil, coal and nuclear power. And it is nigh on impossible to increase that proportion. It's impossible to power ships and aeroplanes with electricity.

Fifth, an awful lot of people rely on gas for their central heating and cooking. If all those people are forced to use electricity for heating and cooking then there is going to be a great shortage of electricity because we are already using up every drop of the stuff that we can make.

Sixth, renewables such as solar energy and wind power provide only a tiny portion of our current electricity needs. We would need to carpet the countryside with solar farms and wind farms to increase that proportion significantly. And without subsidies (paid by consumers to rich landowners) the electricity produced would be horrifically expensive.

Seventh, (and this is a real heartbreaker for the Greens), maintaining windmills and solar panels requires more energy than the windmills and solar panels actually produce. The much loved renewables are actually a negative source of electricity. For example, when there is no wind the windmills have to be turned by electricity to stop them seizing up.

Eighth, there is no evidence that it is a bad thing if the earth is getting hotter. Rising tides would be bad for people with beachfront properties in some parts of the world. But if there is more carbon dioxide in the atmosphere, there will probably be more plants on the planet and then there will be less starvation. Surely we can all agree that would be a good thing?

Ninth, all the bizarre taxes forced upon by the European Union are costing a fortune. Because of subsidies paid to rich farmers operating wind farms and solar farms, ordinary people are having to pay more for their heating and many thousands more are dying in the cold weather. Is that supposed to be a good thing?

Finally, since renewables only produce electricity, we will have to survive on a source of energy which provides just 20% of our current needs. (You can't make oil or gas from windmills or solar panels). And since renewables only provide a quarter of our electricity, we will have to survive on just 5% of the energy we use at the moment. This is a bit of a problem because we can hardly cope on the energy supply we have now.

So, the bottom line is that we can only cope with the Green's demands if we give up: all forms of powered transport (including cars, planes and ships); all forms of entertainment which require electricity (e.g. television, radio, computers, mobile phones etc.); all forms of heating; all factories which make things; all mechanised farming and all fertilisers; all hospitals, medical treatments and all drug production. Of course, the real bummer is that the 5% of our energy which we have left will be needed to maintain and service our solar panels and our windmills. If there is any energy left over we may be able to boil a kettle and make a cup of hot water, though there won't be any tea leaves, milk or sugar to put in the hot water.

Welcome to the Green World.

If the Greens have their way, our planet will plunge into the biggest war of all time. The survivors will be those countries which retain fossil fuels and use them to manufacture armaments and to make and fuel bombers and tanks. The citizens of countries which decide unilaterally to rely on renewables will die. The good news is that our inability to use tractors and fertilisers will mean that most of us will starve to death, so we won't mind too much.

All this is unfashionable but it is quite accurate.

The bottom line, of course, is that the climate change myth, the allegation that the earth is hotting up or cooling down or whatever Prince Charles says it is doing this week, is simply an excuse for the introduction of the hideous and hateful global reset being planned by a bunch of crazed billionaires in order to reorganise the world to give them more power, more control and more money.

Just remember: the self-righteous and ignorant Greens are our mortal enemy.

July 19th 2020

We Are Victims of the Greatest Crime in History

I've done some unusual things in my life.

After I left school and before I went to medical school, I spent a year working as a Community Service Volunteer in a place called Kirkby, just outside Liverpool. I recruited a small army of teenagers and had them painting the flats of old folk. I drove an old Meals on Wheels van too. You may think that sounds dull but the fact that the van didn't have any brakes or lights added a little excitement. I was given about thirty bob a week pocket money as a Community Service Volunteer and so I earned a little money writing drama reviews for a local newspaper.

When I got to medical school, I carried on writing reviews and worked my way up to being a drama critic for a daily newspaper. I also ran a nightclub called The Gallows. I got paid for the reviews but the nightclub was run for a charity. It was good fun and everyone should run a nightclub once in their life.

And I used to write fictional stories for magazines.

I remember that every week the latest instalment would begin with a paragraph explaining to new readers what had happened in previous weeks. It was quite fun trying to cram the events of twelve weeks' episodes into a single paragraph. The paragraph always began with the words 'New readers start here…' though the words also helped remind regular readers what had already happened.

I don't know what reminded me of writing those stories, all those years ago when I was at medical school, and the paragraph entitled 'new readers start here', but it occurred to me yesterday that I was beginning to get a little confused about what had happened with the coronavirus hoax. And it seemed that it would be helpful to write a few words explaining the story so far. The closer you examine it, the less believable it becomes. And, in a strange way, the more believable.

So here goes.

New readers start here…

It all began sort of sometime either at the end of 2019 though no one seems entirely sure when, or even if it began at all and it seems to have started in China. It was not however, until the middle of February 2020 that people started to panic. A bloke working at Imperial College in London scared the living daylights out of millions by predicting that 600,000 people might die in the UK alone. There was talk of millions being taken ill in Britain and of hospitals all over the world being overwhelmed by sick patients.

We were about to be devastated by a plague-like illness that would devastate the world in a way not seen since the Spanish Flu a hundred years earlier.

The media led the panic, as they usually do, and within days people were cancelling holidays and panic buying toilet rolls, soap and loaves of bread. The British always buy toilet rolls, soap and loaves of bread at times of crisis. Photographs were taken of people pushing shopping trolleys piled high with loo rolls. Curiously, the people who were buying the most loo rolls didn't seem to be buying any food though you would have thought that without any of the latter there wouldn't have been much need for the former. The stock market had a nervous breakdown collapsed in a corner, as it always does at times like this, and the chap called Ferguson, who had started the excitement and who was apparently a sort of cross between a mathematician and an astrologer, was interviewed and quoted everywhere sharing his gloomy predictions. People hung on his every word and the BBC and the newspapers encouraged us to be terrified. On 28th February, I reported that we had been told that masks weren't much good.

At this point, back in February, I was puzzled by the fuss being made over what seemed to me to be no more toxic than the flu. So I decided to look a little closer.

When I looked at the figures that were available it was immediately blindingly obvious that something wasn't right. This isn't me looking through the retrospectoscope, that invaluable aid for looking backwards and seeming wise. I expressed my doubts on my website right from the start and pointed out that according to the WHO it was not unusual for 650,000 people to die of flu in a single season.

I started looking for a hidden agenda and came up with several.

On 28th February, I suggested that the virus might be being used to stop unnecessary travel, and to save oil for more important things like Prime Ministerial limousines and fighter jets or for flying Prince Charles to climate change meetings, or to soften us up for a compulsory vaccination. That web entry is in my book, *Coming Apocalypse* which was published back in April.

I was, inevitably, considered to be a lunatic.

On March 2nd I pointed out that the mortality figures which were being quoted were wrong because the authorities were only identifying the people who had the disease in a bad way. They weren't counting the thousands of people who had the disease but weren't very ill. I pointed out that if 1,000 people go to their doctor with the flu, and one patient dies then the mortality rate is 0.1% but if another 9,000 people have the flu but don't go to their doctors then the mortality rate is 0.01%.

No one seemed interested in my thoughts, apart from a few loyal website visitors, for which many thanks, and the panic continued to grow. I predicted that governments would use the crisis to create a cashless society and to get rid of old people.

It all rather reminded me of the AIDS scare. TV and newspapers were united in ignoring the facts and promoting the fear. The BMA warned us that everyone would be affected by the year 2000. I got into trouble for arguing, quite accurately, that the fear had been exaggerated by lobbyists with their own agenda.

On March 3rd 2020, I warned once again that compulsory inoculation would be coming. The panic grew and people were seen walking around with plastic boxes on their heads. Governments also appeared to panic, and in the UK the coronavirus was made a notifiable disease. Within days, doctors everywhere were warning that old people would have to be left to die because the virus was going to kill millions and every hospital bed would be needed for young coronavirus patients. On March 7th I reported that people had been cheering at the prospect of old people dying in huge numbers. 'It will clear hospital beds,' said one commentator.

By March 14th I was still pretty much on my own among doctors in insisting that the coronavirus wasn't going to kill us all. I was reminded of bird flu and swine flu. I had dismissed the scare stories about those two diseases at the time but the authorities had made dramatic claims. The WHO had claimed that the bird flu would kill up to 150 million people. I said that was rubbish. In the end, the bird flu killed less than 500. The UK Government claimed that swine flu would kill 65,000 in 2009 and spent £500 million on medicines that had to be thrown away. Again the total number of deaths didn't reach 500. It wasn't until a little later that I discovered that those wildly inaccurate predictions had been made by Professor Ferguson of Imperial College, London – a college heavily funded by the vaccine loving Bill and Melinda Gates Foundation. Ferguson had also made absurdly inaccurate predictions about mad cow disease – he had predicted up to 150,000 people could die but the total was 177. And it was Imperial College which made terrible predictions about foot and mouth disease.

Ferguson's forecasts, later described as severely flawed, led to six million animals being killed unnecessary and cost the UK £10 billion. Despite knowing all this history, the governments in the UK and the USA and, indeed, much of the rest of the world, listened to Ferguson's predictions, accepted them with enthusiasm and introduced lockdowns and social distancing. It was clear at the time that governments would have done better to have ignored Ferguson and his team at Imperial College, the Eurovision song contest losers from the world of mathematical modelling, and taken advice from Bob the Builder or Postman Pat instead. The world would have been a better, safer place but possibly a less profitable one for vaccine companies.

Angry at the way people were being terrified by a disease which was clearly no more deadly than the flu, I made a video for YouTube on 18th March. I called it 'Coronavirus Scare: The Hoax of the Century'. I've had a lot of abuse over the years, mainly from people hired by drug companies, but this time the abuse was phenomenal, deliberate and cold-blooded and I became the subject of a sneering, libellous, smear campaign so vicious that I regret making that video more than anything else I've ever done. I wonder how many people are put off speaking out because of the viciousness of the mindless, ignorant trolls and fake so-called fact checkers who hide behind stupid fake names, dribble on their keyboards, stalk the internet and attempt to smother the truth with transparent lies. In due course, I intend to identify the abusive trolls and sue them. It will be good to see them dragged into court, wheedling and whining. A little something to look forward to with relish when all this is over. They think they can remain anonymous but they're wrong and libel costs can run into millions. I've been busy with these videos but I am already close to identifying some of them. For example, the Wikipedia administrator, a self-confessed professional nerd in his early 50s who is married, with two children and who works for Dell might like to know that it is too late to put the house into his wife's name because the lawyers are coming for him. He says his wife is tolerant but I wonder if she will be quite so tolerant when they are living in a draughty tent.

I subsequently carried on making videos because I don't like being bullied by abusive thugs, because it was clearly too late to stop but mainly because I was still angry about all the lies being told and the people being unnecessarily upset. The things being done by scientists and politicians seemed to me to be egregious.

On March 19th, the public health bodies in the UK and the Advisory Committee on Dangerous Pathogens decided that the new disease should no longer be classified as a 'high consequence infectious disease'. The coronavirus was downgraded to flu level.

A couple of days after this decision, the UK Government introduced lockdowns and introduced the most oppressive Bill in British Parliamentary history. The Emergency Bill, which was 358 pages long, turned Britain into a totalitarian state and gave the Government and the police unprecedented powers. Public meetings and elections were banned and there were new powers relating to 'restrictions on use and disclosure of information'.

Curiously, even inexplicably, much the same thing happened around the world.

Following Ferguson's guidance, governments introduced lockdowns and social distancing, told the elderly they had to stay indoors, sent thousands of elderly folk out of hospitals and into care homes and cancelled operations and other procedures for millions of cancer patients.

In the UK, the public were ordered to keep six feet away from one another – presumably so that they would cheer when later told they only had to keep three feet away from one another. That's an old psychological trick. Terrify someone with something terrible and then they will rejoice when you remove the terrible and replace it with something merely awful. Brainwashing psychologists have been busy throughout this fiasco.

The disease turned out to be unique in that doctors could make a diagnosis without doing any tests or, in some cases, without even seeing their patients. The list of symptoms associated with the coronavirus grew and grew and the official line was that anyone suffering from one of those symptoms, such as a cough or a sneeze, had the disease. Thousands of patients were sent to care homes to keep hospitals empty so that nurses could learn how to dance and rehearse their clapping. In the UK, doctors got so good at misdiagnosing coronavirus that Britain soon headed the world figures for coronavirus deaths. Months ago, back in March, I pointed out that anyone who wasn't actually riddled with bullet holes was being put down as a covid-19 death and that the death totals were being exaggerated. Little did I know that even the bodies with bullet holes were being listed as covid-19 deaths. Harold Shipman, the mass murderer, would have had a wonderful time. Anyone who ever had covid-19 was put down as having died of it even if they were run over by a bus or hacked to death by a mad politician. Officially, it was impossible to recover from the disease. I suspect that the UK Government, having overegged the pudding, is now keen to reduce the total number of covid-19 deaths. On 30th March I predicted that the lockdowns would kill 100,000 to 250,000 people in Britain. I predicted that the result would be that far more people would be killed by the lockdown policies than would die as a result of the virus. It's in my book, *Coming Apocalypse* which was published back in April. I'm not making this up. And yet I am still being widely banned – yesterday YouTube took down another of my videos – on masks.

Tragically, the UK government has now admitted that this prediction has also been proved accurate. And during the next few years, the number of deaths resulting from the closure of hospital departments will soar to unimaginable levels. Suicides, as I predicted, will soar. Indeed, they are already are. Exactly the same thing has happened in other countries. This is a global crime.

Again, I predicted this back in March.

It has also gradually become clear that the number of people who have died from covid-19 is far less than the number who regularly die from flu in the same time period. The mortality rates from covid-19 and the flu are pretty well identical. The total number alleged to have died from the coronavirus has clearly been wildly exaggerated as people with the virus have been described as dying of it. Some doctors have spoken out but most are too frightened to do so since governments have, for the first time in history, forbidden medical and nursing staff to debate or question official policies.

The coronavirus has infected around 10 million people but the flu can affect a billion people a year. This supports the point I made in March that the virus seemed less infectious than the flu. And, of course, the total number of global deaths from the coronavirus – even with the absurdly exaggerated death totals produced by putting down every death as coronavirus related – is far, far fewer than the 650,000 who can die of the flu in a single season. It is also far fewer than the 1.5 million who can die of TB in a single year – also an infectious disease. Now that it is far too late to make any difference, governments are doing lots of testing and the testing is showing that more people have the bug. Only politicians and the brain dead could possibly be surprised at that. If you test more people – especially if you use tests which are about as reliable as Ferguson's predictions – you will find more people with it but without any symptoms. Many of those now testing positive are young, otherwise healthy individuals who are probably about as likely to die of falling downstairs as they are to die of covid-19. The R number, the rate of infection, is irrelevant. All that matters is the D number – the number of people who die. But nobody is talking about that.

And so now, as the virus becomes less virulent and appears to be disappearing, as the death rate falls dramatically, it won't be long before horse riding, or falling off horses, kills more people than the coronavirus, governments are warning of a second wave, lockdowns are being reintroduced and in the UK the wearing of masks in shops will be compulsory. When the disease was allegedly at its worst masks were considered unnecessary. But as the number dying fell, so it was felt that we needed to be kept frightened until the vaccine was ready. Masks were recommended as a good way to remind us to remain fearful – and look very silly. Anyone who saw French President Macron wearing a mask knew how silly it is possible to look – and how impossible it is to take anyone seriously when they are wearing half a bra on their face. They could have got us all to tie knots in our hankies to remind us to remain fearful but these days most people use paper tissues and it's difficult to tie a knot in a paper tissue.

And in mid-July it appeared that the virus had unprecedented powers. If you catch a disease you will usually acquire immunity. But not, it seems with covid-19. Though this claim was previously dismissed it was again announced that immunity to covid-19 mysteriously disappears after a few months. The answer, of course, will be repeated vaccinations. Maybe we will need vaccinations four times a year. Maybe we will be told we need a vaccination every month. The UK Government has so far agreed to buy 190 million doses of vaccine for a population less than a third of that. Vaccine company shares are going to soar. What a massive surprise that will be to everyone.

And that, I fear, is what it's all about. Not one vaccination. Not annual vaccinations. But vaccinations several times a year.

If the science appears to have gone mad so too are the rules, the regulations, the laws.

The rules now are unutterably stupid, incomprehensible and indefensible. If you told me they'd been written by a five-year-old donkey I'd believe you. The entire world appears to be run by people who are at least one sandwich and a bottle of fizzy pop short of a picnic. You can go into a pub but not a bowling alley. You can have your hair permed and your nails varnished but physiotherapy departments are still closed. If the idea is to keep people confused, miserable and damned near suicidal then it is all working brilliantly well.

Oh, and researchers now claim that a skin rash is another sign of covid-19. Apparently 8.8% of patients with a positive covid-19 test also have a rash. Has anyone realised that if the rash is on the individual's hands then it was probably caused by the damned sanitiser fluid that everyone is being forced to use in absurd quantities?

We are living in a manufactured nightmare.

This is either the most unlikely badly managed epidemic in the history of the world or it is, as I described it in my video made on March 18th, the hoax of the century – with hidden reasons behind what has happened.

If it is the former then we need to sack and arrest everyone involved in the decision making process. And we need to halt all the mask wearing, the social distancing nonsenses still being forced upon us.

If it is the latter then we need to sack and arrest everyone involved in the decision making process. We need to halt all the mask wearing and social distancing nonsenses still being forced upon us. And we need an independent judicial enquiry into exactly who is behind a commercial and political operation which can only be described as genocide.

Back in February, I said I thought that the hoax might be part of a plan to introduce compulsory vaccination.

One large drug company claims it expects to have made two billion doses of a vaccine by September. Will that vaccine be compulsory? What testing will have been done?

And how frequently will they tell us we must be vaccinated?

This nightmare gets more scary every day.

There are moments when I wish I were an ostrich, with my head firmly buried in the sand. Anyone who watches this and doesn't see the truth either works for a government , and doesn't care about himself, his family or the truth, or is a dribbling, dead eyed zombie who dwells in the dark, watches BBC programmes and thinks that Bill Gates is a good, kind person who wants to save the world rather than a grinning psychopath whose plan is to gain world domination and who makes the worst James Bond baddie look like a benevolent Father Christmas. Remember, you're not on your own.

July 20th 2020

Five Battles We Cannot Afford to Lose

The masks we are being encouraged to wear are useless. The virus goes through the mask like a wasp through chain link fencing. So, what is the point?

Are the English being forced to wear masks because Scotland's diminutive dictator made mask wearing compulsory north of the border? Is Boris the Bullock being led by the nose by the Sturgeon woman?

When Sturgeon made mask wearing compulsory in Scotland, she created a clear division between the two countries and threatened to turn the border with England into a quarantine zone. This seemed to me to be political – and part of the Scottish Nationalists' plan to declare independence. So did Boris, desperate to prevent a split, make masks compulsory in England to keep the two countries united? Whatever next? If Sturgeon makes kilt wearing compulsory will Boris do the same? Boris likes to think of himself as Churchillian. He is more a Prime Minister in the Chamberlain mode.

Is it just to humiliate us, oppress us and take away our identity? To create fear and make us demand the new vaccine? Or is it to prepare us for the one world religion, which has long been planned?

Is it a coincidence that July 24th – the day when masks became compulsory in English shops, is the special day of St Charbel Makhluf – a monk and priest who had links with both the Christian and Muslim worlds?

When your own government and the mass media continually lies to you, nothing can be counted as impossible.

Talking of mass media, it is important to realise that the whole of the mass media is now our enemy. I have read articles arguing that the Government and its experts couldn't possibly be wrong because they are all singing from the same hymn sheet. This is such blatant nonsense that it makes me want to weep. Governments everywhere are involved in a conspiracy and they have passed laws forbidding dissent or discussion or the publication of information that doesn't fit the official line.

It is no secret, for example, that in the UK, doctors and nurses working in the NHS are forbidden to talk about anything relating to the coronavirus. All whistle blowing is now banned. Anyone who breaks this law will be fired and probably lose their licence to practice. But what a pity that doctors and nurses have failed to speak out. Any doctor or nurse who still thinks this virus is a plague, should be struck off for incompetence. Health professionals should have the guts to speak out at a time like this. And before anyone accuses me of asking others to do what I need not do, just remember that I have been viciously attacked and lied about endlessly because I have spoken out. And I would add that I have twice resigned from well-paid jobs on principle. I resigned as a GP in the early 1980s because I disapproved of having to put diagnoses on sick notes. And I resigned from a job as a newspaper columnist when my column condemning the Iraq War was censored.

Let me just give a couple of examples of how blatant the mass media has become in distorting or hiding the truth.

First, a few days ago, the British Government admitted that the number of deaths for covid-19 had been dramatically exaggerated. Anyone who had tested positive for the coronavirus and who subsequently died was officially counted as having died of the coronavirus. I've been saying this for months now but it was good to see the Government admit that the death total for coronavirus had been wildly exaggerated in order to bring the total up closer to the annual number of respiratory disease deaths. If you had the coronavirus in February and were then run over by a bus in July, you officially died of the coronavirus not the injuries caused by the bus. This was, in my view, one of the biggest news stories of the whole fiasco. I wonder how many murders were covered up that way. Dr Harold Shipman would have had a great time. But, as far as I could see, the BBC did not even mention the exaggeration on its website. The story wasn't there. The BBC did, however, have a story dismissing those who didn't want to wear a mask as 'socially obnoxious'. The BBC has given up even pretending to be fair or even handed in its reporting.

Incidentally, the BBC has a 'reality check' item on its website. If you go to that part of the website you can find a form on which you can ask the BBC to check on something that seems inaccurate or misleading. I suggest you go there and ask this question: 'How corrupt is the BBC? Has the BBC's bias become more obvious since it forged financial links with the EU and with Bill Gates?'

Second, an editorial in the *Economist* said this about Donald Trump: 'he seems to be wrong about almost everything. He has promoted a dud malaria drug, said the virus would disappear and even that 99% of cases of covid-19 are harmless'. Well, Trump was right about all those things and the *Economist* was, as it usually is, wrong about everything. I think it is vital to swamp all mainstream media with messages reminding their readers that the mass media is often providing a biased viewpoint. Ask their readers to look at these videos to find the truth. Whatever the truth may be I think the war we are fighting against our own governments, and their agents and manipulators, can be divided into five specific battles.

First, there is the battle against face masks. Since the WHO changed its collective mind and started recommended masks, just as infections fell, there has been massive confusion around the world as more and more politicians have followed the party line, defied the science, and made mask wearing compulsory. There is a let out in some countries such as the UK. Anyone who has a physical or mental health problem which makes mask wearing difficult can refuse to wear one. So, if you have a respiratory problem such as asthma or you suffer from anxiety when wearing a mask you are, as I understand it, legally entitled to refuse to wear one. And I don't believe you should have to tell a shop assistant or policeman precisely what your confidential health problem might be. On the other hand if you tell the police officer that you are asthmatic and will suffer if you have to wear a mask then you would presumably have a good reason to appeal against a fine whereas if you insist on not explaining your condition, you would undoubtedly still have to tell the magistrate the nature of your problem.

In the UK, children under the age of 11 don't have to wear a mask and since masks can cause hypoxia and can kill, parents who do put masks on children under 11 should, in my opinion, be arrested for child abuse. Where are the damned social workers when you need them? All sitting at home wearing six masks and with their feet in a bucket of disinfectant since the BBC (the taxpayer funded home of fake news) seems to have suggested that you can catch it through your feet.

Second, there is the battle to retain cash. I think this is absolutely crucial. If they succeed in removing cash from our society then we will all become slaves to the electronic system – easy to track and trace whatever we do and wherever we go. Implanted chips will be the next step and we will all bear a tattoo. The banks have wanted to get rid of cash for a long time and they've been closing branches and cash machines in an attempt to force us to use plastic cards. The solution is to refuse to shop in establishments which won't take cash. If you know a shop won't take cash then take a pile of purchases to the counter and then refuse to pay for them if your cash is refused. The shop will lose the sale and will have to put all the items back on the shelf. And make sure that the manager knows why you are going elsewhere.

Third, we need to make sure that social distancing is ended – particularly in schools. Parents should contact their child's school and make it clear that they do not want their child to attend a school which insists on social distancing. They should make it clear that if a school puts social distancing measures in place then they will hold the headmistress or headmaster personally responsible for any psychological damage their child might suffer. Petty bureaucrats hate being held personally accountable.

Fourth, we don't want any more lockdowns. Now that local politicians and bureaucrats have been given the authority to introduce local lockdowns, we do at least know where we need to put pressure. Contact your local councillor and make it clear that you will never vote for him or her again if lockdowns are introduced in your area. And demand that executive staff be fired if they try introducing lockdowns.

Fifth, vaccines. Why are the authorities so desperate to force a vaccine on us just to deal with a mild disease no worse than the flu? We have to make it clear that we won't accept mandatory vaccinations. We aren't going to be able to end the vaccination programme – it is far too well entrenched within the system – and the zombies will be rolling up their sleeves and holding out their arms in eagerness the minute a vaccine is available. They don't care whether it works, causes brain damage or kills them stone dead. The zombies are as desperate for the needle as heroin addicts after two days of cold turkey. If you don't want to be vaccinated then make this clear on message boards and in letters to newspapers and radio programmes. Point out that in the USA the authorities have paid out over $4 billion to vaccine injured patients. In the UK, the Government has a standard payment of £120,000 for those injured by vaccines. Why pay out all that money for vaccines which are supposed to be perfectly safe? If the authorities realise that there are many people who will not accept mandatory vaccination, in any form, then they will not try to force their damned vaccination on us.

May your God go with you in these difficult times.

July 21st 2020

How to Survive in the Lunatic Land of the Coronavirus Hoax

I'm afraid there is no point in our hoping that things are going to return
to normal. They aren't. Our enemies have made their move and the war
that they've started isn't going to be over in weeks or months. And
make no mistake – we're in a war.

My apologies if this sounds depressing. But I can't see any point in
pretending that things are going to be hunky dory in a matter of weeks.
Only if we accept that we are at war will we be prepared and able to
defend ourselves and to defeat the enemy. Government ministers will
offer promises and assurances but it will all be fake – part of the
misinformation they've been feeding us, part of the psychological
operation to unsettle us with promises and disappointments.

We are living in the worst of times.

It is always difficult to say that, of course.

What about the First World War? Or the Second World War? Or the
Hundred Years War? Or the American Revolution? The American
Civil War? Or the plague?

All terrible times.

But there is something especially strange about these times.

Usually, when there is a war or a major conflict we know the identity
of our enemy. We have leaders we can trust – well, trust a little.

But this time it is different.

Our leaders, globally, nationally and locally, are our enemy.

Ronald Reagan's greatest legacy was, for me, his remark that the most
dangerous words in the world are: 'I'm from the Government and I'm
here to help'. That has now matured into: 'I'm from the Government
and I'm here to make your life miserable and, if possible, to kill you.'

Governments all over the world have been bought and are now
controlled by global organisations such as the United Nations, the
World Health Organisation and the Bill and Melinda Gates Foundation
they want to take from us everything we value – and to turn us into
slaves.

In previous conflicts we could count on the military to protect us.
Not now. Today the military are the enemy. Under orders from
governments which have betrayed the people, their job is to suppress
the truth to protect the lies. Politicians and their advisors have lost
touch with the science, the truth and reality.

And we certainly cannot rely on the media to expose dishonesty, oppression and injustice. Today the mainstream media are siding with our oppressors. They are promoting dishonesty and endorsing injustice and they have encouraged millions to become mortally afraid of death. We may be on our own but we are not alone.

We are the guerrilla army. As someone said during the French revolution, this is not a revolt it is a revolution. And we are the resistance.

The time to prepare for bad times is when no one else is panicking. The zombies are hunkered down waiting for their vaccine but we have one huge advantage: we have some idea what is in store for us. Nothing is ever going to be as it was. For the time being the men and women in black hats, the bad guys, have taken over.

So, how can we prepare?

First, if at all possible you should try to move out of a town or city. The Agenda 21 plan is for us all to live in what they call 'smart cities'. They want us all corralled in apartment blocks because then we are easier to control. In their ideal world, we will live in flats no more than a mile away from our work. Our groceries and other purchases will be delivered and we will spend our evenings shopping, playing games and watching television programmes on the internet.

You may not earn as much if you move out of the city and change your job but your living expenses will be lower – especially if you work at home and don't have to spend a fortune travelling to work, buying smart work clothes and purchasing expensive lunches and coffee. The air you breathe will be cleaner and you will probably be able to grow some of your own vegetables. Try to become as self-sufficient as you can. The TV series 'The Good Life' is now more of a 'how to' documentary than a comedy series.

Should you move to another country? Until the dust settles it's difficult to know. One certainty is that the UK and the USA will be the worst affected by the lying, the manufactured chaos and the lethal policies of corrupt administrations. I wouldn't want to live in France, either. France has been a cauldron of dissatisfaction and unwound racial conflict for years and Macron, vain even for a politician, has made things infinitely more dangerous.

Second, prepare for problems with the utilities such as electricity and water supplies. The climate change movement is based on fake science but it's a fundamental part of the United Nations' Agenda 21. The people behind Agenda 21, the plan for a global reset and a New World

Order, have been infiltrated by green self-styled environmentalists and their plans include a massive reduction in world population, a reliance on non-fossil fuels and the destruction of all aspects of capitalism. The plan is to enslave us, and the coronavirus hoax is part of the programme of control. This is practical fascism in its rawest and most dangerous incarnation. I'll explain precisely what is planned in a future video.

There are probably going to be electricity outages in the coming years. But there are many things you can do to prepare yourself. You can buy batteries, usually sold for campers, which hold a good chunk of electricity and which can be charged from the mains, when it's working, or from a portable solar panel. You should obviously also keep good torches and a supply of batteries. A camping stove and a supply of cartridges will mean that you're independent of the mains supplies for cooking. If you have an open fireplace or a log burner make sure you have a supply of fuel.

I realise that I'm beginning to sound like one of those redneck survivalists who lives in the wild and gets sneered at a good deal. But I don't care. I've been sneered at for decades and I've been right more often than any of the people doing the sneering. So yah boo sucks to them.

Our utility supplies are more fragile today than they've been for decades. This is partly due to neglect, of course, but it is also a consequence of the chaos and damage by the deliberately engineered coronavirus crime. And if you don't think the whole coronavirus crime was deliberately engineered then I'm afraid you haven't been paying attention and you must write out two hundred times 'Bill Gates is the Most Dangerous Person on the Planet'.

To protect yourself from water supplies I suggest that you lay in a supply of bottled water. Keep it out of the direct sunlight. If you can fit a water butt to a downpipe that will usually supply you with a good supply of water. Use water purification tablets or a purification cup and you can use the water you collect.

I've previously suggested that you should lay in a supply of long-dated food – rice, pasta and tinned vegetables for example. Don't rely too much on the freezer because if the electricity goes out you could be in trouble.

Next, you should lay in a supply of whatever medicines you use or may use. Your doctor is unlikely to give you more than a two or three month supply of any essential prescription medicines but you can stock up on whatever supplements and over the counter medicines you might need – dispersible aspirin tablets, antihistamine, a steroid cream, eye drops, antiseptic cream and so on. Just watch the 'use by' dates. Stock up on whatever vitamin and mineral supplements you use. Check out some of the online pharmacies. Reputable ones tend to be properly regulated. Put together a decent first aid kit and know how to use the contents. Buy enough emergency blankets for one each – just in case you have no heat in the winter. Take regular, gentle exercise.

If you need to see a doctor other than your GP, it might be wise to be vague about your age. It is not uncommon these days for patients to be refused treatment if they are over 65. So if you are over that and you accidentally knock a decade off your age don't bother to correct the error. I was now born in 1991 but I think I may have to edge that back a tad. In the UK, the NHS is already unfit for purpose. It's going to get worse and services are going to decline dramatically. GPs surgeries are pretty well closed in many parts of the country and accident and emergency departments will soon require an appointment, so we are told. Learn to take care of yourself to minimise the risk of accidents. Build up your immune system. (My book *Superbody* explains how to do that.)

Look after your teeth and visit your dentist regularly because if there is another lockdown you might not be able to see one. In the UK, there is going to be a massive shortage of NHS dentists and it's my suspicion that the Government plans to close down this part of the NHS. Free eye tests will probably disappear too. Agenda 21 means that governments won't want to spend money on the elderly, the frail or anyone with any sort of health problem. The new global reset, espoused by Prince Charles, means that every citizen must be useful to the State. So that's the end of the Royal Family.

Sanitisers in shops are a growing irritation in more ways than one. (See my video on hand sanitisers if you haven't. It's full of scary truths.)Touching a sanitiser bottle that has been handled by hundreds of dirty hands is daft. The stuff inside the bottle could be something dangerous and it may well irritate your hands and be dangerous. You can always say 'No, thank you' if an assistant suggests that you use their dispenser. Carry one of your own and fill it with something mild and non-irritating.

If you have relatives in care homes then it might be wise to move them out if possible. It is frequently cheaper to live in a hotel than a care home and if someone just needs help with cleaning, bed-making, laundry and meals a hotel will often be just as good. And there isn't the risk that a local hospital will fill the hotel with flu-ridden patients. There is going to be an increase in the average age in populations everywhere and the elderly are going to find that they are increasingly marginalised.

If you have children then it might be worthwhile looking at home schooling – especially if teachers are going to continue to behave irresponsibly. Children who go to schools where social distancing rules are in place will, in my view, grow up to be psychologically damaged.

Don't take holidays abroad while governments are still talking about quarantines. If you do then you might have to spend a fortnight in quarantine in a foreign hotel and then, on your return, have to spend another fortnight in quarantine.

Keep vehicles topped up with fuel for emergencies. Buy a bicycle or get an old one repaired.

Check that whatever investments you have are suitable for the new world. Be prepared for banks and even building societies to introduce negative interest accounts. The commercial world is going to continue to change dramatically. The United Nations plan for the new world which governments everywhere have bought involves the closure of small businesses so if you think you could be vulnerable, increase your savings. Don't take on new debts that you aren't certain you will be able to service. Unemployment is going to be high and stay high for a long, long time. Many people who have spent years acquiring skills and training will find that they have to find new skills. Computers and robots are going to take over many jobs – a lot sooner than most people realise. Try to avoid the mass market media as much as you can. Most of it is biased, misleading prejudicial, hypocritical and downright dangerous. In my view, the BBC is the most treacherous organisation on earth – Lord Haw Haw would work for it today and Goebbels would have been proud of it.

Find local people who think as you do. Make plans to stand for your local council when, or perhaps if, the ban on elections is ever lifted. We have to take back control of our country and starting locally is the best way. We have to fight the sense of depression that has been deliberately created so that we remain strong enough to continue fighting the enemy. This is going to be a long war. May our God go with us in these dark and difficult times.

July 22nd 2020

How They Are Lying to Enslave Us

The lies keep coming. I have never in my life seen so much misinformation being broadcast with such apparent enthusiasm. I spend much of each day trying to understand what we are being told and why.

But the mysteries arrive faster than the explanations. There is a good deal of misdirection, a good deal of exaggeration, much sleight of hand, a good deal of psychological warfare stuff and many attempts to blind us with a small part of a story; to exaggerate in order to influence.

When I was a medical student I ran a night club in the city where I was studying. The club was in a pretty rough part of the town and apart from having a DJ playing music, we showed upside down Buster Keaton films on the ceiling and occasionally mixed them up with colourful histology slides which we also projected on the ceiling. It was the histology slides which got me into trouble when the BBC mentioned them in a broadcast about the club. The medical school Dean was not amused and I acquired a large black mark as a result. Although quite a lot of students attended the club, there was a hard core of youths who would make the roughest and toughest of today's statue toppling Black Lives Protestors look like kids on a Sunday School outing.

Most of them carried knives and weren't afraid to use them and it was, I'm afraid, a rare evening when there wasn't a large puddle of blood on the floor at the end of an evening.

Most of the time, the kids with the knives were decent enough with me and I didn't have problems with them. But then half a dozen new ones turned up and were spoiling to make their mark. They got a little feisty with their knives and although I wasn't cut, I was allowed to take an uncomfortably close look at some fairly intimidating pieces of steel.

So the next day, I went into the city centre and bought myself a stick. It wasn't an ordinary stick, however. It was a sword stick with a long, very pointy blade hidden inside it. In those days you could buy and carry a swordstick quite legally.

The following evening, when the boys with the knives gathered around, there was much jeering at the stick I was carrying.

Until, that is, I pulled the first foot and a half of the blade out of the stick. It was, of course, a considerably larger blade than any of those the boys were carrying. This was a couple of decades before Crocodile Dundee.

The effect was instantaneous –and so was the respect.

The knives were all put away. And they never came out again.

I would never have used my sword, of course. But they didn't know that. The existence of it, and the implied threat, was enough.

It was a crude psychological trick to take control of the situation.

And that's what governments are now doing.

They are using every trick in the book to threaten us and to keep us terrified and awed. Some of the tricks are very crude. Some are fairly subtle. They're the sort of tricks used to defeat a real enemy. Our own governments are using the same sort of tricks which were used in World War II. But this time they're not using them on Nazis – they're using them on us.

And the tricks, and the lies, keep coming because they are working. Our own governments, which are now our enemy, are doing everything they can and they are succeeding in terrifying a good chunk of the population. They are doing so, not because of the science but for political and commercial reasons.

Politicians are obeying the principles of Agenda 21 – more of which in a future video – and trying to satisfy the commercial requirements of an industry which sees a bonanza payday tantalisingly close.

Yesterday, I saw several tiny children wearing masks because their parents had obviously believed the nonsense. One child, no more than four or five-years-old, started to cry when her mask slipped. She was only comforted when the mask was replaced.

And I saw two motorists, alone in their cars, driving while wearing masks. The truth, if that is still considered acceptable, is that masks can cause hypoxia and damage brain function. It won't be long before drivers start having crashes because they are wearing masks. And why are small children being forced to wear masks? There is no scientific point to it.

Why does no one in government point out that the virus is so small that it will zoom through mask material like a fly through chicken wire?

A large car park, run by the council, was still shut but it didn't much matter because there weren't many people about. Many of the shops which should have been open were shut. Some obviously permanently and some shut because staff didn't want or dare to return to work.

Coffee shops were open only for take away coffees. No one seemed to be buying. We went into a restaurant, mostly empty, and they happily served us coffees – pleased to have a couple of customers buying something.

The official estimate is that 0.03 of the population of England have the virus. Can you imagine how likely it is that you will meet someone with the virus? Or that you will catch it? Or that it will do you serious harm?

Am I the only one to see the irony in the fact that last year, in Britain, a man was fined £90 for wearing a mask while walking past a facial recognition camera put there by the police? It's odd how things have changed so quickly. Last year, Hong Kong banned masks to stifle public protests. Laws banning face coverings in public were passed in France, Belgium, Austria and Denmark. In Canada, rioters who covered their faces with masks risked ten years in jail. And in America some states have had laws banning face coverings since 1845. The laws were put in place to try to get rid of bandits.

Cressida Dick, the Police Commissioner for the Metropolitan Police in London has said that the police will only enforce the law on wearing face masks as a last resort. 'My hope,' she is quoted as saying, 'is that the vast majority of people will comply, and that people who are not complying will be shamed into complying or shamed to leave the store.'

How nice of her.

Cressida Dick should know all about shame. She was, of course, the officer who made the decision for the police to shoot a young innocent Brazilian man in 2005. Police apparently shot eleven times from close range. They managed to shoot the entirely innocent man seven times in the head and once in the shoulder.

'I think about it quite often,' Dick allegedly said last year while chatting on a BBC programme called Desert Island Discs. Quite often? Most people, I suspect, would think about it pretty well all the time. I suspect I am not alone in thinking she should have been sacked. Instead she now has a top police job and believes that those choosing not to damage their health by wearing useless masks should be made to feel ashamed. I am not entirely sure that encouraging other shoppers to shame non mask wearers is entirely within Ms Dick's role in the police.

And does this surely damned woman (I use the word damned in its Christian sense) not realise that the Government has made it clear that people with health problems – including anxiety – do not have to wear masks? And nor do young children. Is she suggesting that these individuals, who may be fearful for many reasons, be deliberately shamed? Are the police officially suggesting that patients with respiratory and heart disease be deliberately shamed? Is Dick suggesting that those with mental health problems be shamed? So it would seem. My utter contempt for Cressida Dick is endless.

We should call en masse for her to be sacked. Write to your MP. Write to the newspapers. If you do nothing else today, do what you can to get this woman fired. She is an utter disgrace to the human race. I cannot believe it. Encouraging people to shame the sick and the frail and the anxious and the mentally ill! And shaming children!

It is said that masks are being made compulsory not to protect against an infection but to provide reassurance for people who are too terrified to go to the shops. It seems that the World Health Organisation may have reversed its view, and decided that masks are necessary, because of political pressure. From whom? Was it Gates – now about to be the WHO's main sponsor? Is the plan to keep us terrified until the vaccine is ready?

The masks are not giving confidence, of course – they are increasing the terror among the people who fear that we are living in a plague year. I shall certainly not be wearing a mask, of course.

In many of the shops which were open, there was a real sense of terror. I got stuck at one point on the wrong side of a barrier designed to keep pedestrians in two lines. I moved a barrier just enough to squeeze through and within seconds a guard had appeared from nowhere. He shouted at me and when I ignored him he started screeching excitedly into his portable radio. I have no idea what he was saying or what he thought was going to happen.

I went into several shops to try to buy a top up for my ancient mobile phone. No one would sell me one. In one shop a masked cashier, whom I could hardly hear (he was also sitting behind a plastic screen), started to sell me a top up voucher when a manager rushed over screaming 'No top ups. We don't do top ups'. Why on earth not? What did she, or her bosses, think might happen?

Anyone who talks glibly of a V shaped recovery in the economy needs to get out into the shops. I will be surprised if there are many High Street shops left in the UK by Christmas. And things are getting worse everywhere. Pensions will be devastated because many companies have stopped paying dividends. Everyone who doesn't have a job and a pension with the State will be financially disadvantaged. The State is using over £1 billion of taxpayers' money in the UK to act as a patron for the arts though it is difficult to see why the arts, and the suffering celebrities, shouldn't suffer, make do and be creative to find their way out of the manufactured crisis. Meanwhile, an estimated 250 million people around the world will lose their jobs – largely due to the lockdowns which followed Neil Ferguson's slightly hysterical in my view, and inaccurate, forecasts. The ensuing poverty will create pain and illness.

And the disappearance of High Street shops is, of course, part of the plan. This isn't paranoia. It's Agenda 21 from the United Nations. I've been reading yards of material about the plans they have for our future and to be honest it's terrified me.

This is, of course, all the part of the Global Reset. It has not been kept a secret but they've slipped the plan past most of us and they have sold it, falsely, as a solution to non-existent global warming – the second biggest scam in history and an excuse for the awful things they are planning for us.

The misdirection has been skilful. Governments have made life complicated and unpleasant and threatening in order to distract us and blind us with a threat which doesn't really exist. Doctors and nurses have been forbidden to counter the propaganda – and most have, sadly, obeyed their orders.

Governments have persuaded millions of half-wits to worry about climate change, and also racism and sexual politics of course, when these are not the main danger we face. The spoilt elitists who are trapped in their own concept of history and have energy to waste on worrying about Cecil Rhodes and so on, should try looking forwards rather than backwards.

We are heading for global slavery, organised by the United Nations, the World Health Organisation, the Bill and Melinda Gates Foundation and a bunch of unelected billionaires. The risk for our future is very real and it is a horror coming to your family and your home.

The protestors have, in my view, missed the big picture and, misled and lied to by governments everywhere, they dismiss as a conspiracy the truly frightening elements of the Global Reset they have planned for us.

I know some people won't believe any of this. It's all too much for them.

But let me leave you with one threat that you can easily check.

Part of the Global Reset is a plan to combine all religions together into a new World Religion which may or may not be called Chrislam.

Chrislam, an attempt to combine Christianity with Islam, has been around for some time, in a very quiet sort of way, but it is now progressing rapidly. Pope Francis, the first Jesuit Pope, announced that May 14th is to be World Chrislam Day and is said to have appointed 13 Chrislam friendly cardinals. Last year the Vatican released a Chrislam Logo for Pope Francis.

I wonder if it is a coincidence that churches may now be open but are not providing services.

Oh, and just put Chrislam and ex British Prime Minister Tony Blair into your search engine. Or take a look at the Tony Blair Faith Foundation and the Tony Blair Institute for Global Change.

Blair launched his Faith Foundation in 2008 to work towards global faith. Blair said then that extremists who did not want to join together would be put 'into retreat'. What did he mean by that? I don't know. But I've seen the film of him saying it.

Later, Obama got involved. And in 2012, the Vatican called for One World Order and a Global Government.

The constant excuse was that we needed a global government and a global church to protect us against climate change.

Oh and guess who can be found among Blair's list of partners.

You won't guess if we sit here all day.

The Bill and Melinda Gates Foundation.

And Microsoft.

It's all there, out in the open.

The United Nations 21 plan is for a World Government (with population control near the top of its agenda). The excuse for this is climate change. The UN also says that we obviously need a World Church. It seems that individual religions will disappear into one. But what will happen to Jews, Buddhists, Hindus, Methodists, Evangelical Christians, Presbytarians?

Do any of us have a say in any of this?

Before we know what has happened, the UN will have given us its World Government and its World Church – whether we like it or not.

That is what the climate change campaign was all about – preparing us for a global reset. And that is what the coronavirus nonsense is all about.

Check it out. All the information is available on the internet. I've given you all the clues you need. This is definitely, most definitely, not a conspiracy theory.

The only conspiracy is the one leading towards a World Government and a World Church.

Oh, and think about this: in 1991 the Club of Rome published a book entitled, *The First Global Revolution* in which it admitted to inventing climate change as a common enemy of mankind in order to unite the world.

It really can't get any clearer.

Finally, before I stopped receiving emails, I saw several complaining about the sound quality of these videos and, not surprisingly, offering help with new equipment and professional advice.

Well, thank you but no. I'm not interested and don't have time or energy for upgrading our top level equipment. We use my old iPad, a microphone that cost under a tenner and a cheap camera tripod and anyone who wants better sound quality will need to go and watch something else – I gather the sound quality on those videos about skateboarding hamsters is excellent.

Oh and my thanks to YouTube who have, after I protested, put back up my video entitled, 'Face Masks – Ending the Confusion'. That probably took some courage, so thank you.

July 23rd 2020

The Forces of Evil are Gathering

We older folk talk a good deal about the past, partly because there is a lot of it, and it's something we know more about, partly because it is sometimes easier to make more thoughtful comments about the past than about the present and partly because the future is now much of a foreign, unexplored land than it used to be.

The big advantage of knowing the past is that it gives us a sense of perspective and a better chance to understand where we are going.

So I want to explain how we arrived at the position where we are today – with the whole world seemingly frozen in fear of a virus which has been proven to be no more of a killer than a pretty standard annual flu bug.

In case any of you are still in any doubt about that, let me just remind you of some simple facts. You can check out all these facts quite easily by going to official websites such as the Centers for Disease Control and Prevention in the United States and the World Health Organisation.

First, it is not unusual for the flu to kill well over 600,000 people in a single flu season. Just check out the current death total for the coronavirus, remembering that governments are now admitting that their death totals have been wildly exaggerated. In the UK, for example, patients who tested positive for the coronavirus and then died were put down as having died of the virus – even if they were run over by a bus or battered over the head by a mad axe-man. Once you'd had the disease you could not officially recover from it. This was clearly nonsense. But it was why the total number of deaths built up.

Second, governments everywhere have been talking of the R number. This denotes the number of people who are infected by someone with the virus. But the R number isn't of any great significance. If most people who catch the virus have no or few symptoms and then get better, the disease isn't much of a threat. What really matters is the D number (you won't see that quoted anywhere I'm afraid – it is my own small invention). The D number is the number of people who die of the disease. And it has always been clear that covid-19 is no more of a killer than the flu. The death rates are much the same, and in both cases the people who are most likely to die are the ones who are already seriously ill with something else. It was always a nonsense to lock up the elderly. It was those individuals with pre-existing medical conditions who needed protecting – and this is just as true of the flu as of the coronavirus.

Third, the number of people who have so far caught the coronavirus worldwide is around 10 million. But the number who catch the flu in a pretty standard year can easily hit 1 billion. Even Neil Ferguson, the mathematical modeller who started the chaos, would have to admit that 1 billion is a bigger number than 10 million. So the flu affects more people than the coronavirus. The only reason that the number of deaths with covid-19 seems to be getting close to the total number of flu deaths in a single season is that the number of covid-19 deaths has been massively exaggerated. Let me remind you that in the UK it has been officially recognised that the official number of covid-19 deaths has been massively over-stated because of the policy of counting anyone who ever had the infection as eventually dying of it – whatever they died of. And many people who had flu symptoms were counted as covid-19 deaths. It is also important to remember that total deaths for many countries are just about what they would be in any other year – in some areas fewer people have died this year than died last year for example.

So, what is this all about?

Why have nations around the world deliberately over-stated the threat of a bug which is, it is perfectly clear, no more of a danger than the flu. Why were millions put under house arrest and hospital departments closed? Why have economies everywhere been destroyed?

Well, I don't think it was some sort of global hysteria. I don't think governments everywhere suddenly went pottier than they usually area. And I don't think lots of people made the same mistake in many different countries.

I'm afraid it was, and is, part of a plan.

Malevolent individuals have for centuries dreamt of controlling the world. But their plans have always failed – usually because one mad individual doesn't usually live long enough to see their plans through to fruition.

That isn't to say that there have not been some successes. Mao Tse Tung, Stalin and Hitler all wanted to break down traditional connections so that they could rebuild society and create global citizens. But only China's plan proved really effective – and it was localised to China.

This time, as they say, it is different. This time the takeover of the world involves a good many people and although they have many different aims, they have all taken full advantage of this pre-planned pandemic to further their own ambitions. I know this sounds like a conspiracy theory and if any of you aren't already aware of what is happening then I can only ask you to be patient and to trust me. Unless I am writing fiction I don't make stuff up – though there are inevitably all sorts of lies around on the internet these days. I've dealt with some of the most egregious on my website.

It is difficult to see precisely where everything started but things speeded up when the United Nations got involved, and I think and the first signs of what is happening now may have appeared in 1976 when the UN decided that at some point all private property should be controlled by the United Nations itself.

In the decade or so that followed specific changes were made to education. Instead of teaching children the old-fashioned way, and teaching them to think for themselves, education was redirected and the purpose became to train young people so that they would be useful to society, and to teach them that individualism, and the family, were less important than collectivism.

Anyone who has seen how the teaching syllabus has changed will understand how effective this has been. Children aren't taught real history any more – they are taught a version of history which supports the idea of global living. Nationalism and patriotism have become dirty words and children have been taught to feel guilty for the alleged sins of their ancestors. Colonialism and empire are linked to slavery. For decades now we have been moving slowly towards the idea of social credit for human value. I'll discuss this in a future video but this concept is already alive and thriving in China where individuals get points if they are good citizens and have points deducted if they misbehave. Your rights are then adjusted according to the status of your social credit.

One big move appears to have taken place at a United Nations conference held in Brazil in 1992. The conference seems to have been pretty much under the influence of a variety of powerful groups – the Bilderbergers, the Club of Rome, the Rothschilds, the Rockefellers, the Jesuits and so on. This wasn't a one man plan. For example, it is important to remember that Bill Gates – the number one villain to many was still flogging software in the 1990s. The changes that are now taking place so rapidly were begun when Bill Gates was still running Microsoft – and doing so fairly ruthlessly. The Bill and Melinda Gates Foundation did not exist. At least not publicly.

The ultimate aim was to end national sovereignty, to break down existing, traditional borders and to then restrict movement, to create human settlement zones, to further dumb down education and to set in place actions which would lead to mass global depopulation.

It was, of course, all about power, control and money.

The people who wanted to change the world realised, of course, that they needed something to drive their plan forwards. They needed to start a major panic that they could gradually build up into a fear which would provide an excuse for the changes they wanted to make.

And they decided that they would build their new world order upon climate change – they deliberately created the myth of man-made global warming, carbon taxes and so on. They used the idea of protecting the environment to bring in central global control of all land, private property, energy supplies, production and distribution of food and the control of people.

As I have explained in a previous video, climate change was nothing new even back in the 1990s. The theory had been around since the 19th century and it was always considered pretty potty and nonsensical.

But things really got started in 1991 when the Club of Rome published a book entitled *The First Global Revolution* in which it was boasted that climate change had been invented as a common enemy of mankind in order to unite the world – and thereby bring about the changes required for a world government and a world church.

Everything that has happened in the last thirty years has been a result of that.

And now you understand why so many large corporations and government leaders have, contrary to what you might expect, suddenly become wildly enthusiastic about climate change, global warming, global cooling and whatever else seems fashionable.

People who had never previously shown any interest in environmentalism have suddenly started giving huge amounts of money to green groups and to climate change organisations.

Huge banks and investment groups and hedge funds fell over themselves to line up behind a little Swedish girl who played truant from school and became a figure head for the new global state – though I'm not sure that's what she thought.

The children who had been indoctrinated into believing that the end of the world was just around the corner doubtless believed what they had been told.

In fact, of course, the end of the world as we know it was just around the corner but it wasn't anything to do with climate change. The climate change nonsense was pseudo-scientific gobbledegook that didn't really stand up to examination. People like Prince Charles were brought on board to give the whole thing an air of respectability. The real power brokers did their best to stay in the background.

The fact is that climate change was merely the trigger that would prepare us for the huge changes that the power and money hungry wanted to make.

And they have managed the climate change scare skilfully and with great success. But climate change wasn't moving things fast enough. The United Nations, and those who control it, have a plan called Agenda 21 and they have a number of subsidiary plans – such as Agenda 2030 – which need things to move faster. Agenda 21 is a conspiracy for world domination. It is nothing less than a coup. Many of those who are overseeing the crisis which has been deliberately managed are old. It is fair to assume that they want to speed things up so that they can see some results in their lifetime. And so we now have a plandemic: the coronavirus hoax; the scare story; the biggest crime in human history. And the associated manipulations.Fear has been created globally. Governments everywhere are using psychological warfare tricks to control their populations – if you haven't seen it take a look at my video on brainwashing. The nonsenses about social distancing and masks are deliberately confusing. We are living in a world where our own governments are using psy-op techniques against us. We are being taught and encouraged to distrust our neighbours. We have been deliberately separated from our friends and our families in order to break our spirit and make us accept whatever they force upon us next. Naturally, as I said back in February and again in my first video 'The Coronavirus Hoax', one of the main aims is to trick us into accepting a mandatory vaccination. As yet I have no certain idea why. But I have some theories. And none of them is very nice.

So, that's the basic story; that's a précis of what has happened and why.

July 24th 2020

Vaccination Challenge

Here's a strange thing.

There have, in recent years, been a good many headlines about the dangers posed by kitchen appliances such as refrigerators and tumble dryers.

Newspapers have been full of stories of fridges and dryers suddenly bursting into flames for no good reason at all. There have been headlines, enquiries and questions galore – and manufacturers have been forced to issue recall notices and provide modifications. Consumer magazines have had a field day with reports and scary stories.

There was a story last year that in the UK, half a million owners of tumble dryers were urged to unplug their appliances. One manufacturer who had sold five and a half million appliances was reported to have been responsible for a fault which had caused 750 fires over an 11 year period.

In numerical terms some probably thought the risks seemed to be fairly small – approximately 1 in 7,500 appliances sold.

But that was rightly considered unacceptable.

Now, what I don't understand is that the people who regarded that sort of risk to be a scandal and an outrage and a subject for thousands of column inches of carefully crafted indignation in the press, have not been in the slightest bit concerned by the risks involved in vaccination programmes.

Indeed, the people promoting vaccines never talk about risks at all. They admit that there might be some discomfort, a headache, a fever and so on.

But they don't talk about the big risks: the risk that a patient could be killed or severely brain damaged by a vaccination. Let's put aside the autism risk – which, for some inexplicable reason, seems to drive pro-vaxx defenders into a state of incoherent rage – and concentrate on the risk of death and brain damage.

And here is the surprise: the risks with vaccines aren't particularly small. The serious risks with some vaccines are, of course, fairly low – around one in 100,000 for example.

But the risks with other vaccines are known to be much higher – one in 20,000 or one in 10,000 even.

The figure of 1 in 10,000 for a future vaccine for the coronavirus was mentioned by Bill Gates in an interview in which he said that if seven billion people were, as he planned, given a new coronavirus vaccine then 700,000 people might be damaged.

And with a vaccine, we aren't talking about a need to repaint the kitchen – as might happen after a tumble dryer fire. You can't put vaccine damage right with a few pots of paint, a brush and a new set of curtains.

A paper published in the *Journal of the American Medical Association* reported that seizures occur in about 1 in 640 children with one popular childhood vaccination.

The problems with vaccines are, I repeat, often dismissed as inconvenient symptoms.

But with vaccine damage we can be talking about severe brain damage requiring life-long care. And we're talking about the ultimate side effect – one that none of the pro-vaxxers ever likes to talk about – death.

If you think I am making this up, just ask yourself why the American Government has paid out over $4 billion as a result of vaccine injuries. In the UK, the Government has a standard fee of £120,000 for damage caused by some vaccines. And in the past it has paid out large amounts of money to people damaged by vaccines. And remember that most patients, and their relatives, never make a claim because no one ever admits that the brain damage or the death was caused by a vaccine.

In America, the CDC states that the Vaccine Adverse Event Reporting System receives reports for only a small fraction of adverse events. The quoted figure is that approximately 40 cases of death and permanent injury a year are reported for the MMR vaccine alone but it has been estimated that as few as 1% of serious side effects from medical products are reported. Doctors don't tend to report suspected side effects however serious they are – usually because they are frightened of being sued but also because they don't like to face the fact that a product they have recommended has done so much harm.

Check it out. Do a little research. Ask your political representative – though you may have to wait a while to get a straight answer.

How much fuss do you think journalists and parents would make if it were reported that if a brand of tumble dryer killed or permanently injured 40 children a year?

But journalists concentrate on demonising anyone who dares to suggest that there might, conceivably, perhaps be more problems with vaccinations than is generally accepted. In a number of countries there has been talk of making it an act of terrorism even to mention the fact that vaccines might cause problems.

It is, perhaps, not surprising that Mr Gates has insisted that the manufacturers of any new vaccine against the coronavirus be provided with legal immunity.

If something goes wrong with a vaccine, the manufacturers will be safe. If you haven't already seen it then I urge you to watch my video entitled, 'Would you trust these people with your life?' If you're not terrified, appalled and angry when you've watched it then nothing will ever terrify, appal and anger you.

The bottom line is that the risks with some vaccines are considerably greater than the risk of a fridge or a tumble dryer catching fire.

Why aren't parents and journalists demanding answers and information? Why are so many pro-vaxxers content to remain ignorant and supine?

And there is another problem that dramatically affects the risk.

Most people only have one tumble dryer or one fridge.

But children these days are given dozens of vaccines – one after the other. Vaccine schedules vary from country to country but by the time they're 12, most children will have had a couple of dozen vaccinations. Each one with its own risk.

And there is another hazard.

No one, as far as I have ever been able to find out, has ever done any research to find out how all these different vaccines inter-react in the human body. What do they all do to the immune system? Your guess is as good as anyone else's. No long-term studies are done. No long-term safety tests are done. If they have been done then they seem to have been kept secret – which seems unlikely.

Now, some of the pro-vaxxers will doubtless say that none of this matters because vaccines protect individuals from disease – and save lives.

Well, I am afraid that too seems to be rather doubtful.

The facts show that many vaccinations fail to provide protection for a good many of the people who are vaccinated.

So why on earth are vaccinations so popular? Why are so many otherwise apparently intelligent people so trusting and downright stupid when it comes to vaccines? Are they all just gullible? Rabid? Mad? Or just fanatics who like needles? I honestly don't understand.

But drug companies make billions out of selling them, doctors make tens of thousands each out of giving them, and pro-vaxxers such as the Bill and Melinda Gates Foundation have strewn money about among journalists and a huge variety of apparently independent bodies.

But putting all that to one side, the other reason for giving vaccinations is to provide herd immunity.

Now, the phrase 'herd immunity' has been used a great deal in the last few months. People who have never heard it before now put it into just about every sentence they utter.

Herd immunity simply means that a high number of people in a community have had an infection, or been vaccinated against it, and are therefore considered immune.

If a lot of people are vaccinated, and they acquire immunity to a disease, then there will be fewer cases of that disease in that community.

Not every individual will be protected against disease – because vaccines don't always work.

And some individuals will be damaged because of vaccines.

But the economy will benefit because fewer people will become ill.

Money will be saved because less money will be spent on looking after people in hospital. Fewer people will need to take time off work to look after relatives who are ill. That's the theory and it works as long as there are not more people damaged by the vaccine than are saved.

So the main pro-vaxxer argument is money.

Vaccination costs a good deal of money and kills or injuries some people but it's cost effective.

I am not saying that vaccines shouldn't be given.

I am simply saying that we need more information, we need more testing and we need more truth.

The idea that seven billion people are to be given a new vaccine – when there cannot possibly have been any long-term tests done – terrifies me.

What long-term effects might there be? Could a new vaccine cause cancer? Could it affect fertility?

I have, over the years, offered to debate the issue of vaccination with successive Chief Medical Officers in the UK – live on national television.

The offer has sadly always been met with silence.

So, since that clearly is not going to happen I would now like to talk to or interview the politician at the head of the UK's vaccination programme – Matt Hancock.

Being a politician, Mr Hancock likes being on television. I hate it and don't want to do it. If someone else would like to make the challenge that would suit me fine.

Television companies like good ratings.

Wouldn't this make a worthwhile programme?

I or someone else will simply ask Mr Hancock some simple questions and he could give all the points in favour of vaccination. We could debate the issue and talk about safety and effectiveness. The programme has to be live – not pre-recorded – and it has to be national so that everyone can see it.

I would, for example, like to know why Hancock is so keen to have everyone given a new vaccine when at least 80% of those dying from covid-19 appear to be over 80-years-old and to have many other illnesses. Why, when governments don't seem to care overmuch about the elderly to put it politely, is he so desperately keen to introduce an untried vaccine to protect a small group of people who are usually ignored? The UK Government used the Liverpool Care Pathway to kill off the elderly by starving them and depriving them of fluids. And now they want to vaccinate everyone in the country in order to protect the over 80s? I don't understand.

I'm honestly keen to know what is going on.

And in the US, maybe Dr Fauci would allow someone to interview him live on television – and to debate vaccination with him.

In no other area of life, apart from some areas of national security, is public debate regarded as unacceptable.

Today, it seems that we are back in the days when debate was banned. We have drifted back to the sort of times when Snow, Semmelweiss and Paracelsus were met with dangerous opposition when they dared to question the unquestionable.

Mr Hancock is a fervent supporter of vaccination why wouldn't he want to defend his position on television?

And the public could then decide for themselves.

I'm prepared to put my reputation on the line.

Is Mr Hancock prepared to put his reputation on the line and to defend a vaccine which, it is proposed, will be given to everyone?

If not – why not?

Meanwhile, might I suggest that those reading this might like to include a note on all articles about vaccination in the national press.

Simply ask: if vaccines are so safe, why have governments paid out millions to patients injured by them.

If a tumble dryer manufacturer had paid out over $4 billion in damages wouldn't people want to know why and what for?

Two final small points:

First, I use thousands of books and scientific articles to prepare these short videos. They take every minute of the day. If I were to list all the references for each video there would be only one video a week at most. But the sources aren't difficult to find especially now that the internet exists. Just find reputable sources and don't use the BBC.

Second, I am afraid that there is no longer any available email address for me. So please don't try sending emails. Up to 3,000 people a day were trying to contact me with abuse, questions and comments – and I cannot make videos and reply to emails. If Mr Hancock accepts my challenge then he can simply say so at one of his many press conferences.

July 25th 2020

The Satanic Wars Have Started

We went round the shops when the mask law came in and what a miserable bloody experience it was.

We didn't wear masks, of course, and we had relatively little trouble with shop keepers but we had more than enough trouble from sanctimonious, holier than thou customers who had probably been inspired by the 'shame your neighbour' rhetoric from Cressida Dick, a senior policewoman. If they had been on bicycles they would have doubtless worn helmets with little cameras fitted to them. They listened with surprise when I explained the facts about viruses and masks and mosquitoes and chicken-wire fencing.

I confess that I have never been good with rules. It's something genetic and I can't help it. At school I was always in trouble. Not for fighting but just for refusing to obey the rules. I volunteered for the army cadet force because it was compulsory, and on Fridays we had to wear a horribly itchy brown uniform and parade in the playground. It was raining one Friday so I put my blue gabardine raincoat on top of my uniform. I was shouted at by the sergeant major and made to sit in a warm classroom and read a book. It was a valuable lesson.

On another occasion we went out on an initiative test. We were dropped in a village miles from anywhere and told to answer 20 questions on a sheet of paper we were given. I stopped off at the village shop, bought a bottle of pop and a bag of something bad for me and the lady behind the counter answered all the questions for me. I then sat in a wood and watched the squirrels. I was the only one to get all 20 correct answers and the major in charge asked me why the answers on my sheet of paper were in such neat, feminine writing. I told him the truth. He was very angry. I reminded him that it was an initiative test but I got another black mark and was thrown out of the cadet force. I then had to spend every Friday afternoon sitting in the classroom reading a book. They knew how to punish someone at my school.

When I arrived at university, they told me I had to join the National Union of Students. I said I didn't want to. I didn't know anything about the National Union of Students but I didn't want to join because they said I had to. I quoted some human rights legislation I managed to find and they had to let me not join. It caused chaos for months.

When I went for my first hospital job, an accountant told me that the cost of my board and lodging would be deducted from my first pay cheque. I told them I preferred to give them a cheque. They said they wouldn't do that. I said I'd go home then. They had to reorganise their accounts system.

I've resigned from just about every club I've ever been in and every job I've ever had. Always on a matter of principle.

I tell you all this not out of shame or pride but just to explain why I feel comfortable going the wrong way in supermarkets when they have arrows pasted on the floor. I don't think I've ever gone through a customs post without having an argument with someone and they can be nasty. I can't help myself.

So, we went to the shops the other day and I exchanged words with just about everyone I saw. On the whole it wasn't the staff who were the trouble. With two exceptions they didn't seem to give a damn.

'Where's your mask?' asked one sales assistant.

'I haven't got one on,' I replied with simple honesty, though I did think of saying I was wearing one of the new invisible masks.

'Are you exempt?'

I said I was.

'What's your health problem?' she demanded.

I told her I thought the question was impertinent and irrelevant and intrusive. Shades of Perry Mason.

'Are you planning to discriminate against me because I have a disability?' I asked politely.

'Shall I put down asthma?' she asked. 'That's the usual one.'

And so I think she wrote asthma on her bit of paper.

The next time an assistant asked why I wasn't wearing a mask I said that I was a homicidal psychopath and that my psychiatrist had told me that wearing a mask might trigger an attack.

'But I'll wear a mask if you insist,' I said sweetly.

'Oh no, that's not necessary,' said the assistant very quickly.

On the whole, it was the other customers who demanded to know where our masks were. I took the opportunity on each occasion to explain why masks are useless and dangerous and why our government is untrustworthy.

My only other strange experience was on the pavement outside the greengrocers.

'Are you waiting to go in?' asked a young man.

'They say they're full and I have to wait for someone to leave,' I pointed out.

'Why?' asked the young man, not entirely without reason.

'It's the floor,' I told him. 'It's weak and they're worried that if too many people go in at once it will collapse and deposit everyone in the cellar.'

'Gosh,' he said. 'That's terrible.'

Then, after a pause, he grinned at me. 'I'm very gullible aren't I,' he said.

I told him I had an old lawn mower I could let him have very cheaply. 'It's an antique and probably worth thousands.'

'You can't catch me twice,' he said with an even bigger grin.

It's all very silly.

But it was depressing to see so many people making themselves even more stupid by wearing masks. I saw one young fellow trying to eat a piece of cake with his mask on. He was stuffing bits of cake round the side of the mask. We saw a woman in a mask which matched her blouse. That depressed me. Wearing a mask as a fashion item is akin to slaves wearing Christian Dior outfits while picking cotton.

I saw a bookshop which had a table across the doorway with a notice saying that all customers must use the sanitiser and wear a mask. There were no customers in the shop. I thought about covering my hands with sticky sanitiser and then going into the shop and handling all the books. But I couldn't go in because I wasn't wearing my badge of shame, indoctrination and subservience. A bookshop, for heaven's sake.

In one small shop someone had stuck arrows on the floor to tell us which way to go. Naturally, I went the wrong way. A masked woman, who looked like the Lone Ranger's auntie Flo, had a mild attack of hysterics and jumped sideways into a chocolate biscuit display. One has to take one's amusement where one can these days. We can have no mercy for those who have betrayed us.

A department store refused to take cash printed by the Bank of England so I walked out without buying anything and told an assistant to tell the manager that I had spent thousands of pounds in the establishment over the years but would not patronise them again until they reversed their policy over cash.

At a supermarket, they had a huge poster telling me to be a local hero by wearing a mask. It made me want to weep. Be a slave to terrorism and you are a hero.

Terrorism?

My personal definition of terrorism is 'politics by intimidation without moral restrictions'.

And if you stop and think about it for a moment you will, I think, see that we are all currently victims of terrorism being organised by our own governments and paid for by us.

In the UK our government, which exists to serve the people, is employing the 77th brigade of the British army, which we pay for, to suppress the truth and stifle debate. How can this be legal, let alone morally defensible?

Our lives have been taken over, and are being managed in minute detail, by professional experts in wartime manipulative techniques. The laws we must obey have no basis in reality and are so extraordinarily confusing that no one can understand them. The confusion is, of course, deliberate. The virus is known to affect the frail, the sick and the chronically ill but under the law the elderly were kept prisoner, even though they might have been as fit as fiddles, whereas many of the frail, the sick and the chronically ill were all allowed out as long as they didn't have a picnic or go bowling.

We are put under house arrest, for no logical reason, at the whim of the Government, and kept there until we are allowed out. But when we are allowed out we must keep our distance and we must walk carefully and avoid the cracks in the pavement. We must wear masks if we go into a shop or bank or restaurant but not if we go into an office. We should wear masks in our own homes but only downstairs since the virus doesn't like heights and won't go upstairs. If we go into a department store we must wear masks on the ground floor and in the lifts but not in the restaurant, if there is one or on the higher floors, if there are any. You can stay in a caravan as long as it is more than 18 feet long and only two people at a time can travel in a car which is under 14 feet long. Swimmers must wear masks unless they are drowning. People must not share a mask unless they have been married for at least five years.

In stores the staff do not have to wear masks but the customers must but in restaurants the staff must wear masks but the customers do not have to. If someone goes into a takeaway wearing a mask they must take their food outside to eat it but if they enter not wearing a mask then they can eat food while sitting at a table. We must not talk to friends, sing or do anything that looks like fun. We can play tennis or cricket with one friend as long as the ball we use is wiped with a disinfectant wipe for 30 seconds every time it is handled. If we are

379

professional sports persons, we can play our sport as long as no one watches us. We can enter a place of worship if it is open, as long as we wear a mask and maintain social distancing, but there will be no services, no public worshipping and definitely no singing. We can go into a pub as long as we sit quietly and order our drinks by using our mobile phones, sit quietly at our table and give all our personal details to the person at the door. We cannot play pool, darts or dominoes or take part in quizzes. There can be no live music and we must not approach the bar at any time or for any reason. We can leave our table only to visit the loo and then only after the loo has been thoroughly cleansed and sanitised. We can have our hair cut and our nails polished but hospital physiotherapy departments are still closed. We can visit a dentist if we can find one which is open but we cannot have our teeth filled, so anything aching or painful must be removed. We can go out into the streets to demonstrate for politically acceptable views but we cannot go out into the streets to demonstrate for or against the laws which prevent us leaving our homes. Social distancing laws and laws about wearing masks can be ignored if we are protesting about issues which have been endorsed by left wing politicians but not if we are protesting or campaigning about issues which have been endorsed by right wing politicians. We cannot have picnics with friends or relatives if the picnic is held on the beach, in the park or in our own gardens but we may eat by ourselves in our own homes though we may not go shopping to buy food unless we wear masks. We can jog in a park but we cannot sit on a bench to rest if we are tired. We can have sex indoors with a professional sex worker but if we have sex with a fiancé we must make sure we do it under a blanket and in a garden.

Can you spot which of that is real and which I made up? I'm not sure I can. Nothing makes any sense any more.

We are constantly being warned that there is worse to come. The coronavirus is about to mutate. When it does then it will become far more dangerous. A completely new virus is about to leap from pigs or bats or some other creature and it will kill millions, hundreds of millions or possibly billions. Those who have had the virus do not have permanent immunity and so regular vaccinations will be essential. Next winter's flu is going to be worse than usual. They have said there is going to be much flooding and no doubt when the floods go down there will be massive fires. All this is our fault because we put up too many statues to the wrong sort of people.

We are paying our government and our civil servants to terrorise us.

In the thrall of Satan they and their acolytes are everywhere.
Our world is upside down and it is impossible to guess what will come next.
But meanwhile you and I must continue to aggravate the traitors and the collaborators. It is a war and we are the resistance.

July 26ᵗʰ 2020

BBC Fact Checking Investigated

The other day the BBC's website carried an article entitled:
'Coronavirus: Deadly masks claims debunked'.
The article had two authors with additional reporting by five others.
Only the BBC would have seven people writing one fairly short article.
Their collective aim was to investigate what they called false and
misleading claims about the health risks of face masks being shared on
social media.
Their first target was the claim that masks deprive your body of
oxygen and, surprise surprise, their verdict was this was a false claim.
They quote someone called Professor Keith Neal, described as
infectious diseases expert, who says that 'thin paper or cloth masks
will not lead to hypoxia'. Professor Neal is reported elsewhere to think
that masks or, rather, face coverings may need to be worn indoors.
And they quote the WHO, where the latest view is that 'the prolonged
use of medical masks when properly worn does not cause carbon
dioxide intoxication nor oxygen deficiency'. That view, of course, may
have changed by the time I finish this sentence.
And that appears to be it.
One professor and the WHO – a body which I don't think I am alone in
thinking is about as reliable on health issues as the members of the
Goon Show or the Marx Brothers.
The BBC comes to their debunking conclusion without actually
quoting any research.
Now, I'm sorry children at the BBC, but if you are going to debunk
something you need some proper research.
What about, for example, the fact that the British Government has
stated that citizens don't have to wear masks if they have respiratory
problems of any kind.
Why would they say that if masks didn't make breathing more
difficult?
Breathing, I should perhaps explain to the BBC, involves breathing in
oxygen and breathing out carbon dioxide. It's a natural process –
oxygen in and carbon dioxide out.
And what about the fact that two school boys who were wearing face
masks while running on a track both collapsed and died? It was
surmised that this was probably because the strain on their hearts by
the shortage of oxygen proved fatal. And what about the picture which

appeared on the internet the other day and which showed a lady collapsed in the street with her face mask pulled down from over her mouth and nose.

More significantly, what about the study, involving 53 surgeons, which showed that the longer a mask was worn the greater the fall in blood oxygen levels. It was concluded that this may lead to the individual passing out and it may also affect natural immunity – thereby increasing the risk of infection. It has been reported that an N95 mask can reduce blood oxygenation by as much as 20% and this can lead to a loss of consciousness. Naturally, this can be dangerous for drivers, for pedestrians or for people standing up.

The BBC could have done their own research by buying an oxymeter and a mask. Not scientific but nevertheless revealing.

And there was the study of 212 mask wearing healthcare workers which showed that a third of them developed headaches with 60% needing painkillers to relieve the headache. Some of the headaches were thought to be caused by an increase in the amount of carbon dioxide in the blood or a reduction in the amount of oxygen in the blood.

Another study, this time of 159 young health workers showed that 81% developed headaches after wearing facemasks – so much so that their work was affected.

Sadly, the seven writers working for the BBC didn't quote any of these. Who wants boring research papers cluttering up a debunking? Never mind, how did the BBC do with their second debunking?

This time their target was the claim that masks can cause carbon dioxide poisoning. Their verdict was there was no evidence to support this claim.

Once again they relied on good old Professor Neal who said that carbon dioxide wouldn't be trapped unless you wear a tight fitting mask – which is, incidentally, the type officially recommended. If your mask is all loose and floppy then it will be pretty pointless. Not that masks aren't pretty pointless anyway.

And, er, that seems to be it.

Good old Professor Neal.

However, the fact is that anyone who has a breathing problem will find that a mask makes it worse. It makes sense that some of the carbon dioxide which is breathed out with each exhalation is then breathed in because it is trapped. The problem is that the mask wearer may breathe more frequently or more deeply and if that happens then someone who has the coronavirus may end up breathing more of the virus into their lungs. If a mask is contaminated because it has been worn for too long then the risks are even greater. How long is too long? No one knows. No research has been done as far as I know.

The BBC's third attempt to debunk a claim concerned the claim that masks harm the immune system. I was not surprised to see that the BBC concluded that there was no evidence to support this claim. Once again the BBC's seven writers and fact checkers relied on Professor Neal who said that 'masks may stop germs getting into your mouth or nose so your immune system doesn't have to kick in, but this doesn't mean it is being suppressed'.

Really?

Well, I hate to disagree with the BBC and their one and only outside expert, but if people wear face masks for long periods (months or years) then the absence of contact with the real world might well in my view have a harmful effect on immunity.

Do face masks prevent us developing immunity to particular diseases? This depends on many factors – mainly the effectiveness of the face mask. But in my view if the mask isn't preventing the development of immunity then it probably isn't worth wearing. Not that it's worth wearing anyway. Also there is a risk that the accumulation of the virus in the fabric of the mask may increase the amount of the virus being breathed in. This might then defeat the body's immune response and cause an increase in infections – other infections, not just the coronavirus.

I'm not alone in being concerned about all this. Dr Russell Blaylock, a retired neurosurgeon, reported that wearing a face mask can produce a number of problems varying from headaches to hypercapnia (a condition in which excess carbon dioxide accumulates in the body) and that the problems can include life threatening complications.

Oh, and in New Hampshire, a driver passed out and crashed while wearing a face mask for several hours. The police reported that the driver passed out due to insufficient oxygen intake and excessive carbon dioxide intake.'

And here's something else, from the *British Medical Journal*: 'Face masks make breathing more difficult. For people with COPD, face masks are in fact intolerable to wear as they worsen their breathlessness. Moreover a fraction of carbon dioxide previously exhaled is inhaled at each respiratory cycle. Those two phenomena increase breathing frequency and deepness, and hence they increase the amount of inhaled and exhaled air. This may worsen the burden of covid-19 if infected people wearing masks spread more contaminated air. This may also worsen the clinical condition of infected people if the enhanced breathing pushes the viral load down into their lungs.'

So I think I've got more research on my side than the BBC has managed to dig up.

Sadly, and with great regret, my conclusion is that the BBC is once again wrong, and spreading false comfort which could, in my opinion, be dangerous and potentially deadly.

Their researchers, in my view, really need to look for more than one source.

And, children of the BBC, it is always a good idea to look for a few scientific papers and bits of research to back up your opinions. Ringing up one bloke for a quote isn't really doing your research. The fact is that sadly, not much research has been done into mask wearing. But there is some. Maybe next time you plan on doing a little fact checking you should ask a grown-up to help you.

Please send your complaints to the BBC – which has known financial links with the British Government, the European Union and the Bill and Melinda Gates Foundation.

And if you want the real facts about wearing masks look at my two videos entitled 'Face Masks: Ending the Confusion' and 'Masks (part 2) – The Reasons They Want Us to Wear Them'.

YouTube took down the first of my mask videos but when I protested that it contained nothing but real facts, and that taking it down was a political act, they kindly put it back up.

Oddly, I suspect that the BBC's team of researchers didn't look at my videos or my website. What a surprise that was. I was terribly disappointed and quite shocked.

Finally, once again, my researches show that the BBC is unreliable in my view. If this article had been written by primary school children for a school newspaper I would have given the seven authors 7 out of 100 – for spelling their own names correctly. (I am rashly and magnanimously assuming that they managed this.)

I firmly recommend that if you are British, you avoid giving any money to this terrible and untrustworthy organisation.

You must not do this illegally, of course.

The basic rule, as I understand it, is that you must have a TV licence in the UK if you watch, record or otherwise consume live television. If you don't watch live television then you don't seem to need a licence. I have no idea what streaming is but if you start doing it before a programme ends you need a licence but if you start streaming after a programme has ended you don't need a licence. I checked all that with an article in a rag called, *The Guardian* because I thought that *The Guardian* would not be rotten about the BBC – after all they both have links with Bill and Melinda.

I wish I could stop paying the BBC licence fee myself.

Sadly, I can't do this because I haven't paid the BBC licence fee for years.

July 27th 2020

It's Our Bloody Country – and We Want it Back

So, who are the people who seem now to be running our lives and our world?

I have made a list of some of the people who would go onto my personal list of the most dangerous people on the planet: the folk who I wouldn't like to have round to dinner, if I were the sort of person who liked having strangers round to dinner which I am afraid I am not.

Well, first of course is our self-appointed medical expert Mr Gates, who has more fingers in more pies than anyone would have thought possible for anyone with the normal number of fingers. The other day we asked our TV set if Bill Gates is a psychopath. The answer, from the voice inside the TV was: 'On Wikipedia he is referred to as a pure psychopath.' That was our TV set's opinion not mine but what can you say. It seems that even TV sets have a view on Mr Gates these days.

If there is something nasty and threatening going on anywhere in the world the chances are high that Gates has invested in it.

Gates has been funding scientists at Harvard who are trying to block out the sun's rays in an attempt to stop global warming.

If you haven't heard of this before just stop and think for a moment. The scientists want to spray millions of tons of dust into the stratosphere to stop the sun's rays reaching the earth.

One plan is that every day more than 800 large aircraft would lift millions of tons of chalk dust to a height of 12 miles above the Earth and then sprinkle the dust to stop the sun's rays getting through.

Another plan is to send up hot air balloons to release powder into the atmosphere.

There are, you won't be surprised to hear, a couple of problems with this.

Obviously, the first is that no one has yet proved that global warming is taking place and is anything more than a natural phenomenon even if it is. Moreover, there are a lot of scientists who believe that we are heading into a phase where the planet is actually cooling.

And there are those who think that the Gates' money and the scientists throwing powder into the sky could help create droughts, hurricanes and mass deaths. It seems fairly well agreed that altering the atmosphere to cool the planet could have unpredictable effects. In 1815, a volcanic eruption created crop shortages and disease outbreaks.

Some might say, of course, that all this could be considered a bonus by a man who wants to reduce the world population.

No one seems to have told him, by the way, that 800 large aircraft taking off every day and flying to 12 miles up, would require a good deal of aviation fuel. And what sort of dust are they planning to have sprayed? Well, some say calcium. But I have also heard talk that barium, alumina and strontium might be used. Whatever it is won't improve the quality of the air we breathe. Bottom line is that this seems to me to be a way to reduce the world's population rather than protect it – all in the guise of dealing with the climate change hoax.

And then there is George Soros.

Let me tell you something about George Soros. He is a man who has apparently admitted that he is here to make money and he's done well at it. He's alleged to have 25 billion dollars in his piggy bank. The mainstream media describe him as a philanthropist though to be honest if he still has 25 billion dollars he hasn't given too much of it away.

One of the most chilling interviews I have ever seen was in 1998 when Soros was interviewed for the `60 Minutes' programme. I found it scary. Soros admitted that when he was a teenager he worked with the Nazis to confiscate property from the Jews.

'Did he feel bad about it? Was it difficult?'

'Not at all difficult,' he said. He felt no guilt.

I can't remember whether he actually said it or not but the implication was clear: if he didn't do it someone else would have done.

These days Soros is rumoured to give money to the Black Lives Matter and to Antifa.

Now why would he do that? Is there, perchance, profit to be made?

Could it be, perhaps, that he is deliberately trying to stir up trouble so that it is easier to break down society ready to accept the global reset he and his co-conspirators are so keen on?

Who else would make the list?

Well, the seemingly brainwashed little Swedish girl, of course. Her bleating and whining about the end of the world has proved enormously useful to those pushing Agenda 21 and the Global Reset and the plans for a New World Order.

Personally, I think she has been used very cleverly by the black-hearted folk who needed a seemingly innocent front for the climate change nonsense – they needed someone who seemed innocent and honest and whom it would be very difficult for critics to question or to attack.

How the devil can you ask serious questions of a little Swedish girl who looks to be about seven-years-old and very earnest?

But she, and all the other Greens, definitely go onto my list of people I don't like.

Oh, and I include Greenpeace in there too. Let me tell you a little something about Greenpeace – gold medal winners of my Sanctimonious Organisation Year Award for the last 287 years.

Greenpeace campaigns to have the world's oil left in the ground.

But in 2014, a Greenpeace senior executive was reported to have been commuting by plane for two years. The employee, who had been flying regularly from Luxembourg to Amsterdam, was defended by the Executive Director of Greenpeace UK who seemed to think it was acceptable for the employee to fly so much so that 'he could balance his job with the needs of his family'.

In February 2020, Greenpeace bought a full page advertisement in the *Financial Times* to reprint a letter that the Executive Director of Greenpeace UK had sent to BP, the oil company. The letter, demanding an end to the use of fossil fuels, was, in my view, the most arrogant letter I have ever read.

I can only assume that Greenpeace would nevertheless like BP to continue making a small amount of fuel available for planes used by its employees.

That level of hypocrisy seems to me to be so great that it is impossible to measure.

Next on my list, and something of a newcomer, goes the boss of the Metropolitan Police in London.

On the day before it became the law that English citizens had to wear masks in shops (for no very good reason that I could think of), Cressida Dick, the Police Commissioner for the Metropolitan Police in London, and not as far as I know a doctor of medicine, was reported to have said that the police will only enforce the law on wearing face masks as a last resort.

'My hope,' she was quoted as saying, 'is that the vast majority of people will comply, and that people who are not complying will be shamed into complying or shamed to leave the store.'

Of course, as we should all remember, Cressida Dick should know all about shame. She was, of course, the officer who made the decision for the police to shoot a young innocent Brazilian man in 2005. Police apparently shot eleven times from close range. They managed to shoot the entirely innocent man seven times in the head and once in the shoulder.

'I think about it quite often,' Dick allegedly said last year while chatting on a BBC programme called Desert Island Discs. Quite often? Most people, I suspect, would think about it pretty well all the time.

I suspect I am not alone in thinking she should have been sacked after an innocent citizen was shot and killed. I certainly called for it at the time.

Instead she now has a top police job and believes that those choosing not to damage their health by wearing useless masks should be made to feel ashamed. I am not entirely sure that encouraging other shoppers to shame non-mask wearers is entirely within Ms Dick's role in the police.

And does this woman not realise that the Government has made it clear that people with health problems – including anxiety – do not have to wear masks? And nor do young children. Is she suggesting that these individuals, who may be fearful for many reasons, be deliberately shamed? Are the police officially suggesting that patients with respiratory and heart disease be deliberately shamed? Is Dick suggesting that those with mental health problems be shamed? Does she want us to run after the disabled who cannot wear masks and smother them with abuse? How precisely would she like people to shame their fellow citizens?

My contempt for Cressida Dick is endless.

We should all join together to demand that this woman be officially shamed and sacked. An apology isn't enough.

Write to your MP. Write to the newspapers. If you do nothing else today, do what you can to get this woman fired. She is an utter disgrace to the human race in my view. I cannot believe it. Encouraging people to shame the sick and the frail and the anxious and the mentally ill! And shaming children!

It is, I believe, at least partly as a result of her urging that I have seen non-mask wearers being shouted at in shops.

A civilised society discusses complex issues by debate. But in our society debate is banned. And instead of discussing the issues with the opposition, the Gates and Soros supporting, mask wearing, line toeing folk, encourage the routine shaming and humiliation of those who do not agree to click their heels and salute those who would run our lives, control our every moment and enslave us with an unending variety of laws which have little or no basis in science.

Finally, on this short list of a few of those whom I hold in contempt, are the collaborators: the mindless millions who are willingly wearing masks and kowtowing to the dictators who want to rule our lives and are using, as an excuse a virus which is no more deadly than the flu.
How many of those who are currently wearing masks in shops wore them last year to protect themselves against the flu?
And, if they didn't wear masks to protect themselves against the flu, why didn't they?
The risks were then much as they are today.
Our main enemies in this war are not Soros, Gates, the little Swedish girl, Dick or the rest of them.
Our main enemies are the collaborators who are too damned lazy to seek out the truth for themselves.
I reserve my greatest contempt for them.
It's our bloody country and we want it back.

July 28th 2020

Why There Are So Many Zombies

'Getting and spending we lay waste our powers,' wrote William Wordsworth, the Lakeland poet in a rare moment when he wasn't being mesmerised by daffodils.

These days he would have to rewrite that, changing it to: 'Worrying and obeying we lay waste our powers'.

That's what is happening today.

The new abnormal, whereby our every movement, small ambition and thought is controlled and constricted by laws which make about as much sense as an episode of Patrick McGoohan's magnificent TV series, The Prisoner (of which, I confess, I am constantly reminded these days) deteriorates daily, advancing into ever more absurd realms of Orwellian fantasy.

Those of us who know for certain that something is wrong now waste much of our time trying to unravel the complexities of the new world order which has been foisted upon us; the Gordian knot of our times. We venture down rabbit holes, into dark caves and up beanstalks looking for clues.

The fact, of course, is that many people are responsible for the confusion and the fear which now rules our lives.

The politicians, the medical and scientific advisors, the global organisations with their agendas and the billionaires who apparently want to gain ever more riches, control and power would be at the top of most people's lists of suspects. And then there are the drones of Common Purpose, carefully brainwashed into thinking that they are in control, the new top rank citizens, when in reality they are merely in place as facilitators; present to ensure that the will of their masters is carried out without question.

And, of course, the idiots who don't bother to question anything they are told but who merrily wear their silly masks, maintain social distancing and obey every new damned silly law as though their lives depended upon it, are also on the list. They will soon wear their masks all the time – indoors or out of doors. They will willingly put on gloves every time they leave home. They will wash their hands ever more frequently in a vain attempt to rinse away a threat that almost certainly isn't there to be washed away. Their pathetic compliance has strengthened their own enemies but they trust what they are told and so they are doomed. The danger is that they will drag us down with them.

They think they are behaving sensibly but they are collaborators, traitors to the human race, guilty of stupidity and ignorance more than anything else. Their misplaced trust and their contemptible weakness are enabling the enemy.

Without their obedience the people who are trying to destroy our civilisation would get no-where.

The protestors tearing down statues, attacking buildings and attempting to destroy every artefact and memory of our history are playing straight into the hands of those who want to destroy the past, good or bad, in order to rebuild a new world of permanent slavery. By denouncing those who do not appear to think acceptably about racial or gender issues they are aiding and abetting the greatest enemy the human race has ever faced.

The climate change protestors who make so much noise and who are filled with a sense of self-righteousness, self-satisfaction and unparalleled smugness are behaving like crazed lemmings – taking us over the edge of the cliff and down onto the rocks where the survivors will fall into the hands of a bunch of truly evil men and women whose motives may be cloaked in the false colours of philanthropy or well-meant desires to eradicate poverty or hunger but which are, in truth, no more than selfish yearnings for the traditional triumvirate of power, control and money.

The problem, of course, is that simple-minded citizens who wear their masks with so much pride that they pick out colours and styles as though they were choosing any other new accessory, don't understand that they are being lied to.

They are suffering from something called cognitive dissonance: they cannot believe that they are living in a world where nothing is as it was. The lie is simply so huge, so complete, that they cannot accept that anyone would be so evil as to tell it. Maybe they haven't heard of Goebbels and Hitler, who believed that if you told a big enough lie no one would believe it to be a lie because they wouldn't be able to conceive of people being prepared to tell it.

You can see them walking around anywhere these days. They look and behave like zombies, as though they are under a spell.

But there is another group which is helping to make all this work: the mass market media.

Without the media, the manipulators would not have been able to pull off their coup.

And they are at it everywhere in the world.

In *The Spectator* magazine the other day I read an article on the coronavirus by someone called Matthew Parris who tossed into his article the words, 'it's killing millions worldwide and threatening to overwhelm health provision'.

With rubbish like this in print it's hardly surprising that there are so many zombies or covid fearing idiots around.

The total death number for covid-19 has officially passed half a million – but that is now recognised to be an absurd exaggeration. And I really don't think anyone other than Mr Parris seriously believes that covid-19 is now threatening to overwhelm health provision.

However, I doubt if any organisation is quite so adept at control through misinformation as the BBC – once known for its integrity and reliability but now, I believe, hated and reviled in Britain as never before.

And rightly so.

Distrust the Government, Avoid Mass Media and Fight the Lies.

July 29ᵗʰ 2020

Global Nightmare: Staying Sane During the Madness

The lies and the widespread fear-porn promoted by governments and mainstream media have terrified millions.

But they're terrified of the wrong things. They're terrified of something proven to be no more deadly than the flu.

The coronavirus is worthy of respect. All infective organisms need to be respected.

But the coronavirus was never going to destroy our world.

Today, the real terrors are far greater than a pesky virus. Paranoia is no longer a medical condition to be suspected and feared. It is the only way to live.

The collaborators, the mask wearing zombies who are playing their part in this deliberate takeover of our lives have never heard of Agenda 21, of course. They think the United Nations is a benevolent, well-meaning organisation which does good things around the world. They believe that the World Health Organisation is independent and honourable. They have no idea that a group of global organisations are now reaching the final stages of their long-planned aim to take over the world. They don't understand that the myth of climate change has been steadily built up over thirty years simply to provide an excuse for the Global Reset that the enemy talk about with such enthusiasm.

They don't realise that the Bill and Melinda Gates Foundation is helping to fund a plan to block out the sun – a plan that will help destroy traditional farming. They don't realise that the Bill and Melinda Gates Foundation has also invested heavily in Monsanto – the company which makes genetically modified seeds – and in a company which makes artificial meat. They don't see the links.

They don't realise what chemtrails are for – or, even, that they exist at all.

There are millions who still believe the lies printed daily in the mainstream media and broadcast daily and worldwide by treacherous organisations such as the BBC.

The truth is that if you aren't angry, bewildered, overwhelmed and terrified out of your wits then, as my old Aunt Agatha used to say, you haven't been paying attention.

The simple-minded believers sigh with relief when their politicians tell them that it will all be over by Christmas. They believe it. But the only way it will all be over by Christmas will be if we are all walking around with our masks and gloves on and our sleeves rolled up begging for vaccinations.

(The gloves will, I suspect, be their next move in the humiliation process. Our government's aim is to destroy our strength, our will, our humanity. If you need some light relief watch my video entitled, 'New Law: Everyone Must Now Hop and Wear Galoshes'.)

Ah, yes, the vaccines.

If you haven't seen my video entitled, 'Would you Trust These People With Your Life?' then I beg you to watch it. If you've seen it watch it again. Insist that everyone you know watch it and then watch it again. I described in the video the backgrounds of the companies making our new vaccines.

Consider GlaxoSmithKline – also known as GSK.

GSK is one of the world's biggest pharmaceutical companies and in my view if it made toasters you'd never buy a toaster from them.

In 2014, for example, GSK was fined $490 million dollars by China after a Chinese court found it guilty of bribery. In 2006, GSK paid out $160 million for claims made by patients who had become addicts. In 2009, GSK paid out $2.5 million to the family of a three-year-old born with severe heart malformations. And in Canada, a five-year-old girl died five days after an H1N1 flu shot and her parents sued GSK for $4.2 million. The parents' lawyer alleged that the drug was brought out quickly and without proper testing as the federal government exerted intense pressure on Canadians to get immunised. In 2010, GSK paid out $1.14 billion because of claims over a drug called Paxil. And they settled lawsuits over a drug called Avandia for $500 million. In 2011, GSK paid $250 million to settle 5,500 death and injury claims and set aside $6.4 billion for future lawsuits and settlements in respect of the drug Avandia. In 2016, GSK paid out $6.2 million in Canada.

In 2012, GSK pleaded guilty to federal criminal offences including misbranding of two antidepressants and failure to report safety data about a drug for diabetes to the FDA in America. The company admitted to illegally promoting Paxil for the treatment of depression in children and agreed to pay a fine of $3 billion. That was the largest health care fraud settlement in US history. GSK also reached a related civil settlement with the US Justice Department. The $3 billion fine also included the civil penalties for improper marketing of half a dozen other drugs.

GSK is one of the top earning vaccine companies in the world. And in 2010, there were reports of narcolepsy occurring in Sweden and

Finland among children who had the H1N1 swine flu vaccine. It is reported that not all the safety problems were made public. I have seen a report that by December 2009, for each one million doses of the vaccine given, about 76 cases of serious adverse events were reported though this was not made public.

The British Government paid out £60 million to patients who had been damaged by GSK's Pandemrix vaccine which was then said to affect one in 16,000 individuals. GSK had demanded that the Government indemnify it against claims for damages.

In Ireland, the Irish Government kept inviting people to get vaccinated even when it was clear that the pandemic was on the wane and it was nowhere near the catastrophe portrayed by influenza researchers, governments, industry and the media.

Clare Daly, a member of the Irish parliament, called the adverse effects after Pandemrix a 'completely avoidable catastrophe'. She reported that: 'The Health Service Executive decided to purchase Pandemrix and continued to distribute it even after they knew it was dangerous and untested.'

Most people in Britain will, I suspect, have heard of Sir Patrick Vallance. He is helping to lead the fight against the coronavirus. Vallance is the Chief Scientific Adviser in the United Kingdom and, I suspect, a key figure in dealing with the coronavirus in the UK and the plans for a vaccine.

And yet how many know that Vallance worked for GSK between 2006 and 2018. By the time he left GSK, he was a member of the board and the corporate executive team. All of the fines and so on which I have listed took place while Vallance was working as a senior figure at GSK.

Check it all out. And share the information with everyone you know. Spreading the word will help us survive – both individually and collectively.

I find that every new answer brings with it a host of new questions. Every realisation arouses another barrage of questions. Trying to understand the big picture is like trying to do a jigsaw puzzle while sitting on a playground swing.

We know that part of the Global Reset is a plan to combine all religions together into a new World Religion which may or may not be called Chrislam.

As I described in my video entitled, 'How they are lying to enslave us', Chrislam, an attempt to combine Christianity with Islam, has been around for some time but it is now progressing rapidly.

I wonder if it is a coincidence that churches may now be open but are not providing services. Is it a coincidence that cathedral and church choirs are being shut down – and not just because the coronavirus doesn't like us to sing. Is it just a coincidence that Notre Dame cathedral in Paris burnt down. And that the same thing happened to the cathedral in Nantes.

The coronavirus hoax is the biggest crime in history. But the climate change nonsense is close behind. The whole recycling nonsense was introduced simply to keep us busy and under control. It was a prelude to the mask wearing. If they'll wash out their empty yoghurt cartons with fresh water – known to be the world's most essential, valuable and rarest consumable – then they'll put up with anything.

The stuff that was sorted into half a dozen different containers was never sensibly recycled. Much of Britain's recycling went to China to be dumped. Then it went to Poland. Most recently it was being dumped in Turkey. And it wasn't being dumped in special pits – it was being dumped by the roadside. If you dump stuff near your home it's called littering or fly tipping. If it is dumped for you in another country then it's called recycling.

In Europe, the whole recycling nonsense was an EU initiative. It was and is part of the process of suppressing and controlling us. The EU has for years been linked to Agenda 21 and the United Nations' plan for global control. It is no surprise that the individuals who opposed Brexit, and who supported the EU with some unprincipled venom, are now coming out as keen supporters of Agenda 21.

Things are happening very fast now and before we know what has happened the UN will have given us its World Government and its World Church – whether we like it or not.

All the information is available on the internet. I've given you all the clues you need. This is definitely, most definitely, not a conspiracy theory.

The only conspiracy is the one leading towards a World Government and a World Church.

And underneath it all there is the huge nonsense called climate change. In 1991, the Club of Rome published a book entitled *The First Global Revolution* in which it admitted to inventing climate change as a common enemy of mankind in order to unite the world.

I wonder if young Greta knows of that. I wonder if Prince Charles has even heard of it. Somehow I doubt it.

But it really can't get any clearer.

That is what the climate change campaign was all about – preparing us for a global reset. And that is what the coronavirus nonsense is all about.

Our world is in turmoil. History everywhere is being turned upside down as national identities are deliberately destroyed. Racism is being deliberately built up by aggressive well-funded agitators. Gender choice is destroying everything we know about society and about our past, our present and our future. People now have to put he/him or she/her after their names in order to denote their choice of sex. Anyone who doesn't toe the officially approved line on all these issues quickly becomes a non-person, an unemployable pariah.

You'd have to be mad as a March hare not to be deeply disturbed and genuinely depressed by what is happening.

Those of us who see through the lies are enraged both by the lies which are told and by the fear of what is going to come next.

Personally, I would rather we were fighting a traditional war. I genuinely believe that the risks to physical and mental health would be lighter.

Anxiety and sleeplessness are commonplace. I know I am not alone in having difficulty sleeping. The nightmares are a regular part of my nights.

I spend nearly all my time researching and thinking about what is happening, and analysing how best we can deal with the mental and spiritual effect of this outrageous removal of our civil and human rights, our freedom and our freedom of speech.

Meanwhile, we at least have the knowledge that we are none of us alone.

Millions of people around the world are as enraged as we are.

We have to turn that rage into determination to overcome those who are determined, for whatever reason, to remove our basic rights as citizens.

And when we have won the war we all have to make sure that we make changes to our entire political system so that nothing like this can happen again. They've been planning this takeover for decades. We have to start planning now.

Meanwhile, I believe that the best way to tackle the depression is to do everything possible to defend ourselves, our history and our humanity.

For example, in the UK the law states that citizens must wear masks when entering shops. But, as I speak, we don't have to wear a mask if we have a valid reason not to – a physical or mental condition for example. Asthma or anxiety are apparently acceptable reasons.

So, if you have a valid reason not to wear a mask then go out with a naked face. But if possible don't go alone. Go with friends. Look for people you can go shopping with and who also don't need to wear a mask because of an exemption. Don't break the law, of course, though you will have to check what the law is on an almost daily basis because laws seem to change with the wind.

And if you positively have to wear a mask because there is only one shop in your village and they won't let you in without a mask then wear the damned thing but protest politely and explain why masks are useless and dangerous.

If my wife has to go to hospital and they change the rules and let me in then I will wear a mask if that is a condition of my entering the building. At the moment, the hospital physiotherapy department is still shut because of the coronavirus. Hairdressers, pubs, restaurants, gyms and so on are open. But some hospital departments – including physiotherapy – are still closed. There is no good reason for this so it must be a bad reason.

Try to find people you can talk to, people who think the way you do. We have to stick together. Take time out to enjoy books and films which entertain and relax. Spend time on old hobbies and pastimes and find new ones. We have to protect and treasure some of our life – or they will win anyway.

And if you are alone then tune in here at around 7 p.m. each evening. We'll try to put up a new video each evening about then. If there isn't a new video then hunt around for it, because they do seem to get hidden. And if you still can't find one go to my website where we will hope to be able to put up news.

July 30th 2020

We Are Prisoners of War

The politicians and the psychologists are running what they think is a clever game. They are trying to confuse us by changing the laws and giving very little warning.

I hope, for example, that viewers took note of my advice not to take a holiday abroad this summer. Those who flew off to Spain and suddenly found themselves having to go into quarantine for two weeks will wish they'd gone to Bridlington instead.

We have to remember that there isn't anyone in the Conservative Government who could remove the childproof top from a bottle of aspirin tablets. They aren't the brightest of God's creatures and most of them have IQs smaller than their hat size. The armies of scientists, mathematical modellers and psychologists and lunatics let out of the asylum for the duration, are screwing up our world with the sort of determination you might expect of a bunch of hooray Henrys trying to put toothpaste on their own toothbrushes or, heaven forbid, tie their own shoe laces.

Prince Charles, enthusiastic climate change nutter and aficionado of the Global Reset, will know what I mean about the toothpaste on the toothbrush. He is said to have always had a valet to do that for him so the stuff would doubtless be on his shoes and the ceiling if he had to try to do it all by himself. And he'd probably strangle himself if he tried to tie his own shoelaces – thereby proving that there is plenty of mileage in the old adage, much favoured by my Aunt Agatha, who once worked as a Lady in Waiting in one of the European monarchies: 'There's no tosser like a Royal tosser'.

The chaos our would-be leaders are deliberately creating is being helped along by the fact that up in Scotland the Sturgeon woman is doing everything she can to ensure that everyone realises that Scotland is not the same as England. The bloke who claims to run Wales, and whose name I cannot for the life of me remember and can't be bothered to look up because to be honest who gives a damn, seems to be doing much the same thing.

So, I discovered the other day that whereas blood donors in England must wear masks at all times, or they won't be allowed to give blood, the people in Wales who are generous enough to offer half an armful of blood must remove their masks for safety reasons so that if they go pale and start to faint this can be spotted.

I have to say the Welsh theory makes far more sense than the one being favoured in England.

I have no idea what the law is in Scotland at the moment. I wouldn't mind betting, however, that it will be something different to the laws in England and Wales. And probably something a little barking. Maybe in Scotland blood donors have to wear a Tam O'Shanter over their faces, or wear a kilt in the Sturgeon tartan and pull it up over their faces as they are being phlebotomised.

You would have a job to find a better example of the lunatic way this whole psy-op is being managed.

No one can possibly take such madness seriously. I know we have to take them seriously because they're trying to take over the world but honestly it's difficult not to laugh at them all.

Everywhere I look I find evidence that governments are talking absolute gibberish – and treating their citizens the way you might expect them to treat a full blooded enemy.

Look at what has happened in Quatar for example. Quatar is one of the richest nations on earth but when they introduced a contact tracing app, many low earning workers had to borrow money in order to buy the sort of new, up to the minute phones needed to download the app.

And why did they bother buying the phones and downloading the app? Simple. Not having the official app installed on your phone could lead to a fine of up to $55,000 or three years in prison.

The app, developed by a private firm, requires access to the files on the phone and permanent use of the GPS and Bluetooth.

And the police have apparently been stopping motorists to check that they had their phones with them and that the required App was up and running.

And that created a problem for some citizens who didn't have the phone required to run the app.

They didn't dare leave their homes to buy one in case they were stopped on their way to the phone shop.

Three years in prison for not having an app on your phone.

Back in the UK, mask wearing has become the law and there are still politicians and scientists telling us that we should wear masks to save the community. Be a local hero by wearing a mask.

But there is absolutely no decent science to prove that masks are of any help.

Indeed, on the contrary, the evidence shows that they probably do more harm than good. I have already detailed the evidence about masks in several videos but here is another piece of scientific evidence.

At the beginning of what was a hoax and has now morphed into a crime, it was decided that there was no evidence that wearing a mask would help healthy individuals avoid infections with viruses such as covid-19.

On 6th April, the World Health Organisation said that there was no evidence that masks would help. Numerous medical experts repeated that.

There has been no evidence since then that could have persuaded the WHO to change its collective mind. I think the change was political. Indeed, I have been reminded of yet another paper, published in the BMJ Open in 2015, which I quoted some time ago and which seems to suggest cloth masks are, shall we be polite and say, offer limited protection against respiratory infection.

The study, led by the University of New South Wales, but covering medical workers in Vietnam studied 1,607 workers, some wearing heavy duty medical masks, some wearing ordinary cloth masks and some just wearing usual hospital protection. The study showed that the subjects wearing cloth masks had higher rates of infection than anyone – including the control group. The researchers also measured the masks to see how many particles got through – they found that cloth masks allowed 97% of particles through.

And as I have shown in other videos on mask wearing, the evidence shows that wearing a mask can lead to illness and, possibly, worse.

As I showed in my video about the BBC's fact checkers, masks can cause real health problems. Hypoxia, low blood oxygen levels, is a very serious problem which should not be dismissed.

You'd have to be an idiot not to be able to see that masks do far more harm than good.

The only possible conclusion, of course, is that we are being pushed into wearing masks for simply political reasons. Masks are part of the oppression.

Why, then aren't all doctors screaming out about the pointlessness and danger of forcing people to wear masks for many hours a day?

So why are so many doctors so silent?

Fear and cowardice, I am afraid.

Doctors have been ordered to keep quiet about anything relating to coronavirus which is critical of the Government's line.

This is pretty well a global clampdown.

If doctors had found the courage to ignore the orders they were given and to speak out, in order to protect their patients and save lives, then this whole criminal enterprise would have been over weeks ago.

But doctors have feebly followed the philosophy 'keep your head down' and 'don't rock the boat'. Or, to stick in another piece of nauseating, nautical self-protection: 'don't make any waves'.

It surprises me, and saddens me enormously, that members of the medical and nursing professions have accepted this takeover of our lives.

Even if they don't think there is anything sinister behind what is happening they must by now realise that the whole response to the coronavirus has been wrong.

Hospitals have been closed. Patients with cancer and other serious disorders have been denied essential treatment. Thousands of patients in care homes have been murdered as a result of inept policies and management. Schools have been closed and the lives of millions of children have been ruined. They know that is no exaggeration. The Government has been employing brain washing techniques to control us and to create a fake affection for the health service.

Doctors and nurses all know this is true. They know that the clever three word, three phrase slogans, the encouragement to take part in weekly clapping sessions and the advertising were all designed to build up the fear and to create a sense of national obedience.

Medical doctors and nurses know that the spin doctors have been doing everything they can to exaggerate the number of deaths. Patients with the coronavirus were listed as having died of it.

If the truth about what has happened ever emerges then the medical and nursing professions are going to be embarrassed and humiliated to put it kindly. People in both professions are going to go to jail, I think. It is time to insist that hospitals and clinics are opened immediately without any of the social distancing which every thinking person knows was never necessary.

The media has found many curious heroes in the last three months, mostly as part of the propaganda process I'm afraid. Now is the time for the professions to earn their plaudits. The nation needs to have its health service back. It would be a big step forward on the road back to real normality – and it would destroy the not so hidden agenda of the United Nations, Bill Gates and company.

It hurts me to have to say this but I have nothing but contempt for the doctors and nurses who have kept silent through all this. Their cowardice in refusing to stand up to the politicians and the bureaucrats has already led to millions of deaths worldwide. And things are getting worse by the day.

'I'm just doing my job,' say the silent ones. 'I have my family to think of.'

Where have we heard that before?

And no doctor today is going to be executed for speaking out.

It isn't just doctors who have betrayed us, of course.

The majority of the professions have done so.

Teachers betrayed their pupils and their responsibilities to them by insisting on absurd and inhuman social distancing rules. And I gather that some are now demanding that pupils wear masks when schools finally reopen in the autumn. There is absolutely no scientific reason for pupils to be required to wear masks or to obey any daft social distancing rules. If teachers would make the effort to look at the science they would realise this.

The clergy have betrayed us too. By closing churches and by agreeing not to hold services they have betrayed their parishioners and their God. Now their leaders are negotiating for a universal global religion which makes as much sense as combining all sports into one. Can you imagine the fuss if it were suggested that football, cricket, golf, tennis, hockey and so on should all be combined into a single sport? Well, that's the madness being promoted by Tony Blair and senior churchmen.

The people who have come out of this with my great respect are the postmen and women, the delivery drivers, the rubbish collectors, the shop assistants and the transport workers – all of whom have done their jobs throughout.

Henry David Thoreau has long been one of my favourite authors. He is best known, of course, for Walden but I have been re-reading his short book 'On Civil Disobedience' which, not surprisingly, contains much advice which seems well suited to our peculiar, current circumstances. Here's one quote: 'It is not desirable to cultivate a respect for the law, so much as for the right. The only obligation which I have the right to assume, is to do at any time what I think is right.'

And then there is this: 'Law never made men a whit more just; and, by means of their respect for it, even the well-disposed are daily made the agents of injustice.'

And finally, for now: `All men recognise the right of revolution; that is, the right to refuse allegiance to, and to resist, the Government, when its tyranny or its inefficiency are great and unendurable. But almost all say that such is not the case now.'

But, of course, it is the case now.

We have to stand up to our tyrannical governments.

And if doctors and nurses stood up together and told the truth – that's all they have to do – tell the truth – then the people would see the extent of the lies, governments would fall and the coup would be over. If it doesn't happen soon, it will be too damned late.

July 31st 2020

Why Genetic Engineering Must Stop!

Science has, during the last few decades, presented us with a steadily increasing and apparently endless variety of moral dilemmas and practical threats. The subject of genetic engineering is a perfect example of how politicians have betrayed us all and are, through their refusal to take on big industry, threatening our very future.

In just a few decades genetic engineering has evolved so rapidly as a branch of science (if science is the right word for a form of alchemy which seems to pay little or no attention to logic or research) that the future of our species is now threatened. Genetic engineering enables scientists to transfer genes between species in an entirely unnatural way. Human genes can be transferred to pigs, sheep, fish or bacteria. And genes from bacteria, slugs, elephants, fish, tomatoes and anything else can be put into human beings.

Genetic engineering started in the 1970s. The technique involves putting genes from one species into another species. In order to do this, the genetic engineers put the genes they want to move into viruses. They then put the virus into the animal or plant which is to be the recipient.

It is important to understand that genetic engineering is nothing at all like conventional breeding techniques.

Listen to the boastful, extraordinarily arrogant claims of genetic scientists and you might believe that they had all the answers to hunger and disease. They talk grandly about eradicating starvation by creating new high yield, pest resistant versions of existing foods and manipulating genes to banish physical ailments, aggression and depression. They will, they say, be able to control the overpopulation problem, purify water supplies, remove crime from our streets and deal with deforestation.

Genetic engineers have even talked of modified strains of bacteria able to eat up plastics, heavy metals and other toxic wastes.

Vast amounts of money have been poured into identifying the human genome (the genetic blue print for human life). There has even been talk that we will be able to clone ourselves so that we need never die. Moral and ethical questions have been brushed aside as the unnecessary anxieties of ignorant Luddites who either do not understand what is going on or are temperamentally opposed to progress.

But if it all sounds too good to be true — and all rather reminiscent of the sort of cheap promises with which confidence tricksters make their money — that is because it simply isn't true. Genetic scientists don't have the answers to any of our problems. On the contrary, they have created a hugely successful money making myth which keeps them in fat grants and huge salaries. It is important not to underestimate the importance of money in the world of genetic engineering.

None of this would matter too much if what they were doing was harmless. But fiddling around with genes is an exceedingly hazardous business. Messing around with genes can cause cancer.

It is time that the insane burblings of the geneticists were exposed for what they are. I have been writing about the horrors of genetic engineering for over 40 years but most doctors, critics and journalists have so far been too frightened to oppose the torrent of undiluted praise for genetic engineering.

When genetic engineering first hit the headlines, the public was promised that there would be strict rules about just what could and could not be done. But the rules that were intended to protect us have been bent, pushed aside and ignored. Regulations were, it was claimed, slowing down progress, interfering with the competitiveness of the developing new industry and getting in the way of individual scientists keen to get on with their plan for improving the world.

Genetic engineers claim that there is no need for caution and that only the narrow-minded and the reactionary have reservations about this exciting new branch of scientific endeavour.

But the fact is that the genetic engineering industry has succeeded in 'persuading' politicians and administrators that there is no need to segregate genetically engineered produce from naturally grown produce and yet the risks associated with genetic engineering are numerous and widespread.

There is little doubt that genetic engineering is at least partly responsible for the problem of antibiotic-resistant organisms. And there is even less doubt that genetic engineering is responsible for some, and possibly many, of the new infective organisms now threatening human health.

Under normal circumstances, viruses are species specific. A virus that attacks a cat will not attack a human being. But the genetic engineers have changed all that. They have deliberately glued together different bits of viruses in order to cross species barriers. These genetically engineered viruses can then become virulent again. Genetically engineered viruses are extremely infectious. None of this happens by accident — this is how genetic engineering works. I first warned about this hazard in a book I wrote in the early 1990s.

Naturally, the men and women in white coats who were convinced that they knew best ('Trust us — nothing can go wrong') have been releasing genetic material that they have been fiddling with into the environment for decades.

We thought that the dumping of waste chemicals was bad news. And it was. But the dumping of genetic misshapes and off-cuts will, I believe, create a problem infinitely larger than the dumping of chemical waste or even nuclear waste. Genes, once they start moving and reproducing, can keep spreading, recombining and affecting new species forever. Once the door has been opened, it cannot be shut. And the door has been opened wide.

'Don't worry!' said the genetic engineers. 'Genetic material is easily digested by gut enzymes.'

Sadly, they were wrong about that too.

Genetic material can survive a journey through an intestine and find its way, via the blood stream, into all sorts of body cells. And once inside a new body, the genetic material can begin to affect host cells. If you eat a genetically engineered tomato, the foreign genes in the tomato could end up in your cells. Cancer is an obvious possible consequence of this. Exactly what are the risks? I'm afraid that your guess is as good as mine. And our guesses are just as good as the guesses made by genetic engineers. They don't have the foggiest idea what will happen. But they know as well as I do that something terrible could happen. What about the altered genetic material in new types of food? What happens to genetically altered food when it is eaten?

Will the altered genes find their way into our own genetic material? Could genetically engineered food cause cancer?

Could genetically engineered food affect the human immune system? Asking the questions is easy. But no one knows the answers.

Genetically engineered foods have already been shown to be toxic. One major hazard is that plants which have been genetically engineered to be resistant to disease may be more likely to produce allergy problems. A soya bean genetically engineered with a gene from a Brazil nut was found to cause allergy problems when eaten by people sensitive to Brazil nuts. A strain of yeast, genetically altered in order to ferment more quickly, acquired cancer inducing qualities.

Contaminants in an amino acid led to 1,500 people falling ill and to the deaths of 37 individuals.

And yet politicians have done nothing to protect the public. The people paid to look after the world have rolled over before the big cheque books of the companies which mess around with genes.

No one tests genetically engineered foods to see whether or not they are particularly likely to cause allergy problems. The new food is tested when it is put onto the market. You and I are the unwitting test subjects. Even drug companies have to do some tests before they can launch new products. Food companies seem to be entirely free of controls.

Amazingly, the politicians and administrators whom we pay to protect us allow the manufacturers to get away with the argument that it would be impossible to separate and identify genetically engineered foods. 'Segregation of bulk commodities is not scientifically justified and is economically unrealistic,' said the industries involved in genetic engineering. 'Certainly!' said the politicians and the bureaucrats. 'If you say so.'

The problems are only just beginning but already they are frightening. Potatoes were genetically engineered to be resistant to herbicide. The resistance spread to weeds within a single growing season. Thanks to the irresponsible overuse and abuse of pesticides, and the widespread introduction of crops genetically engineered to produce 'natural' insecticides, more than 1,000 agricultural pests have now acquired so much resistance that they are immune to chemical control. Crops which have been genetically engineered to tolerate herbicides have already begun to make weeds immune to the same herbicides.

If the big seed companies and the politicians have their way then farmers throughout the world will be growing the same variety of genetically engineered soya, the same type of genetically engineered potato and the same genetically engineered corn. That is not a prediction which is difficult to make. It is exactly what the big seed manufacturers are planning. And when the world's single crop of soya/potatoes/corn is destroyed by an insect or plant disease which is immune to every pesticide known to man (and remember there are already 1,000 insects and plant diseases which satisfy that requirement), countless millions around the world will die of starvation.

It's time for all the messing around with genes to be halted. This isn't Ludism, it's common sense and self-preservation.

I leave you with one final thought.

Monsanto is one of the best, known companies turning out genetically modified seeds.

And guess what: The Bill and Melinda Gates Foundation is a big investor in Monsanto.

I have always regarded Monsanto as the most evil company on the planet and I've thought of it this way for several reasons.

First, Monsanto has long been a leader in the development of genetically modified plants. These terrify me because as far as I have been able to find out they have never been properly tested to see what long-term consequences there might be. What damage could there be to crops in a few years' time? Could they become more susceptible to disease? And are there any risks to the people who eat genetically modified food? For some years now, Monsanto has taken to patenting its seeds and as a result small farmers who have traditionally grown their crops from their own seeds have found that they have been unable to do so. There are said to have been many thousands of suicides as a result of this – as farmers found that they weren't allowed to grow the seed they had saved from their own crops but had to buy seed they couldn't afford to buy. I have reported on this many times in the past. And, of course, Monsanto is the manufacturer of Roundup – a doubtless effective but equally doubtless nasty weed killer.

Unfortunately, there have been a number of claims that Roundup causes cancer and there were 125,000 lawsuits as a result. The German company Bayer bought Monsanto a little while ago. Bayer is alleged to have paid $63 billion for Monsanto and to have paid $10.9 billion to settle the claims relating to Roundup.

The bottom line is that I cannot imagine why anyone who really cares for people and the planet would put any money into Monsanto or Bayer.

Oh, and Bill Gates funded research to create genetically modified mosquitoes. If that doesn't keep you awake at night then you haven't been paying attention.

July 31st 2020

We're the Good Guys – and Good Guys Win

The longer this goes on the clearer it becomes that we are being abused, manipulated and, in many cases, murdered by our own governments.

So, for example, in the UK, there were 66,000 deaths in care homes between 2nd March and 12th June this year.

Last year there were 37,000 deaths in care homes in the same period.

Take 37,000 from 66,000 and, with the aid of my Neil Ferguson approved calculator, I worked out that there had been 129 million extra deaths in care homes this year. The calculator, if you're interested is a snip at £99 and is made by the Bill and Melinda Gates Foundation.

When I did the sums in my head, however, the difference came to 29,000 extra deaths.

So, it isn't much of a stretch to deduct that the British Government's policies over the coronavirus led to the deaths of 29,000 people who might otherwise be alive today and who almost certainly died as a direct result of the lockdown, the closure of hospitals and the panic and hysteria over covid-19.

Take the 29,000 deaths from the total number of deaths alleged to have been caused by covid-19 and you are left with around 20,000.

So that's the unofficial official figure for the number who died from the coronavirus.

And that 20,000 includes many patients who didn't die of covid-19 because, as the Government has admitted, anyone who was tested and found to have the coronavirus and then subsequently died, was assumed to have died of covid-19 even if they fell off a cliff or were shot by policemen.

And many cases of flu were erroneously put down as covid-19 deaths.

It's pretty fair to conclude that the total number of deaths from covid-19 in the UK so far this year, during the worst of the infection, was considerably under 20,000 – and probably less than half that. The more we look, the more we learn the lower the real figure goes.

So the big question is: how many people died of flu in Britain?

It varies, of course, but the answer, is that in the last year for which figures are available it was around 50,000.

So there you have it.

Proof, if proof be needed, that the coronavirus has killed far fewer people in Britain than would be expected to die of the flu in the same period.

Now will the doubters believe that the coronavirus scare was a hoax? And will all those people who were so abusive when I recorded my video entitled, 'Coronavirus scare: the hoax of the century' on March 18th now write and apologise?

Maybe the Government would like to know why an assessment made by an old bloke in a chair was considerably better than their guess.

And why my predictions turned out to be far more accurate than theirs – even though their guess was based on the work done by vast numbers of no doubt well remunerated advisors and so-called experts – including of course, the work done by Professor Ferguson and his team at Imperial College whose track record is hardly stellar.

None of that will happen, of course.

No one will apologise. Because trolls never admit that they are wrong. If you collected together 1,000 trolls you would find them incapable of organising a piss up in brewery. They wouldn't have a functional brain cell between them.

More significantly, no-one in the Government will want to know how and why they cocked it up so badly.

Because, of course, they didn't cock it up.

This whole lethal, soul destroying farce has been stage managed to perfection. And the evil minds behind Agenda 21 and the Global Reset must be sniggering and guffawing at the fear they have created and the ease with which they have succeeded in turning billions of people into willing slaves – ready to do whatever they are told to do. They have been brainwashed into damaging their brains by wearing masks which reduce their blood oxygen levels.

I call these people collaborators or zombies. I know some people call them sheep, and I understand that, but I have kept sheep and they are intelligent, thoughtful animals who are very good at protecting themselves. So I prefer the words collaborators or zombies.

Those of us who believe it is a scam have all the facts on our side – as I have just demonstrated.

But facts are of little consequence these days and those who believe it is a new plague prefer to believe what their governments tell them.

I don't really understand this, by the way. Governments always lie. Politicians can't open their mouths without lies coming out. And around the world there are hundreds of health advisors who are closely linked with the drug industry in general and the vaccination industry in particular.

Of course, these days, governments have specialist psy-op experts advising them on how best to demonise those of us who know the truth – and they are very good at it.

In the UK, they are using exactly the same tricks which they used during the Brexit campaign.

During that campaign, which they lost let me remind you, they tried to demonise Brexiteers by describing them as stupid, ill informed, treacherous and selfish.

Those were interesting insults because you didn't have to be a genius to realise that they were, in truth the faults of the Remainers – the people who wanted Britain to remain in the European Union which was always part of Agenda 21 and the plan for a Global Government. The Remainers were not very bright people, they were led by established traitors and people like Blair, and they were terribly ignorant about the facts, they were betraying their country and their history and they were worried more about whether or not they were going to be able to continue to buy French cheeses and go skiing in Italy than they were about the economic and social consequences for their fellow citizens.

It is interesting, is it not, that those who seemed to have fought hardest to oppose Brexit, and are perceived by a large proportion of the UK population as having betrayed the voters, are now being well rewarded. Theresa May, former Prime Minister, is receiving huge sums for giving lectures – though to be honest I can't imagine her having anything to say worth listening to and I can't imagine her being terribly charismatic about it. And Boris Johnson nominated the former chancellor Philip Hammond, who seemed to do everything possible to stop Brexit, for a peerage. He also nominated Kenneth Clarke, also a staunch EU lover.

And the same, now rather tired, insults are being dragged out to try to demonise and condemn those of us who can see that covid-19 is not a new plague.

There is, a school of thought that says that governments are deliberately trying to divide us into two groups – those who believe that covid-19 is a huge threat to us all and nothing less than a re-visitation of the plague – and those who know, without any doubt, that the whole thing is a scam.

And from that knowledge, comes the belief that those of us who believe the whole business is a scam should not argue with or fight those who believe everything the Government says – and who happily wear the masks, avoid using cash and so on.

I understand that point of view.

But I think it is absolutely wrong.

If we do and say nothing then we too are collaborators.

Think about France in World War II for example.

When the Germans were swarming over Paris and France, the brave souls who opposed Hitler formed a resistance movement which fought hard to oppose the Germans, to make their lives difficult and to make their occupation uncomfortable. The British Government sent brave agents over to France to help and equip the French resistance. And there is no doubt that the French Resistance were quite ruthless in their dealings with collaborators and traitors. Nor is there any doubt that that the Resistance helped to defeat Germany.

And we now are the resistance movement – a world-wide resistance movement.

If we do nothing then we are lost; if we don't rebel (peacefully) then we are lost. The enemy – our governments – will have won and will have control of every aspect of lives for eternity.

There is a line in John Ford's film 'Stagecoach' in which John Wayne says: 'There are some things a man can't run away from'.

And there is a similar line in 'Absolute Power', scripted by William Goldman. After discovering what a two-faced hypocrite the President is, Clint Eastwood abandons his plans to run away with the line, spoken to an image of the President on television: 'I'm not about to run from you.'

Well, I'm not about to run from the bunch of second-raters now making a concerted effort to turn me into a slave and pretending to be doing it for the sake of mankind. It was, I think, Albert Camus who said that the welfare of humanity is always the alibi of tyrants.

Society has always been a work in progress. There has always been lots wrong with it. There has always been much room for improvement.

But we, as independent human beings, were doing our best to improve things. We made huge mistakes but we moved forwards – it may have been slow but it was a sort of progress.

Now, the enemy – the United Nations, the WHO, a bunch of unelected billionaires and assorted other evil organisations – want to eradicate democracy, remove our freedom, take away our freedom of speech and turn us all into slaves. They have bought our governments. And it is difficult to find an advisor of any kind who doesn't have links to the drug industry or the Bill and Melinda Gates Foundation or both.

It's happening. And it is happening fast.

The people who want to control us, and run every aspect of our lives, want to do it without asking our permission. They think they are too important and too clever to need our approval.

But we are winning important battles.

It is, for example, becoming clearer each day just how much the greens have lied about climate change. I have detailed some of their lies in other videos.

The other day the BBC, in my opinion the most accomplished provider of fake news on the planet, warned that polar bears will be wiped out by the end of the century unless more is done to tackle climate change. I really do find myself increasingly angry at the BBC. They get worse. It is, it seems to me, a racist, sexist, ageist organisation – anti-white, anti-English and totally fascist. It is controlled by thousands of well-connected, privileged, superior, ignorant liberal lefties whose only talent is the ability to meld hubris and ignorance, ignore the facts and create an apparently unending diet of fake news to its gullible viewers and listeners.

In fact, the paper the BBC quoted didn't actually say that about polar bears.

The prediction was based on a worst case scenario which imagined what would happen if coal burning increased fivefold between now and the year 2100.

That wouldn't be easy because it's reported it would mean burning more coal than there is on the earth.

Polar bears are, for some reason, always used by climate change hoaxers as a warning sign of doom. Their demise and disappearance has been predicted many times. And scientists who have dared to point out that these predictions are nonsense have often been fired.

So, for example, zoologist Susan Crockford who wrote a book entitled, *The Polar Bear Catastrophe that Never Happened* was allegedly relieved of her post as Adjunct Assistant Professor at Victoria University.

The fact is that polar bears aren't going to disappear. And even if they did it wouldn't be because of climate change.

That wasn't my favourite BBC headline, however.

My award goes to this one: 'Climate Change: Summers could become 'too hot for humans'.

That is a headline for which the word 'bollocks' is entirely inadequate. Why, I wonder, does the word 'scaremongering' spring to mind and refuse to go away?

What next? A plague of man eating Martians are living in London sewers. Giant Ants Living in Volcano. Dr Mengele Found on Moon Living in Caravan. They all sound like perfectly plausible BBC headlines.

I would love to see just a little bit of science pretending to assert that summers are going to be too hot for humans.

Do not, I beg you, do anything illegal, but please don't pay the BBC licence fee. You can find lots of advice on how (legally) to avoid paying the BBC on the web – including my website.

More and more former enthusiastic supporters of the climate change hoax are coming out and admitting that it was a load of baloney – and that the 20% of British children who are having nightmares about climate change really need not be worried.

So, Michael Shellenberger, a green activist for 30 years and someone who has advised the Intergovernmental Panel on Climate Change – the IPCC – has admitted that he has been as guilty as anyone of contributing to the panic and now admits that the truth is that climate change is not even our most serious environmental problem. It is, he says, not making natural disasters worse and carbon emissions are falling. He says that for financial, political and ideological reasons, we are all being badly misled. And he adds that it's hard to avoid the impression that the public have been duped.

All this is crucial, of course.

Because, as I and many others have shown, the climate change hoax was created and used to provide the basis for Agenda 21 and the need for a global reset.

For more information, read my essay entitled, *How Greens Will Destroy the World.*

The opposition, the proponents of Agenda 21, are rich and powerful and totally ruthless.

But we have the truth on our side.

And we are going to win.

We're the good guys.

August 1st 2020

Zombies and Trolls

I could weep for what has happened to the human race. There are too many pathetic, terrified individuals around with their heads buried deep in the sand. Our governments have lied, deceived, bullied, cheated, threatened and oppressed.

Governments appear to have forgotten the words of John Locke who said: 'The people cannot delegate to government the power to do anything which would be unlawful for them to do themselves.'

We pay our governments to protect us not to destroy us.

There is no doubt that the masks are part of the process of oppression and have made people even more scared than they were. It is, of course, deliberate.

There are few smiles around these days. And not many laughs to be heard. Celebrities are behaving very strangely. Peter Ebdon, the world snooker champion, is the only one I know who has had the courage to question authority and to tell the truth.

Hypocrisy is everywhere.

The other day I reported that Tom Hanks had announced that he would not respect anyone who didn't wear a mask. But then someone called Tom Hanks, together with his wife, turned up standing with the Greek Prime Minister. Not a mask in sight. No social distancing. It seemed at first that Mr Hanks is that thing at the end of the intestinal tract…the word escapes me…begins with the letter A and ends in hole. But then I realised that it must be another Tom Hanks. There are probably dozens of them in Hollywood.

And people are turning their symbols of slavery into fashion items. The *Daily Mail*, a British tabloid, ran a picture of the Duchess of Cornwall who had, they drooled, 'opted for a bold, printed mask, decorated with turquoise, gold and navy peacock feathers'.

Worst of all there are stories that when schools reopen in September some children will be forced to wear masks and maintain social distancing. This is beyond obscene. Parents should threaten to sue the headmistress or headmaster responsible for such child abuse.

Unless we rise up and rebel the masks will never go away.

The plan is very precisely defined.

In the UK, the Government has given people a loophole. For example, anyone who has a respiratory disorder or a mental disorder doesn't have to wear a mask. Also, children under 11 don't have to wear masks.

But there's a snag: no one can get an exemption certificate. Astonishingly, GPs have been instructed not to provide exemption certificates for anyone. The absence of officially signed exemption certificates will make it easy to progress to the next stage when mask wearing will be compulsory for everyone.

Now that Cressida Dick, the boss of the Metropolitan Police in London, has cruelly told mask wearers to shame those not wearing masks, the pressure on those who are physically or mentally ill will be unbearable.

And so most of those people will put on their masks – even if it makes their breathing more difficult or causes them enormous distress.

Soon the masks, symbols of oppression and slavery, will be mandatory for anyone who wants to go into a shop to buy food.

And then the next step will make it compulsory for people to wear masks in the street or even in their own homes. The cameras in our telephones and televisions will identify those who are breaking the law.

The collaborators who have been wearing masks on public transport and in shops may grumble but they will accept the extension of the law – particularly when it is reinforced, as it will be, with more threats about a second wave and a mutated, more deadly virus.

Those who object will be vilified.

So what next?

Well, having pushed us into wearing masks all the time they will want to push us a little further as part of our training.

And so then we will have to wear plastic or rubber gloves all the time.

And the punishments for not wearing a mask will gradually rise.

Within a very short time the punishment will be imprisonment. Anyone not wearing a mask and gloves will be sent to prison.

I am astonished, and rather saddened, that so many people around the world have accepted mask wearing without protest. Although it is perfectly understandable when the punishments are draconian as they are in some countries.

To me the real tragedy is that now that they have been softened up by their house arrest, and the constant fear making propaganda, millions actually want the regulations to be tougher. They want more lockdowns and stricter laws about mask wearing.

What the devil is wrong with these people?

Why are so many not questioning what is happening? Can't they read and think for themselves? The answers sadly are clearly No and No. Of course, in some countries there have been effective protests and mask laws have been withdrawn. In one American state, local sheriffs refused to arrest people who demonstrated against house arrest.

But sadly, Britons have become the biggest wimps on the planet. Whatever happened to the British phlegm that got us through World War II?

One explanation is that the problem is something called cognitive dissonance. Many people just cannot believe that governments could tell so many lies and that politicians could be so deceitful. The zombies and the trolls aren't very bright and are unable to see the big picture. They aren't bright enough to see things in perspective. They don't believe anyone could tell such big lies.

The zombies and trolls have never been properly educated; they are content to believe what they are told or what they read on a lavatory wall; they are incapable of thinking for themselves. Actually, they are incapable of thinking at all. The education process devised by the United Nations over the last few decades has been designed to enforce a belief in collectivism. And that is what has happened. These are people who watch or listen to the BBC and believe what they see or hear and who believe that *The Guardian* is a newspaper – and do not realise it is a propaganda sheet built on money from slave trading and pushing us ever onwards to a new slavery.

Brighter folk can see through the lies and they can understand what is happening.

Another explanation is the zombies and the trolls have a sense of entitlement that closes their eyes to the world around them.

A toxic mixture of reality television and social media has created life goals that are far removed from reality. It is salutary that many zombies and trolls don't have 'friends' or 'contacts': they have 'followers' and 'fans'. There is little proper debate on social media for disagreement. If a troll comes across someone with a point of view that differs from their own their only response is to resort to abuse and a sense of outrage that someone should hold another point of view.

I wonder how many trolls know that the personality traits which trigger heart disease (and which are just as potent as smoking and fatty food) include hostility and extreme self-involvement?

There is going to be a veritable epidemic of heart disease in another decade's time and thousands of zombies and trolls will be demanding instant heart transplants. They won't get them, of course. Transplants will be reserved for the elite.

And there may be another reason why there are so many zombies and trolls around.

I have been pointing out for 30 years that our drinking water is enriched with female hormones. It is clear that those hormones are now having a dramatic effect on the human race. There's more about this, incidentally, on my video entitled, 'Is Tap Water Safe to Drink?'

The problems started in the 1960s when millions of women started taking the contraceptive pill. The hormone residues from those pills are excreted in their urine.

Look at what happens then:

After going through standard purification procedures, waste water containing the hormone rich urine is discharged into fresh water rivers. Drinking water is often taken from rivers.

The water is then purified again – but water purification programmes cannot remove hormone residues.

By the 1990s, it was clear that our drinking water contained female hormones. A report from the UK Environmental Agency concluded that 57% of roach in one river had changed sex. And it is also now known that human male fertility has fallen in recent years.

It is the hormones in the water which explains why so many members of both sexes are constantly confused about their sexuality. Like teenagers struggling with a hormone maelstrom they aren't sure whether they are male or female. Many want to change sex. Some then want to change back. This explains why male zombies and trolls tend to be effeminate and stupid and female zombies, trolls and mask wearers tend to be stupid, confused, irritable and sulky.

And I think the zombies, the trolls, the mask wearers have all been drinking too much tap water. Too many cups of tea, perhaps?

This explains why male zombies and trolls tend to be effeminate and stupid and female zombies, trolls and mask wearers tend to be stupid, confused, irritable and sulky.

So, there you are. The small, poorly developed brains of the trolls and the zombies have been permanently damaged by watching the BBC, reading *The Guardian* and drinking tap water.

There are millions of zombies and trolls around because they are naïve, gullible, poorly educated, unintelligent, immature and self-important but ultimately terrified of authority because the hormones in the drinking water have turned them into permanent teenagers.

They may be beyond our help.

The other day I made a video about the BBC fact checkers and mentioned not paying the licence fee – because if you give the BBC money it is, in my view, akin to supporting terrorism. I just want to add that if you live in England and the BBC's gestapo knock on your door to see if you have a TV set, you do not have to speak to them, open the door or let them in unless they have obtained a court order and/or have the police with them. You don't have to pay the licence just because you own a television set. Check out the rules. It isn't difficult to not have to give the BBC money.

Finally, I can demolish the whole coronavirus nonsense in less than three minutes. Everything in this list can be verified.

Many doctors, including Dr Fauci, the American coronavirus supremo, have admitted that the risk of dying with coronavirus may be similar to the risk with the flu.

The flu can kill 650,000 people a year around the world. Even though governments everywhere have admitted fiddling their totals, the covid-19 death total is similar to the global flu total.

Here's how they fiddled the figures. In the UK, for example, anyone who tested positive for the coronavirus and subsequently died was officially a covid-19 death – whatever else they had wrong with them. The vast majority of those dying with the coronavirus were over 80 and had many other health problems. The risk for fit, young individuals is very small. The risk for children is smaller than the risk of being hit by lightning.

Research has shown that masks are dangerous, don't prevent the spread of infection and almost certainly do more harm than good. The virus can go straight through the material of a mask. And mask wearing affects blood oxygen levels. At least two people have died through wearing masks. I've quoted figures and papers on my website www.vernoncoleman.com and in other videos.

Many of those promoting the coronavirus horror story are linked in some way to the vaccine industry or the Bill and Melinda Gates Foundation – which itself has strong financial links to the vaccine industry. For example, the Chief Scientific Advisor in the UK was formerly a senior executive at GSK – one of the big vaccine makers.

The British Government has admitted that at least four times as many people have died as a result of the lockdowns and other control measures as will have died from the coronavirus. The remedy has been much deadlier than the disease. Millions are waiting for cancer tests and treatment because hospitals were closed. And some hospital departments in the UK are still closed.

Neil Ferguson, the man whose predictions led to the lockdowns had produced a number of inaccurate predictions before he made wildly pessimistic predictions about the coronavirus. His track record is appalling. The college where he works has financial links to Bill and Melinda Gates Foundation and vaccines.

Exactly the same mistakes have been made in almost every country in the world. For example, sick old people were taken out of hospital and dumped in care homes – resulting in tens of thousands of deaths in each country. That couldn't be a coincidence – so it had to be a plan. If you remove the care home deaths from the UK total, you end up with a maximum of around 20,000 deaths (though that is a massive exaggeration because they included flu and anyone who tested positive) which is much smaller than the annual flu death total.

The number of people who have caught the coronavirus worldwide is now said to be around 10 million. But the flu can affect 1 billion in a single year.

These are facts which cannot be disputed, though they are being suppressed. Print out the list and give copies to doubters. I find it difficult to believe that anyone could still want to wear a mask once they were aware of these simple facts.

August 5th 2020

The Plan to Create Unending Misery

The psy-op specialists must be proud of themselves.

Their plan, of course, is to make us miserable and confused. They know that if we are uncertain and bewildered and frightened we will be more pliable; more manageable.

And so, in countries all over the world, the psychologists working for the people pulling the strings are treating their citizens like prisoners of war. The brainwashing specialists have devised, and are constantly updating, a barefaced plan to create unending misery. We have to be dominated, turned into slaves and controlled.

They know that their plan will split the country – though not into equal parts.

One part, inevitably the largest, will consist of the weaker, more gullible individuals who will accept any lie they are told as long as it is told frequently and loudly. In the UK, these are the people who swallowed the global warming nonsense and who voted Remain because they believed the lies they were told about the European Union.

The rebels, the resistance movement, the people who reject the lies and who see through their governments' deceptions, are fewer in number but mostly quite determined. In the UK, these were mostly Brexit voters and they mostly thought the climate change hysteria a massive piece of manipulated pseudoscience. They pose a significant threat to the manipulators and the plan now is to demonise them and isolate them and to turn the majority against them so that eventually they are broken and will do as they are told.

So, for example, those who dutifully wear masks in shops will be praised as good citizens, as local heroes, as people who care for their community. There is no science showing that mask wearing is of any value, of course, but that doesn't worry the manipulators. Besides, anyone who is symptomatic, and likely to spread any infection, is already under strict instructions to isolate themselves.

The dutiful citizens, compliant in every respect, have been co-opted as part time police officers and guardians of the State. They have been officially instructed to shame those not wearing masks; to embarrass them and to make them feel uncomfortable and guilty.

Everywhere you look politicians, civil servants and the mass media are busy doing everything they can to create and spread news fear while constantly making sure that the old fears were kept alive.

In one of my brainwashing videos I mentioned that in the guidance given to the British Government it was pointed out that 'a substantial number of people still did not feel sufficiently personally threatened'. That's us they're talking about. We are not sufficiently personally threatened. Why would they want us to be so threatened? What ulterior motive could there possibly be? Could I have been right back in March when I suggested that one of the reasons for the hoax was to get us ready for mandatory you-know-what?

Their effective, clinical winding up of the fear process has been designed to cause the greatest harm. It's a barefaced plan to cause misery and despair.

When we are under stress our bodies produce a hormone called cortisol. Lots of stress equals lots of cortisol in our bodies.

And guess what: patients who have lots of cortisol in their bodies are more likely to die from covid-19 than people who are calm and relaxed. And, of course, since elderly, frail people with illnesses are more likely to die anyway, they are the ones who are going to be most affected by stress.

So there we are: one of the reasons why the Government has been deliberately terrifying us is because they know that we will have more cortisol in our bodies and they know that the extra cortisol will push those who have co-morbidities over the edge.

It's yet another type of mass murder.

(Incidentally, why is covid-19 commonly written as Covid-19? Why the initial capital? We don't write 'Malaria' or 'Tuberculosis' – both of which, incidentally, kill far more people than covid-19). Is this merely to make this modestly significant disease appear more important than it is? I confess with embarrassment that I fell for this myself once or twice.)

All these things are quite extraordinary. No western democracy has ever worked against its own people so cruelly and with such steely determination.

The immediate intention is to make us all frightened and miserable. It doesn't matter if the rebels appear feisty or even angry. The brainwashing specialists know that in due course they will, if given a little time, succeed in breaking the free thinking citizens.

All round the world people are fighting their own governments. In the UK, for example, Johnson, Hancock and company have made themselves our enemies just as Hitler and company were our enemies in 1939 and the 1940s. Johnson seems to me to be a gullible simple-minded buffoon who is dancing on the end of a piece of string being jiggled by Cummings. Hancock seems to me to be just a pompous, half-witted prefect who would be out of his depth if he were a small town mayor. But they have behind them billionaire manipulators, global organisations, the Bilderbergers and the might of the world's press. Before them, doing the dirty work for them on a day by day basis, they have a small army of Common Purpose trained bureaucrats. The thought is always of the State. Everything is done in the name of collectivism. Individuality and democracy are as out-of- date as cloche hats and feather boas.

The only hope for us, the rebels, is that we can succeed in converting some of the fearful and dutiful citizens to our point of view. To do that we must counter the misinformation as best we can. We have to hope that in the fullness of time we will be able to gather to our side enough citizens so that we become a majority or, at the very least, a sizeable and vocal minority.

It's tricky, of course, and it is going to get ever more difficult because those of us who see through the absurd lies and spot the manipulations, are facing the entire might of the State apparatus, combined with and supported by a compliant media which has willingly suppressed the truth.

The reporting of this massive take-over of the world has been a disgrace. The mass market media has been bought and simply does it best to ramp up the fear and drive the yearning for a vaccine as the only way out of the chaos. The media have been paid to promote the lies and by slanting the news and consistently repeating the same threats, they're doing their job very effectively.

The British Broadcasting Corporation has always been a propaganda machine and an utter disgrace, as untrustworthy as a junkyard dog, but I am surprised at how cheaply the rest of the mainstream journalists have been bought.

During the lockdown, newspapers and magazines were full of articles by journalists writing about their experiences under house arrest. They described how brave and resourceful they were. They gave us intimate details of their dinner parties and productive business meetings conducted by zoom, they showed us film of their silly dances and they gave us lists of all the books they've read, the films they'd seen and the foreign languages they had learned. They wrote about the coronavirus crime as though it had been a great adventure: a weekend's glamping expedition in darkest Snowdonia or a sleepover with chums.

Now the same writers are showing us how to turn our masks into fashion accessories. They are trying to normalise the distinctly abnormal. They are pouring verbal acid on anyone who goes into a shop without a mask. They say nothing about the contradictions, the absurdities and the way the science is being ignored whenever it is considered inconvenient to the billionaires. They lie about the dissenters and when that doesn't seem to be working they simply ignore whatever truths are unearthed.

Each morning, I wake up thinking I must have imagined what has been happening. And then when I realise that I haven't, I feel as though I am living in a bad science fiction movie. The nightmare in which we are living cannot possibly be true. Is this purgatory or some dark hinterland between life and death. I wonder often how many million people are contemplating suicide as the only way out of this obscene piece of global manipulation.

The mass media announced with great excitement that retail sales rebounded since the end of the lockdown. Imagine that! Shops are open and people can leave their homes and the chattering classes are surprised, amazed and delighted that retail sales have gone up a little. The plan, of course, is to get rid of all High Street shops and shopping centres so that we do all our shopping online. In the UK, planning laws have been changed to make it easy to turn a shop into flats.

The social distancing will help destroy bricks and mortar shops. The absurd markings on the floor, the inconvenient one way systems which vary from the impractical to the incomprehensible to the downright annoying, the bottles of hand sanitiser placed by the door with the command that the goo be used before entering, the queues outside as shop staff limit the number of customers within the shop, the growing refusal to accept cash – with advice being given to shops on how to take advantage of all the ways to sell things without using cash. (I predict, by the way, that the one country in the world where cash will remain popular will be Columbia – where some businessmen have huge stocks of the stuff to get rid of.)

And the masks.

Oh yes, those nasty little masks.

There are some shop staff who now refuse entry to those not wearing masks. Others insist on questioning customers, demanding details of their medical history. It's impertinent, it's humiliating and it is going to drive shoppers away. Shop owners and shop assistants who don't realise what is happening will be closed before Christmas.

When you shop online there are no queues, no social distancing commands, no nasty skin sanitiser to give you a skin rash and no need for a mask. You have to pay by card, it is true, but you probably have to pay by card in a shop too.

And you can make yourself a coffee whenever you feel like one.

The Global Reset requires us to do all our shopping online. The plan is to get rid of all small businesses – especially shops. And it's working, damnit; even charity shops are closing their doors.

Incidentally, an aside, some shop assistants have been ordered by their bosses to wear masks. And some have been very distressed; unable to breathe, especially on warm days. Eight hours in a mask is not pleasant. I cannot believe this is legal. I strongly suggest that assistants told they must wear masks contact their trade union for clarification.

And there is no room for fun in our future, either.

That is why the rules governing pubs and restaurants are so utterly absurd. Anyone wanting to visit a pub will be told to order their drink on a phone app so that the Government will know what you order. Presumably, those of us who wouldn't know an App if it stood up and barked will have to do without.

In hotels, guests will be advised to have meals delivered by room service. Oh what a lot of fun holidays and weekend breaks will be. I feel for all those folk who love putting on posh clothes for dinner. Getting all spruced up to sit on the bed to eat your dinner just won't be the same.

There is no room for pleasure in the new world order. We will be living in high rise apartments, close to our employment. Our shopping will be delivered. Our entertainment will be provided by the box in the corner of the room. No laughing, no thinking.

If you think I am exaggerating take a look at Agenda 21 and the plans for the Global Reset. It's absolutely terrifying. And the same sort of things are happening everywhere.

In India, over 122 million people lost their jobs in the month of April alone. In Qatar, there is or was a penalty of three years in prison for not wearing a face mask in public. Who can keep up? And in Panama, where the lockdown allows men and women to leave their homes on alternate days, transgender citizens were apparently complaining that they couldn't go out on either day.

If I put this stuff in a novel I'd be stoned to death by the readers.

A few years ago, there were a lot of threats about ID cards and iris scans being introduced. I wrote about them and helped campaign against them.

The public thought about it, considered the evidence and said a very loud, 'no thank you'.

We need some of that good sense and determination again.

They want to destroy freedom and democracy.

Well the bastards aren't going to win.

We are the resistance.

If you meet people who aren't yet on our side please ask them to watch the video entitled, 'We are the victims of the greatest crime in history' – it's a good introduction to the whole bizarre story from the beginning up until today.

August 9th 2020

How Many Billion Could the Covid-19 Vaccine Kill or Damage?

'The search for new vaccines for old diseases is endless. Some plans are imaginative. Scientists have apparently developed a banana vaccine by creating genetically engineered banana plants. There are plans to develop bananas which 'protect' against hepatitis B, measles, yellow fever and poliomyelitis. Other scientists have developed a genetically engineered potato designed to be used as a vaccine against cholera. The active part of the potato remains active during the process of cooking, and so a portion of genetically engineered chips could soon be a vaccine against cholera. There is a planned genetically engineered vaccine which will provide protection against 40 different diseases. The vaccine, which will contain the raw DNA of all those different diseases, will be given to newborn babies to provide them with protection for life.'

I wrote those words for my book Anyone *Who Tells You Vaccines are Safe and Effective is Lying.* And I wrote that paragraph in 2011.

Predictably, I was attacked with some vehemence by many people inside and outside the medical and nursing professions.

There was much shaking of heads and wagging of fingers and critics fell over themselves to condemn me for revelations which were regarded as more suitable for a science fiction novel than for a serious book about vaccination.

But lo and behold, the covid-19 fraud has provided an excellent opportunity for scientists everywhere to start shouting publicly about their wonderful new plant based vaccines.

And food based vaccines are now on their way.

The absolutely excellent Christian Westbrook, whose website Ice Age Farmer is a better source of information about all aspects of food than anything on the mainstream media and in my opinion approximately a million times more honest and useful than anything ever broadcast on the BBC, recently produced a video detailing the latest news about vaccines in genetically modified tomatoes and other foods. The plan is, of course, to modify the DNA of the foodstuff so that as it grows it produces the appropriate vaccine. And since covid-19 is the fashionable disease of the moment, and the fraudulent reason for bringing Agenda 21 into your home and your life, then the vaccines are, of course, designed for covid-19. You won't need a jab – you'll just have to eat a specially grown and genetically modified tomato. Or whatever fruit or vegetable they choose for their vaccine. Tobacco plants are apparently excellent for growing vaccines. Incidentally, I'm not sure what would happen if you were, over a period of time, to eat 12, 24 or 36 vaccine contaminated tomatoes and I don't think there is any point in trying to find out because I doubt if anyone else knows either.

Naturally, the pharmaceutical industry is constantly searching for more and more new vaccines and wherever they spot the beginnings of a market, a demand, they will do their best to serve up something appropriate. I have lost count of the number of times I have read of researchers working on a vaccine to prevent cancer.

Meanwhile, the drug companies continue with the old faithfuls; the profitable cash cows which keep the billions pouring in. Every year, new flu jabs appear on the market.

I don't know about you but I can no longer keep up with what is going on. I have long since abandoned trying to work out which vaccines are very dangerous and which are just a bit dangerous – and to whom. The only certainty is that manufacturing (and giving) vaccines is big business. The people who sell vaccines make a lot of money. And the doctors who give them (or who authorise nurses to give them on their behalf) make a lot of money too. That, by the way, is one of the reasons why doctors rarely if ever criticise vaccination programmes. (The other reason for keeping quiet is that doctors who do dare to speak out about vaccine hazards are likely to lose their licence to practice.)

Vaccination is a big, and very profitable, industry. Covid-19 is vaccine bonanza time for drug companies and doctors. At the latest count there were over 100 companies and other groups hurrying to be the first with a covid-19 vaccine – and the chance to sell seven billion doses once, twice or even four times a year. This is bonanza time for the vaccine companies and for the doctors who will give the vaccines.

I am not sure, by the way, just how keen doctors will be on vaccines in foods. As I have pointed out, doctors make a fortune out of giving vaccines. Will they be able to make money out of prescribing tomatoes? Quite possibly. I can hear it now. 'Take one of these tomatoes once a day every three months.'

What happens, incidentally, to those people who are allergic to tomatoes? Or who just hate the damned things?

It will be easy to manufacture and sustain reasons for the vaccine to be needed.

The testing programme currently being used for covid-19 is woefully inaccurate. It is at best, less than 50% accurate and it produces a good many false positives. And even if there aren't any real cases of covid-19 around, the testing will, by producing false positives, sustain the myth that the disease is still around and still dangerous.

Indeed, if the authorities want to close down a town or even a single establishment – a pub where the landlord has been seen to be lax about enforcing the rules for example – all they have to do is increase the amount of testing. Even if no one has the disease there will, inevitably, be lots of positives. So then the new gestapo can close down the town or the pub or whatever.

Let me now tell you something about vaccine testing and the side effects. This is the scary truth that no one has mentioned. You will never hear this from any government hired doctor or scientist. But I promise you this is true.

Serious side effects may occur with drugs or vaccines after a considerable number of patients have taken the drug or had the vaccine.

So, for example, it may be that a vaccine only kills or seriously damages 1 in every 10,000 people. It may kill or seriously damage 1 in every 100,000. Or it may kill or seriously damage 1 in every 1,000. The numbers vary.

But the initial testing programme will probably never show up those dangerous side effects.

And here's why.

Developing and testing a new vaccine usually takes 10-15 years and the whole development programme has been well established over decades. In the US, the regulations for vaccine development were first created in 1902 – and were the forerunner of the National Institutes of Health. In the EU, there is the European Medicines Agency. And of course the WHO has recommendations. All these rules are considered necessary because there have over the years been many vaccine calamities. Doctors and governments don't like to mention how often things go disastrously wrong but I detailed some of the bad examples in the book I mentioned. It's enough to say that governments around the world have secretly paid out billions of dollars to patients and relatives injured or killed by vaccines. Bill Gates has, of course, insisted that vaccine developers who produce a covid-19 vaccine will be immune from legal action. They could produce a vaccine that killed 50% of the world's population and not have to pay a penny in damages.

The first stage in developing a vaccine usually lasts a few years and it involves experimenting with various possible antigens – that might trigger a response and provide protection against a disease.

Once a possible vaccine looks promising it is tested on animals.

I have, for over half a century, argued that animal experiments are pointless and misleading. Drug companies always ignore the results if a product is shown to cause cancer in animals for example. They dismiss such inconvenient results by arguing that animals are different to people so the results don't matter.

The experiments on animals usually last a couple of years and many vaccines never get past this stage. Either the vaccine doesn't work or it turns out to be remarkably lethal.

With covid-19 however, governments have allowed drug companies to skip the animal testing and go straight into testing on humans.

Once animal tests have been done, or in this case, not done, the next stage is to test out the vaccine on a fairly small group of people – usually no more than 100. Attempts will usually be made to give the infection to the people taking part in the test. If the vaccine does its job then some, at least, of the brave souls involved in the trial won't get the disease.

If those tests are successful then Phase Three can start.

In Phase Three, the idea is to give the vaccine to more people – certainly several thousand. And the vaccine will be tested against a placebo.

And if all goes well then the manufacturer will apply for a licence and, no doubt, organise some sort of celebration.

Once a vaccine has been produced it will be regarded as suitable for mass use. Technically vaccine manufacturers may continue to test their vaccine for efficacy and safety if they would like to do so.

The idea is to see if lots of people who had the vaccine suddenly go blind or die a year after being vaccinated. And in an ideal world it would be nice to know if the vaccine interferes with other vaccines or prescription drugs or even with genetically modified foods. Who knows? When you start putting stuff into people's bodies the sky is the limit as far as side effects are concerned. With a drug taken by mouth you can at least stop the drug if serious problems develop. That's a bit more tricky with stuff that has been injected into the body with the idea of creating some sort of reaction.

But these long-term tests are voluntary.

So you can imagine how often they are done.

You can, however, see now why testing a vaccine usually takes a decade or more.

But with the vaccine for covid-19 the plan is to get the licence in months.

And in my view the vaccine will not be safe in that time period. Despite the claims made by pro-vaxxers, which is to say just about every politician, doctor, journalist and buffoon in the world, vaccines are not entirely safe.

Doctors don't have to report problems with vaccines and patients hardly ever do because they don't usually realise the connection. Even so, around 30,000 adverse vaccine events are reported every year. And of those, 3,000 to 4,500 are serious – which is to say they cause permanently disability or death. And that's just in the United States. There are three huge problems with the covid-19 vaccine.

First, there is the problem that it is possible that not enough volunteers will have been given the vaccine to test it for safety. And, remember, once the testing is over the vaccine will be approved for distribution. Statistically, you have to test on a lot of patients if you are going to spot serious side effects. If a serious side effect occurs in 1 in every 10,000 patients – and I think that was a figure which Bill Gates mentioned – then you will really need to do tests on many more patients. One important text book on vaccines suggests that in order to detect a significant difference for a low frequency event, a trial would have to include 60,000 subjects – half of them in a control group, receiving no vaccination.

So, it's fair to say that the phase three testing for each of the 100 or so new vaccines will need to involve 60,000 people. That means finding six million people prepared to be guinea pigs for a new vaccine because you can't test more than one vaccine on the same person. I can't see them finding six million guinea pigs. So I suspect that the tests will involve fewer patients.

It's no wonder that Gates had demanded the drug companies making the vaccines have no legal liability.

By the way, individual doctors and nurses can, of course, still be sued and damages will, I suspect, run into billions. Medical insurance companies will go bust and so will thousands of doctors and nurses. They might like to think about that.

A fatality risk of 1 in 1,000 for a drug that may save your life is very acceptable.

One in 1,000 is rotten odds for a drug or vaccine you don't really need.

The second problem is that governments will be tempted to roll out the vaccine very quickly. They've been promoting the vaccine very hard and promising that once there is a vaccine we can all get back to normal. That was obviously a lie but that's what they said so they'll want to get on with things and they will doubtless give the vaccine to too many people too quickly

And, remember, you need to observe patients for quite a while because some problems will only occur later, much later. It may be months or years before serious side effects are seen – especially if the vaccine is prepared using new techniques.

So, if a new vaccine is rolled out and given to nearly seven billion patients in a matter of weeks, the serious problems will only be seen after all the individuals have been vaccinated.

And if, say, 1 in 1,000 people die or are brain damaged then there will be seven million people dead or brain damaged as a result of the vaccination programme.

Arch pro-vaxxer Bill Gates suggested that there might perhaps be problems with 1 in 10,000 people (and he doesn't know whether it will be 1 in 10,000 or 1 in 1,000 or 1 in 100) then there will be 700,000 dead or seriously damaged people. That is 700,000 previously healthy individuals. And, under these exceptional circumstances, I believe that's pretty much the best case scenario. And it is, of course, far more than the total number of people alleged to have been killed by covid-19 around the world.

The third problem is, of course, that serious problems might occur a long time after the vaccine has been given. Who is going to monitor all those patients? My guess would be no one.

Those are all usual, fairly standard problems with a vaccine which has taken 10-15 years to produce.

The covid-19 vaccine will probably be in use within months of being made. Indeed, companies are already making millions of doses of vaccines which have not yet finished their tests. The UK government has already bought well over 100 million doses of vaccine and a huge supply of needles and syringes.

So far it's all sounding a little iffy.

And to all these risks must be added the fact that Gates' doesn't seem to have any entirely trouble free history as far as his various adventures are concerned. His genetic modification of mosquitoes is terrifying many. And there is all that talk about his polio vaccine – which I discussed in previous videos.

There is also the fact that results of a test of one vaccine for covid-19 showed that many volunteers reported mild or moderate side effects. Over half experienced pain, 16% had fever, 28% had headache and 34% suffered from fatigue. Patients who had a higher dose of the vaccine suffered even worse with 57% having pain, 32% having fever, 29% having headaches and 42% having fatigue.

As one analysis reported, the level of mild and moderate symptoms with this covid-19 vaccine is markedly higher than that associated with the covid-19 infection itself. How many people will be keen to have a vaccine when there is a good chance that they will suffer more than if they develop the disease? And, remember, a lot of people who develop the covid-19 disease have few or no symptoms.

And there was another problem with the vaccine that I've just mentioned. Older patients didn't develop very good levels of immune response. And, of course, the vast majority of those who died of covid-19 were over 80-years-old.

Still, it is perhaps reassuring for British citizens to know that Neil Ferguson is acting director of the Vaccine Impact Modelling Consortium at Imperial College. This consortium, by the way, is funded by, among others, GAVI, the vaccine alliance, and the Bill and Melinda Gates Foundation.

But with covid-19 vaccine there is a fourth problem – the biggest problem of all.

Some manufacturers are using a brand new method of making vaccines called third generation vaccines. These contain DNA or RNA technology and are injected into the body and taken up by the cells to change the immune system. The technology is designed to turn your body's cells into viral-protein making machines.

Instead of injecting a piece of a virus into the human recipient, synthesised genes are used. It's gene therapy. Those having the vaccine will be genetically modified like a soya bean or one of Bill Gates' mosquitoes. The artificial gene will be incorporated into your DNA and you will become a different person. Forever. Serious, possibly deadly side effects, might not appear for years or even generations. No one knows how dangerous this vaccine could be because it's new. Drug companies admit they don't know what will happen or what could go wrong. It is a massive experiment.

Here's what the WHO has to say:

'Many aspects of the immune response generated by DNA vaccines are not understood. However, this has not impeded significant progress towards the use of this type of vaccine in humans, and clinical trials have begun.'

That's the World Health Organisation.

Governments and YouTube tell us we must listen to the WHO so I will repeat that:

'Many aspects of the immune response generated by DNA vaccines are not understood. However, this has not impeded significant progress towards the use of this type of vaccine in humans, and clinical trials have begun.'

Naturally, the drug companies making these vaccines know that they could be very harmful. Moderna, one of the drug companies involved, has admitted that there could be significant adverse events.

The fact is that if you have a DNA or RNA vaccine you will become a genetically modified human being. You will be an experiment.

The vaccine might prove to be absolutely lethal.

Can they guarantee that everyone who has it will not drop dead in eighteen months?

I don't believe they can.

And what if they decide to give you a food with a vaccine inside it?

The tomato or the potato or the banana or whatever that I mentioned at the start of this video and first wrote about in 2011.

How safe will that be?

I have no idea, and I would welcome an honest and disinterested appraisal by experts not connected with the vaccine industry or with the Bill and Melinda Gates Foundation.

Though to be honest I'm not entirely sure where they would find such experts.

And, of course, thanks to Bill Gates, the companies making this new covid-19 vaccine will have full legal immunity. If things go wrong they will not be legally liable.

Now if the disease for which the vaccine was being prepared was killing millions then the risk might be worth taking.

But it has been proved time and time again that covid-19 kills no more people than the flu. The lockdowns and other procedures have killed more people than the disease.

So, how deadly will the covid-19 vaccine turn out to be?

As far as the medical establishment is concerned you should remember that I am persona non grata. They and the mainstream media think I'm dangerous though despite many lies about me, they can't point to anything I've got wrong. So they largely settle for abuse, lies and distortions.

I believe that everything I have told you is true.

I do not believe that the new covid-19 vaccine will have been properly tested. I do not believe a vaccine is necessary. I worry about what it might contain. I worry about the fact that those recommending vaccination will not debate with me. I worry about the past record of the major drug companies – take a look at my other videos. And I worry endlessly that they want to give the covid-19 vaccine to every living soul on earth.

And all that is before I start to worry about what might have been added to the vaccine, how much it may change my genetic make-up – and whether or not a vaccine might be designed to in some way change my conscious state or my personality.

Gates is pushing Moderna's RNA vaccine although, or perhaps because, it seems possible genetic changes could be passed to future generations. And yet back in January 2020, the Geneva Statement, a group of the world's leading ethicists and scientists, called for an end to experiments involving editing of the human genome. Dr Suhab Siddiqi, Moderna's former Director of Chemistry allegedly told CNN that he would not allow the virus to be injected into his body.

Having looked at all the evidence, I believe a DNA or RNA vaccine could alter my mind, my moods, my personality and my humanity. It could change the way I deal with and respond to the people around me. I would rather be dead.

How many people will the new covid-19 vaccine kill or seriously injure?

I have no idea. And I don't believe anyone else has either.

Bill Gates has no idea.

Dr Whitty has no idea.

Dr Fauci has no idea.

And UK Minister Matt Hancock, a keen pro-vaxxer, doesn't know.

And none of them dares debate with me or, presumably, anyone else.

If I'm wrong why not debate with me, crush my arguments and make me look stupid?

Could it possibly be that they're frightened to debate because they know I'm right?

Incidentally, as an aside, I don't want to debate with anyone. I have no financial interest in these videos and I certainly don't want to be a public figure. I'm an author, no more and no less, and I'd rather stay here in my comfy chair and look after my wife and the wildlife in our garden and write another book about Bilbury or Mrs Caldicot's adventures. I'd much prefer it if someone else opposed to this vaccine took on the pro-vaxxers.

It may sound crazy but I would rather be dead than have one of these absurd, unnecessary vaccines for covid-19 that could alter my body, my mind and my soul. In my opinion that would be a fate worse than death. I will not accept the covid-19 vaccine.

I do not believe that those enthusiastically promoting the covid-19 vaccine understand what is involved. Those who do understand and who agree to have themselves vaccinated should, in my view, be certified insane.

But, nevertheless, everyone should be allowed to choose for themselves whether or not to accept the vaccine. I don't believe in mandatory vaccination and I don't believe in telling people not to have a vaccine.

I just believe in giving people the facts so that they can make up their own minds.

If governments try to make this vaccine mandatory or essential in any way, then those of us who don't want to be vaccinated will have to fight in the courts and hope that the judges aren't on the payroll of the Bill and Melinda Gates Foundation. We will have to fight on the grounds that the vaccination cannot possibly be proved to be safe or effective and that it is being used for a disease known to be no more deadly than the flu.

I think this video is vitally important. Please send it to as many people as you can. YouTube is taking down my videos almost as fast as we can put them up these days. The other day they took down my video entitled, 'Coronavirus: Will Social Distancing Be Permanent?' which I recorded in the middle of May.

So, please, I beg you, share this video or ask people to read the transcript on my website. Print out the article and send a copy to your family doctor. If this video were not accurate I could not and would not say any of this.

There will be no complaints from drug companies or governments – but, one way or another, they will doubtless try to suppress what I have said.

Oh, and one final thought for this video: the American Government and Yale University are collaborating in a trial to determine the best words and phrases to use in order to persuade Americans to accept the covid-19 vaccine.

So watch out for more psychological warfare – everyone questioning or refusing vaccination will be demonised.

August 12^{*th*} *2020*

Forbidden Truths

I struggle each day to understand what is happening. The only certainty is that the world has gone quite mad. We were always rather reclusive but the events of the last few months have made the reclusiveness almost complete.

I cannot bear to go out because the people in masks fill me with a sense of deep and painful despair. Everyone in a mask is a sign of impending slavery. I find it difficult to understand why anyone with more than two brain cells to rub together could possibly take this contrived lunacy seriously. Everything is false and unpleasant, hostile and unwelcoming. There is a strange madness abroad in the country – with tens of millions now firmly believing in the threat from covid-19 despite the fact that evidence proves without question that they are wrong.

The global prize for scaring its citizens most – and providing the most misinformation – goes to the UK where the Government and the BBC have successfully terrified the population.

Only one third of Britons have gone back to work in the UK – with the remainder working at home or sitting on Bournemouth beach. This compares poorly with the rest of Europe where, on average two thirds of workers have gone back to their offices.

Most startling of all, a recent survey showed that the average Briton believes that 7% of the British population has died of covid-19. That would mean a death total of 4.2 million in the UK alone. The real figure, of course, is probably less than 1% of that.

Still, it's not surprising that people are bewildered and wrong. *The Spectator*, a British magazine, recently published an article reporting that around the world millions had died of the coronavirus. I tried to persuade them to print a correction but the silence was deafening.

In America, Joe Biden, US Presidential candidate for the Democrats, recently claimed that over 120 million Americans had been killed by covid-19. That was clearly absurd but people believe this nonsense. We shouldn't be surprised at this. Outside the USA, the UK probably has closer links to Gates and the big vaccine manufacturers than most other countries.

At the pavement level, it is nothing more or less than hysteria. At higher levels, I am painfully conscious that there are dark clouds of evil hanging over us all. Manipulative crooks play with our lives with a scandalous lack of respect for the truth, our honour or our dignity.

Children are more likely to be hit by lightning or be neglected to death than to die of covid-19 but there is still talk of keeping schools closed. There has even been talk of closing shops and hostelries so that schools can open. If there is a shred of sense in that I can't find it. You might as well say that schools won't open unless everyone stands on one leg and sings Auld Lang Syne all day.

Mind you, parents who are brave enough to send their children to school should think about saying goodbye to them every morning because they may never see them again. The authorities have given themselves the right to test children, with a test which is about as reliable as Bill Gates, and if the test is positive, they'll snatch the child and run off with them. It used to be called kidnapping but these days it's called public health. They'll ask the child if they had ever coughed and the child will probably say yes I coughed last November and then the poor kid will be labelled as having covid-19 and whisked off to hospital where they'll doubtless pick up one of those nasty special bugs that hospitals specialise in breeding. The parents won't be allowed to see the child alive and they won't be able to see them if they die. You think I'm exaggerating? Remember what happened in care homes?

These are strange times. If the politicians told us to paint our faces blue and carry a bucket of toads with us, there are millions who would do so with enthusiasm. It is a mercy that the loonies at the World Health Organisation are unfamiliar with Macbeth. Double, double toil and trouble. Fire burn and cauldron bubble. Fillet of a fenny snake in the cauldron boil and bake. Eye of newt and toe of frog. Squirt of sanitiser and tongue of dog. Adder's fork and blind-worm's sting. Facial mask, strong plastic gloves, six feet apart and test and trace. Scale of dragon, tooth of wolf. Add thereto a Gatesian vaccine to the ingredients of our cauldron.

It is said that covid-19 can now have medium to long-term effects on some patients. And that, of course, is just the same as the flu – which can cause depression and tiredness for months afterwards. Viruses do things like that.

They are threatening, I kid you not, to knock down care homes and private houses if any residents had the coronavirus while dwelling therein. In theory this is to stop a second wave. Politicians aren't interested in the fact that in many areas there haven't been any deaths for ages.

This demolition nonsense fits neatly with the United Nations Agenda 21 plan to get rid of all private property and to move us all into smart cities. They didn't knock down houses after the plague hit Eyam in Derbyshire. Indeed, the plague ridden houses are still standing and occupied. Houses have never been knocked down because the occupants had tuberculosis or rabies. Or a virus no worse than the flu. I suspect they will not, however, be knocking down 10 Downing Street where Johnson coughed and suffered – though perhaps they should. This reminds me that the EU wanted to knock down Victorian homes in England because they didn't satisfy EU building requirements. I always assumed that by this they meant that Victorian building standards were so much higher than current EU requirements that modern builders were embarrassed to see 150-year-old houses still standing proud while EU approved homes were falling apart after six months. The EU, never forget, has always been part of Agenda 21.

In the UK the Premier League, some sort of football competition I believe, is looking at introducing app based clinical passports for fans. We all know what that means. I hope fans won't let themselves be suckered in. Let the football clubs go bust. It will do them good. No footballer deserves to be paid more than £12 a week. If £12 a week was good enough for Stanley Matthews it should be good enough for anyone.

The politicians and the vaccine soaked scientists are still terrorising the public by warning that the number of cases is still high. What a surprise. You test more people and you find more cases. What a shock that must have been. Most of the people identified are asymptomatic and as fit as fleas. Fitter than fleas were when they were carrying the Black Death.

And, of course, the tests they are using are pretty useless. Governments and their advisors haven't got round to mentioning this but the chances of a test accurately detecting covid-19 are notably less than 50 per cent. In the UK, the Office for National Statistics admits that they don't know the true sensitivity and specificity of the test. The guess is that around four out of five people who actually have the virus will test positive. So one in five who has the disease will test negative. And some people who don't have the disease will be told that they do have it.

In America, the tests seem to be even worse. The current US Centers for Disease Control test kits can produce up to 30% false positives. Some cheaper tests being used are probably ludicrously inaccurate. What all this means in practice is that covid-19 is probably never going to disappear because as long as tests are done there will be false positives and politicians will respond by ordering completely unnecessary lockdowns – even though no one has the disease. Those predictions that we are going to have to live with covid-19 for years are accurate. But there may not actually be any covid-19 – just a lot of positive tests. And, of course, spurious justification for vaccinating seven billion people entirely unnecessarily.

In an attempt to be of assistance I have devised a valuable new alternative test for covid-19 which could be far cheaper and possibly less confusing than the tests currently being used by governments everywhere. My test can be done at home at no cost whatsoever. All you need is a coin. You toss the coin into the air, catch it and examine it. If it's heads then you've got the disease. If it's tails then you haven't. I shall offer my test to the World Health Organisation as an alternative to the ones currently in use. Since my test will probably show that 50% of all those tested have the disease I suspect that governments everywhere will be thrilled. The test has to be worth at least £1 million but I'll offer it free as an item of public service. Unlike the BBC and the *Guardian* newspaper I don't want any money from the Bill and Melinda Gates Foundation.

Meanwhile, the fraud thrives and the lunacy continues.

People who would have never dreamt of wearing a mask last year, to protect them from the flu, now wear their masks with enthusiasm to protect them from covid-19 – an infection no worse than the flu. No one has ever suggested that we wore masks to protect us from tuberculosis – a far more significant disease. And yet, in America there is serious talk of people being told to wear their masks in their own homes. Madness. Mask wearers are breathing in toxin filled air rich in carbon dioxide. It's no surprise that the incidence of lung infections is rising. The only logical conclusion is that mask wearing is part of the Agenda 21 plan for a reduced population. How many will die as a result of the mask wearing fetish? A thousand? Ten Thousand? A hundred thousand? Your guess is as good as anyone's. There have already been mask related deaths and there will be more.

The lunacy is global, the same daft rules being introduced everywhere on earth. And people are waking up, of course. There have been demonstrations in England, America, Australia and Germany. Not that you'd know this if you'd confined yourself to the mainstream media. I didn't see much talk of demonstrations on the BBC website. Nor did I see much about the various enterprises backed by Gates: the spraying of dust to block out the sun or the experiment with genetically modified mosquitoes. If there were a competition for fake news, deceit and misguiding the public then in my view the BBC would win all the prizes. Still, what do you expect? This is the organisation which did a deal with the UK government, agreed to provide free TV licences for the over 75s and then reneged on the agreement and is now reputed to be spending £38 million on chasing pensioners – with the intention of sending those who do not pay to prison. This is the broadcaster which has ignored its responsibilities for decades. Bent as a paperclip. Don't do anything illegal but please don't give the BBC any of your money. Avoiding the licence fee isn't difficult. And don't buy DVDs, CDs or books published by the BBC. Tell your MP you want the BBC defunded. If the BBC has to stand alone without money from unwilling viewers it will soon disappear.

Despite the evidence, governments, local councils, quangos and officials of all kinds are still doing their very best to irritate and to make life difficult for everyone but particularly for those who are still daring to refuse to accept the lies being told about the coronavirus, covid-19, masks, vaccines, cash and Uncle Tom Cobbley's refusal to maintain social distancing when consorting with his mates in the pub. But we're at war with them so I suppose that is what we must expect. They are lying and suppressing the truth every time they see it. It's like the whack-a-mole game. If they see the truth pop up then they smash it down with a big hammer.

The truth, as we must constantly remember, is the first casualty in war. Distractions are everywhere as the mainstream media put effort into their attempts to make us forget the stupidity of what is happening. Many of the distractions are just plain silly.

Campaigners, eager to distract us from Agenda 21, the only game in town for those who care about the future, and laughably out of touch with reality, are now demanding that we get rid of phrases such as Achilles's Heel and Adam's Apple. These medical terms are allegedly misogynistic and therefore offensive and unacceptable. I really don't understand people who have so little going on in their lives that they can afford to be upset by such an amazing load of balls.

Come to think of it, I don't suppose I'm allowed to say that either. If I do then this channel will doubtless go tits up.

The world is crumbling and these cretins are fiddling.

Meanwhile, the cruelty, the sadness and the despair are everywhere. I spoke to a shop assistant who was terribly upset because her employer forced her to wear a mask. I could hardly hear a word she said and she complained that she couldn't breathe properly. She had clearly been crying. She wasn't in a trade union and I don't expect anyone else would help her. What a stupid damned world we are living in. My only advice was that she should ask to wear a visor rather than a mask. Visors are probably as useless as masks but are unlikely to produce the same levels of hypoxia. Incidentally, if you look at a box containing masks you'll probably see a warning that the masks won't stop viruses getting through. They should print that warning on each mask. They print health warnings on cigarette packets. Each mask could have a printed warning saying: 'This mask is entirely useless for the purpose for which it is worn. The wearer is a moron'.

It occurs to me, in passing, that if a shop tries to force you to wear a mask, and you have no alternative but to go there to buy essentials, then you could take down all the details of the person telling you to put on a mask and write down the date and the time. Then point out politely that you are taking notes in case you fall ill while in the shop and need to take legal action against them. Get names and addresses. They'll say they're doing it because it's the law. But in the UK, for example, you don't have to wear a mask if it makes you anxious or upsets you physically. They are lying and exceeding their authority if they say you must wear a mask.

And the mainstream media is, of course, carefully promoting the Government line and demonising those who refuse to wear masks as social and not caring about others. This is wicked nonsense but it will slowly have an effect on people – and will eventually marginalise those who understand the truth, and force them to the very edges of society before throwing them out altogether.

Why aren't doctors screaming out about the pointlessness and danger of forcing people to wear masks for many hours a day?

Some, I know, have tried to speak out and been silenced or lost their jobs. There is no such thing as freedom of speech these days.

A few brave doctors have succeeded in making their voices heard. I have tremendous admiration for two surgeons, Mr Black and Mr Narula, who reported that they had stopped using surgical masks 20 years ago after a series of controlled trials showed that using masks either had no effect on, or actually increased, the risk of post-operative infection.

They point out that it is difficult to see how insisting on a measure shown to be useless or worse will give the public confidence. I sincerely hope neither of these brave surgeons feel the cold hand of the General Medical Council on their collars.

But doctors speaking out are in a minority. They still aren't doing post mortems for heaven's sake. And some hospital departments are still closed. You can, I believe, have a tattoo but in some areas you still can't get physiotherapy.

If doctors really care about what is happening, and the way that patients are being murdered by governments, why don't a hundred get together and write letters to all the newspapers?

Or why don't they just announce that they will resign on a particular date unless the nonsense stops?

Why not just insist that their trade unions speak out against the lies being told?

Why aren't more retired doctors speaking out? They know this is lunacy and they have nothing to lose. Don't they care? Are they are all cryptorchid?

If enough doctors had found the courage to ignore the orders they were given and to speak out, in order to protect their patients and save lives, then this whole criminal enterprise would have been over weeks ago.

I have nothing but contempt for the doctors and nurses who are still keeping silent through all this. Every doctor knows that what we are seeing is a political conspiracy designed to force everyone to be vaccinated with a vaccine which has not been properly tested. Their cowardice has already led to millions of deaths worldwide. And things are getting worse by the day.

One of the disappointments over the last few months has been the scarcity of celebrities showing good sense and questioning the coronavirus hoax – now better referred to as a crime or a fraud.

One or two celebrities have said a little but then quickly withdrawn their comments when they were held up to ridicule by mask wearing zombies desperate to defend the UN's plans for world domination and eternal slavery .

The only celebrity I know of who has had the courage to stick to his guns is Peter Ebdon, the former World Snooker Champion. He's proved to be an absolute star and has resolutely maintained his position despite the inevitable sniping from small-minded morons. I have enormous respect for him. It ain't easy being a target for small-minded, quarter-witted poltroons.

August 16th 2020

Is This Fraud Ever Going to End?

I sometimes envy the zombies who believe that the only problem is an infection which causes a disease called covid-19.

They get up in the morning, check in the mirror to make sure they haven't died in the night, munch their chocolate flavoured bran flakes, choose a mask that goes best with their chosen outfit for the day and venture out into the world a little nervous but confident that their government is doing its best to protect them in these tricky times.

As they go about their business, they disinfect their hands at every possible opportunity, carefully obey the social distancing rules and wait impatiently for the vaccine.

In a way, I occasionally envy them their ignorance. They are like not very bright goldfish swimming round and round in one of those glass bowls.

People sometimes refer to the ignorant as sheep but this isn't fair.

I have kept sheep and they are far more intelligent than most people imagine. Hardly anyone has bothered to do any research because, like cows and pigs, sheep are just farm animals, and farmers and vets don't have much interest in studying animals whose destiny is to be slaughtered, chopped up and eaten.

For example, the books will tell you that sheep are colour blind. They aren't.

I used to have a four wheel drive vehicle which was the same model as the vet's. My car was blue and his was green. When the sheep saw my car coming they ran towards me because I always gave them biscuits. When they saw the vet coming, they ran away because he always wanted to check their feet and they didn't like that. I later tested with different coloured feed buckets, and I can promise you that sheep are not colour blind. They are actually very bright animals. And they are brave too. My sheep once frightened a sheepdog so much that the dog's owner begged me to call my sheep off his dog.

So, to me, the ignorant thickos who still believe the coronavirus is the new plague are zombies or collaborators.

The vigilance of the collaborators means that every trip to the shops has become something of an ordeal.

The staff in the supermarket are always fine and actually a few seem genuinely sympathetic. But there is invariably one customer who worships Bill Gates, probably has his picture above his bed, and who feels it is his duty to confront any intelligent people he sees with naked faces.

This morning I hadn't got more than three feet into the supermarket when a pompous, sanctimonious mask-finder general, one of Commander Dick's shame police, rushed up to my wife and rudely and aggressively demanded that she put on a mask. That's Commander Dick of the Metropolitan police.

My wife was startled and upset and politely told him that she was exempt. He still scowled and I thought he deserved more. And with my wife's permission I explained that it wasn't really any of his business but that she'd had surgery for breast cancer and a month's radiotherapy which has caused damage which makes breathing difficult. Thanks to the absurd coronavirus hoax, the hospital physiotherapy department is still closed so she is in pain most of the day. I wish someone would explain that to me, incidentally. My wife can have a tattoo, were she so inclined, or her hair done, but she cannot have physiotherapy because the physiotherapy department is still closed. I pointed out to the mask-wearing prefect that nurses at the hospital told her to remove her mask after she almost collapsed with palpitations caused by her condition.

You might have thought a human being would have been embarrassed. Not a bit of it. The Dick police specials are shameless. The cretin, utterly indifferent and uncaring, just shrugged and demanded to know why I wasn't wearing a mask.

I always explain to the thickos that the mask they are wearing does absolutely no good, that mask wearing is dangerous, that they didn't wear a mask last year so why are they wearing one this year and that covid-19 has killed fewer people than the flu.

I do this because I think these zombies need to be educated before they accost an elderly or frail person and cause serious upset.

Sadly, however, in my now generous experience, the mask promoting lunatics always run away when you reply to their muttered, 'where's your mask' mantra. The collaborators compound their selfishness and their ignorance with good old-fashioned cowardice: without exception, they run away. Say something, anything, in reply and they scoot away back to the hole in the skirting board.

And that's what happened with this coward. He ran off. All mouth but no guts.

'You are an idiot!' I shouted at the retreating mask wearer.

Not witty, I admit, but adequate.

The collaborators will destroy our lives as well as their own unless they are brought to heel.

I had trouble in the bank, too. There was, inevitably, a lengthy queue outside which was fine because Bill Gates's cloud of calcium carbonate hanging in the sky was keeping the sun at bay though I wonder how many people will freeze to death when the weather becomes a little chillier. All part of the Agenda 21 plan to get rid of the elderly and the frail?

Eventually, when I got a foot in the door, a girl whom I could identify as a staff member only because of her uniform, asked me where my mask was and wanted to know if I was exempt. I smiled and nodded and she offered to get me a lanyard with a label to hang around my neck to show that I was exempt. Since I don't want a lanyard with a label any more than I want a mask, I just smiled and said no thank you and explained that masks are entirely useless because viruses go straight through the material.

'I know,' she said. 'But wearing a mask gives people confidence.' What madness. She knows that masks are useless but she thinks they give people confidence. Does she think all their customers are half-witted five-year-olds? The answer is obviously yes.

And talking of five-year-olds, when is someone going to start arresting parents who force small children to wear masks? In England, children under the age of 11 are exempt from mask wearing. (Look at the Government website for the latest information because the rules change almost daily.) There is much talk of authorities taking children away from parents who disapprove of vaccination. I think they've got it the wrong way round. They should be taking children away from parents who force children to wear masks or let them get vaccinated.

Just before we left town, we saw a maskless man come out of the supermarket. Like conspirators we chatted for a few moments. He was quite awake and aware of the fraud being perpetrated upon us. He told us that he watched UK Column and the 'old man in a chair'. He didn't have the faintest idea the old man, without his chair, was standing just two feet away from him. We didn't mention it.

You and I are involved in a war where we are not quite sure whom we are fighting or precisely what their final aims might be – other than the fact that we are destined to be drones, slaves, proles in a world run by a new self-appointed aristocracy.

The minute we think we have worked it out and know what the rules are they change the rules. It is a world which appears to have been designed by Lewis Carroll to make Franz Kafka feel comfortable.

The only stable currency is the lie.

It is no exaggeration to say that it is fair to assume that everything anyone in authority says will be a lie. They do it so naturally that I sometimes wonder if any of the politicians and their advisors realise just how much they are lying. Maybe it's just like breathing. They do it without thinking.

I think we perhaps all misunderstand how vile politicians are. Auberon Waugh once said that the only thing that any of them is really interested in is the chance to make decisions and see them put into effect – to press a button and watch us all jump.

He was right, but the politicians have recently been joined by an army of advisors, hangers on and confidants who are also in it for the power, and who have very real views on how the world should be but who cannot be bothered to stand for election. I suspect that the Rothschilds, the Rockefellers, Gates, Soros and so on are all too arrogant to expose themselves to the ballot box and I fear they all hold us in contempt.

It is often said that the truth will set us free but the one certainty these days is that long before we get there we will be disappointed, frustrated and not a little angry.

They say we must be prepared for a second wave.

A second wave of what?

Did we actually have a first wave? Covid-19 killed fewer people than the flu. What sort of wave is that? More of a ripple really.

How can there be a second wave without a first wave?

We could, I suppose, have a second ripple.

Take out the hundreds of thousands of old people who were murdered in care homes around the world, and the hundreds of thousands who were put down as dying of covid-19 but actually died of something else, and the total number who have allegedly died of the coronavirus can hardly be called a wave. It certainly wasn't much of a pandemic.

In England and Wales the excess number of deaths has fallen below the five year average for the fifth week in a row. Moreover, the figures now show that more than 90% of covid-19 deaths occurred in people over 60 and 90% of those who died in hospital had existing health conditions before they got infected. In due course, the real figures will be available and they will, I suspect, show that over 90% were in their 80s or older, and had two or three co-morbidities.

There are regions of England where I suspect that more people are dying from falling off horses than are dying from the coronavirus. Does that mean that we're having an epidemic of deaths caused by people falling off horses? In many parts of the world anything that actually kills people is a bigger threat than the coronavirus. Is rabies now a global pandemic? How about falling off mountains? I would bet that there have been more suicides, caused by fear and despair for the future than covid-19 deaths in some places in the last month.

Nothing much makes any sense any more, does it?

And yet, as hypnotherapist and author Colin Barron points out, many of the so-called experts on covid-19 don't have any medical qualifications. Neil Ferguson is a mathematician and yet his predictions were used as the basis for the global lockdowns.

Everyone with a certificate in basic woodwork has suddenly become a medical expert.

The other day, the Scottish Daily Mail printed a letter from someone called Professor Greg Philo of Glasgow University who warns, 'the fear is real and we need a strategy to eliminate the virus'.

So, what is Professor Philo's medical speciality? Medicine? Surgery? Epidemiology? General Practice?

None of the above.

The only Professor Philo I could find is a professor of communications and social change.

And if you've got any idea what that means then you have my commiserations.

Why do such people assume the right to pontificate about whether or not a specific virus infection is a particular threat?

As Dr Barron says, there was a time when only taxi drivers were experts on everything. These days even professors of communications and social change want to share their conclusions about a complex piece of global manipulation.

We have reached the strange position where paranoia is no longer a medical condition. It is a rational state of mind. Governments have lied about lockdowns, they have lied about the number of deaths, they have lied about the need for masks and they have lied about social distancing. Trying to dismantle the lies and find the kernel of truth is like playing three dimensional chess, and if that isn't the most mixed up metaphor in history then I'll try again another day.

I can't remember the last time a politician said anything that bore even a faint relationship to the truth. You'd be mad not to assume that everything the dishonest, deceitful cynical politicians and the advisors say is a barefaced lie. We're being ruled by crazed psychopaths who have somehow succeeded in encouraging the collaborators to believe that it is possible to remove all risk from human life.

Politicians and their advisors should be forced to wear logos on their suits to list their sponsors, allegiances and connections. They'd have so many advertising logos they would look like race car drivers. All BBC staff should have EU and the Bill and Melinda Gates Foundation logos on their clothing at all times. *The Guardian* too. Anyone with links to a drug company should be banned from any sort of public role. As I have shown in previous videos the world's drug companies are more dishonest and dishonourable than tobacco companies. We would be better off if the world were run by a cabal of Columbian drug barons than the pirate crew currently striving for global control.

Telling lies is the new normal in our world.

They say that wearing masks will provide protection. This isn't true. What evidence there is available shows that masks are entirely pointless and potentially dangerous. Only the clinically insane and people with IQs in single figures think masks are of any value whatsoever. Why don't footballers have to wear masks when they're playing? Because masks impede their breathing. Why do even politicians and government advisors agree that those with respiratory problems don't have to wear masks? The answer is obvious – because masks impede breathing.

They say that it will be necessary to introduce more lockdowns to prevent more deaths. But even governments now admit that lockdowns cause more deaths than they prevent. So the only possible reason for having more lockdowns is to kill more people.

They say they need to introduce new laws to avoid a second wave of infections and deaths. The truth is that it was the last lot of laws – the social distancing, the lockdowns and the masks – which have caused the deaths. More laws will result in more deaths.

They say we have to close our borders to keep out the virus. This is bollocks. In March I suggested closing airports to control the infection rate. But airports were left open. Now that the death rate has collapsed, they want to stop people travelling. They are desperate to stop anyone travelling or having a good time. They are deliberately creating fear to sustain their corrupt, satanic ideology.

They say that testing is showing up more cases. This is so deceitful it's worthy of Bernie Madoff. The tests which are being used throw up so many false positives that they are about as much use as a castrated ram in a field full of sheep. And even the politicians and their advisors must realise that if you test ten times as many people then the chances are that you will find more people who have or have had the infection. Tracking and tracing is simply an infringement of our civil liberties. It is of no value whatsoever.

They say the only way we will ever get back to normal will be with a vaccine. This is the biggest lie of all. Worst of all, they say that the new vaccine will be safe. They cannot possibly know this. The dimmest, most stupid person you know can judge whether their new vaccine will be safe as well as they can.

Politicians, advisors, commentators and professors of golf course management claim that the world will not get back to normal until there is a vaccine available.

There is of course, another unspoken option: that the majority will realise that the coronavirus scare is a hoax; a massive fraud deliberately and arranged by people with malignant intentions.

And that's what is going to happen.

I will leave you with a quote from the Robert Donat film version of the Count of Monte Cristo: 'They call me mad because I tell the truth.' What more can I say?

August 18th 2020

Nothing is Now Impossible

It may seem like hyperbole to compare what is happening to us now to what happened in Europe during World War II.

It's different, of course.

We aren't being bombed, for example.

But the threat to us all, and the world in which we live, is now just as great as it was in 1939 and the 1940s.

In some ways the threat is greater.

Then, we just had to beat a small bunch of deranged psychopaths. And we had the support and leadership of our governments. We had Winston Churchill.

Today, in a bizarre turn, our enemies are our own governments. We are being manipulated, threatened and punished by dictators. We are living in totalitarian states. We have no democracy and very little freedom of speech.

We are fighting people who want to turn us into slaves. The plans of the United Nations and the World Economic Forum are worse than anything thought up by Hitler or Stalin.

We are oppressed by individuals who are just as evil as any of those who slaughtered the innocent across Europe, laying the foundations for the development of the European Union.

The EU: conceived by Nazis, built by Nazis and now loved by Nazis was the first step towards a World Government – the first fascist super state. It was quickly absorbed by the UN into the Agenda 21 plans.

Today, the enemy doesn't wear jackboots or do the goosestep. And this time we have elected and financed our own enemy. Our political leaders are the enemy. We are paying for our own oppressors. In New Zealand, concentration camps have been set up for the tiny number of people who have tested positive. They don't call them that, of course. I think they're holiday camps in newspeak. Or quarantine camps perhaps.

We all have a number of choices, of course.

The easy option is always to join the oppressors – to become collaborators. That's what millions have done. They accept the lies about covid-19 because they cannot believe that their own political leaders would lie so much. They socially distance, they wear the masks, they put themselves under house arrest when ordered to do so. Some have probably even managed to convince themselves that the lies must be true. How could anyone lie so much? How could anyone be as totally incompetent as they say that nice Professor Ferguson is? And doesn't the BBC say that smiling Mr Gates does a lot for charity? Some people just keep quiet. They say and do nothing for fear of the consequences. They hope that the evil will pass. Or that someone else will speak up and change things for them.

And then there's us.

There are always some difficult buggers who refuse to lie down and accept unjust and absurd laws.

It happened in World War II. The resistance movement played a major part in defeating the Nazis.

And today the resistance movement is all we've got.

It's us. We're the resistance movement, and we're missionaries to the Truth Deniers.

And we're in a war.

You know how, if you bend a paperclip you can never get it back to the way it was? Well, that's our political system. It is bent and cannot be mended. I have long distrusted the party system and it is now clearer than ever that it doesn't work. Our political system, our administration, our local government, our health care system – they are all rotten to the core. Destroyed by unbridled ambition, greed and the dead hand of the brainwashed, indoctrinated hand-maidens of Common Purpose.

We are watching, first hand, as the pseudoscientists and crooks who run the climate change fraud are leading an assault on God, nature and mankind.

Nothing is as it used to be nor as it seems to be. Everything is controlled from afar by people we can't see and over whom we have no control. In the US and Europe, everything is controlled by lobbyists – tens of thousands of them spending billions a year – and ensuring that the principles of Agenda 21 (if we can call them principles) are introduced, adhered to and thoroughly exploited by the rich and the mega rich – cruising the world's seas in huge self-contained super yachts.

Everywhere I look there is deceit and manipulation. Nothing is what it appears to be. So, for example, it seems to me as though every position the World Health Organisation has taken, based on the available scientific research, has been reversed. A couple of months ago, the WHO thought that wearing masks was pointless and unnecessary. The available evidence said they were right. And then suddenly, without the science changing, the WHO changed its mind and masks became mandatory. The only difference? Could it be that Bill Gates had become a major 'shareholder' in the WHO? That's the pro-vaxx organisation not the rock band by the way – though the rock band would probably give better health advice.

On the 28th May 2020, Dr Fauci, the American coronavirus supremo announced that masks are little more than symbolic. They were derided as virtue signalling. And then, suddenly, there is Dr Fauci standing next to President Trump wearing a mask. In the UK, the Government's medical advisors had dismissed masks as unnecessary. And then suddenly, for no apparent reason, the Government changed its tiny mind and anyone not wearing a mask suddenly became liable to a fine of up to £3,200. The odd figure, incidentally, came from a bizarre and unprecedented system whereby non-mask wearers would be fined £100 for an initial offence with the fine doubling for each subsequent occasion.

Incidentally, what is going to happen to the millions of dumped single use masks? How many people know that if you wash a cloth mask it becomes more useless every time you wash it? And if you don't wash it then you are putting a cloth containing bacteria, fungi and viruses next to your mouth every time you put it on. Legionnaire's Disease is a real and lethal risk. What will happen when vaccines come in? Will those who refuse vaccination be forced to continue to wear a mask as a sign of shame? Perhaps they could issue masks containing yellow stars – just to make the point. And why do so many people wear masks in the street when they don't have to? Just about all the pictures I saw recently of teenagers campaigning for better exam results, showed them wearing masks when they didn't have to. Why? Were they stupid? Or were the photos staged?

Mask enthusiasts often say that masks must be fine because surgeons wear them. This simply displays their ignorance. Not all surgeons do wear masks because studies have shown that wearing them does not reduce infection. Moreover, surgeons usually work in air conditioned, cooled operating theatres. They do their work standing or sitting and they wear masks for relatively short periods of time.

Terrorism, let me remind you, is, according to my definition, politics by intimidation – without any moral restrictions. We are being terrorised by our own governments. Masks must be worn and pubs must be shut.

Is this in homage to the new global religion –Chrislam? The Archbishop of Canterbury provided Christians with a short talk from his kitchen but virtue signalled by shutting churches. What sort of leadership was that?

There is no logic to anything anymore.

Theatres are closed and will stay closed though thespians and artists who behave will receive grants to buy their allegiance. If plays are performed actors will have to respect social distancing rules so no plays by Shakespeare will ever again be performed. There will be no choirs and no opera.

And yet we are allowed to climb into aeroplanes where the air is constantly recirculated, and whatever viruses one traveller has may be shared by everyone by the time the aeroplane lands.

Racism is now so much a part of our lives that no one takes any notice – and if they do then they keep quiet about it. Biden, the Democratic Presidential candidate, who at one point said that 120 million Americans had been killed by covid-19, announced that he would pick as his vice president a woman of colour. No one thought this sexist and racist, though it clearly was.

Ironically, the woman he picked had apparently accused him of being a racist and of sexual assault. It says a good deal to me about opportunistic politicians that the two have, nevertheless, buried any principles they might have had and agreed to work with each other. Incidentally, Biden has supported just about every war America has started for 30 years.

Politicians and advisors are now talking about our needing to wear masks, and maintain social distancing, indefinitely. That is the sort of indefinitely which means forever. The collaborators who are merrily wearing their fashion masks in the open air in countries where it is not a legal necessity are going to kill humanity.

I wonder how many people know that the phrase, 'If you're not with us you are against us' originated with Jesus Christ and not George W. Bush.

The mass of people have unwittingly joined a conspiracy against themselves. Never before have ordinary people been so cowed, so curiously deferential. Children are frightened because they don't know any better. But the adults who believe the crap they are being fed annoy me enormously. How can anyone have got to adulthood without wanting to question the blatant lies we are currently being fed? The lies are grotesque, inexplicable and indefensible. Those of you with a mischievous sense of humour might be amused by two of my early videos – 'New Law – Everyone Must Now Hop and Wear Galoshes' and 'Everything You Are Allowed to Know but I Can't Tell You What about'.

Inspired by appalling policewoman Dick, who encouraged public shaming, the collaborators happily join their masters in demonising, monstering and abusing those too ill to wear a mask or brave enough to think for themselves. I still think the Dick woman should be arrested and charged with something – inciting harassment, perhaps. If that isn't an offence it should be.

Millions who have never taken any interest in protecting themselves from heart disease or cancer now seem so desperately afraid of covid-19, as harmless as flu let us not forget, that they have happily abandoned their freedom and their rights. Sweden proved that the lockdowns and the masks and the social distancing were all unnecessary but those are facts and facts are no longer popular.

Millions of Britons have enjoyed a summer free of work – on furlough, paid by taxpayers. They've been enjoying themselves on their country's beaches; though I hope they observed the ruling that they should remain six feet six inches away from the lifeguards – so presumably any rescuing had to be done at a distance. I wonder if they will feel quite so jolly when they prepare to go back to work and discover that their jobs have gone. The UN recently estimated that half of the world's jobs will disappear. People who find themselves unemployed this autumn will probably never work again. Ever. I wonder whether people will be angry when they realise just how much the damage is going to affect their lives. Economists and commentators say the recovery will be quick. It won't be. This is not a temporary inconvenience. The coronavirus fraud is going to lead to permanent changes in every aspect of our society from jobs to health care and from pensions to education – and those changes are being made cold bloodedly and deliberately and globally. Millions of people are going to die in the next year because their illnesses weren't treated because of the lockdowns.

Health care is going to change dramatically – but not for the better. GPs now seem too lazy or too afraid to see patients. Instead care assistants with modest training see patients in tents or on the pavement or in the car park. You can have a tattoo – which involves a stranger piercing your skin with a needle – but if you do agree to a vaccination it will be done on the pavement because it is too dangerous to do it in the GP's surgery. Assessing patients on the pavement is apparently happening in America too. One patient who had suffered from hay-fever and had visited a nearby town where there have been positive tests, was refused treatment by a doctor but offered a telephone conversation with a physician assistant. Some doctors are, it seems, too frightened to offer even telephone consultations. It must be a relief to them that the golf courses are now open.

You can go into a pub but you can't go to an AA meeting because that would be too dangerous. Education will soon be done exclusively on the internet – using the excuse that it is too dangerous for children to go to school and sit together in classrooms. No one in government cares a damn about the evidence that letting children go to school is probably safer than keeping them at home – as long as you forget about the unnecessary social distancing and the mask wearing nonsense. Surely, even the most unimaginative must soon be able to discern patterns with a purpose.

It's not difficult to see that this is part of a global plan – Agenda 21 to give it a name.

Most of the people who have died of covid-19 have been over 80 with at least two or three other serious health problems – and many lived in care homes where they were murdered.

If old people had been murdered in care homes in one country, then that might have been a result of incompetence. But when exactly the same mistake is made in just about every country in the world then it becomes clear that the deaths are a result of official policy.

It is now allegedly routine to put Do Not Resuscitate notices on everyone over the age of 60. No one is denying it. In Scotland, it is rumoured that the cut off age is 45. No one is denying that. And DNR notices are routinely put on those with mental illness or physical disabilities whatever their age. That is the default position. The elderly and the frail and the disabled must be eliminated. It's part of the Agenda 21 plan, the move towards a community based world where the individual must be subservient to the needs of the greater good.

Nothing will ever be the same again. Savers and investors face a dark and dismal future. One bank with which I have an account, recently told me that my balance earns interest at a rate of 0.00001 % and I consider myself lucky that the interest hasn't yet gone negative. None of this is accidental. It's all deliberate.

I'm told that there are still thousands of people who get their news from the BBC! How can this be? If the BBC ever published an honest fact, the whole bent organisation would go into meltdown and have to issue an immediate retraction and apology. 'We are terribly sorry about the fact we broadcast the other day. It was a mistake and won't happen again.'

Sadly, the BBC isn't the only untrustworthy news organisation.

It has for some time now been the case that magazines, newspapers and broadcasters have been beholden to advertisers.

This wasn't always the case.

I can remember when editors would fly into a rage if an advertiser or advertising director tried to influence a publication's editorial content or policy.

But as circulations fell, the balance of power moved from readers to advertisers and for some time now publications have done little but publish press releases. The sacking of experienced journalists, to save money, and replacing them with naïve, dishonourable youngsters has helped the decline. Today, mainstream media are supine. They promote the governmental hysteria apparently without embarrassment. They use the word pandemic as though it were an accurate appraisal of the situation.

Occasionally, however, there are some bright spots of hope, and I think the pressure from the resistance movement may be having an effect. The usually rather untrustworthy (in my opinion) *Times* newspaper recently ran a headline which read: 'Flu and pneumonia killed five times more than covid last month'. Very true and it's nice to see it in print.

In 2019, the WHO studied influenza pandemics and came to the conclusion that contact tracing is not useful from an epidemiological point of view and (and I quote) 'is not recommended in any circumstances'.

Talking of flu, by the way, scientists still don't know if having the flu vaccine makes people more likely to develop covid-19. Come to think of it, maybe that's why there is such enthusiasm about giving the flu vaccine to as many people as possible this autumn.

Despite the WHO view on contact tracing, governments around the world (most of which were claiming to take their lead from the Bill Gates funded organisation), introduced track and trace systems – largely using a system devised by Google and Apple. The Google and Apple nonsense was pumped into three billion mobile phones and was apparently designed to record and store all contacts – not just those considered medically relevant. A German IT expert described tracing apps as a Trojan horse. I think we all know what he meant. And I'll just remind you that the WHO condemned contact tracing as not recommended in any circumstances.

Never before has science been dismissed with such a cavalier attitude. It is clear that our mobile telephones are due to play an ever increasing part in our lives. In 2011, just 3.5% of payments in China were made with mobile phones. Today, 85% of all payments are made with mobile phones. It is a very small step from a mobile phone which runs your life to a far more convenient chip placed under the skin in your arm. It is hardly surprising that the boss of Microsoft has boasted that 'we've seen two years' worth of digital transformation in two months'. Gates, incidentally, has been funding the development of micro implants to give multiple doses of a vaccine or drug over an extended period.

Using a temperature gun is about as useful as asking someone their astrological sign and then isolating all those born under the fishes or the scales. But temperature guns are now seen everywhere.

Back on 23rd April, Neil Ferguson, the Oliver Hardy of mathematics, but without the charm or loveability, was reported as saying that a second wave, worse than the first, was virtually certain to happen. Politicians seem desperate for him to be proved right. If he is proved right it will possibly be a first.

We have for years been living under the eye of Big Brother. But soon Big Brother will be inside us, controlling us. Trans-humanism plans will develop further. Mobile phones will be replaced by obligatory under the skin controls. The people who happily give all their personal details to phone apps will no doubt be eager to have a chip under their skin.

Millions innocently accepted smart meters for their electricity supplies because they believed what they were told. Anyone was suckered into accepting one should now demand that it's taken out of their home. Just as the authorities can use the smart meter to turn off your electricity so they will switch off your access to money or food or work simply by controlling the chip under your skin. And then there will be accidents that will occur and probably result in millions of deaths. And the hackers. Oh, don't forget the hackers.

Talking of deaths, I see that in Ireland there have, in recent months, been fewer total deaths than in any of the previous three years. I suspect that will change both there and elsewhere in the autumn. The deaths caused by the lockdown will start mounting then. When thousands start to die of treatable cancer and heart disease there will, I suspect, be a little more anger among those who are still naïve enough and ill-informed enough to believe that covid-19 is a serious pandemic. Hundreds of thousands of extra deaths are going to mar nations for months if not years – all avoidable, all caused by the lockdowns and all predicted from this chair months ago. Hundreds of crooked politicians and advisors will doubtless try to persuade us that the deaths have been caused by the coronavirus. They will only be able to get away with this if doctors continue to falsify death certificates.

Unless we stop this nonsense quickly, it is going to get worse.

They are pushing us to see how far they can go. What will they try next? Wearing masks in the street, in offices, in schools and at home. Wearing goggles and gloves perhaps? I now find it impossible to imagine an insult they would not regard as appropriate. They have closed the dentists and there is no effective health care for millions. Most people are rightly now terrified of seeing a doctor or going into hospital. Do not resuscitate notices are routinely put on anyone over the age of 60 and on individuals of any age who have mental or physical problems. I find it difficult to believe it is happening – but it is and there's no point in sticking our heads in the sand, under the blanket or anywhere else.

I am glad to see more and more protests around the world – mostly ignored or demonised by the mainstream media.

In the UK, Piers Corbyn and StandupX are brilliant. Piers Corbyn, clearly a gentle man, has been arrested 45 times for standing up for our freedom. He has been arrested for the modern crime of telling the truth. By now he has probably been arrested 46 times, 47 – who knows. The police should give him a season ticket.

The new normal as they call it is nothing more than the new world order – the global reset so beloved by fascist extremists and wicked hypocrites such as the utterly appalling Prince Charles – what a bloody family that has turned out to be. They're like something out of a bad soap opera. They, like the BBC, should be defunded. The BBC doesn't deserve public money and the royals don't need it.

The internet has, despite all the bans and shutdowns and the activities of the state financed trolls, been a revelation – and our only hope of salvation. Listen to the Richie Allen radio show and watch, among others, UK Column, Amazing Polly, Dr Judy Mikovits, Ice Age Farmer and The Corbett Report.

When all this is over, every political leader who has put citizens under house arrest and maintained the evil myth of this pandemic must be tried for treason. We'll try them before hanging, drawing and quartering them because that's the way civilised people do things.

Remember: decisions are made by those who speak up.

And what's the point of a life if you sell your soul for a little peace and quiet?

Share this video quickly because it contains a lot of truths. YouTube quickly took down my recent video entitled, 'Forbidden Truths' – presumably because it contained truths which are forbidden. Naturally, in this Kafkaesque world they didn't explain precisely what my crime was.

YouTube has also now recently taken down and banned my video entitled, 'Coronavirus: Mental Health Problems Will Now Soar' which was published in May and in which I predicted that government policies would result in an increase in anxiety and depression. Figures just published confirm that the prediction was, sadly, accurate. I don't know whether the video was taken down because I predicted what would happen or because it has now happened.

August 23rd 2020

Guarded Secrets and Blatant Deceits

Our house needs painting but what's the point? We really can't get excited about it. We are living in the middle of the greatest threat to human life since, well, since ever. As far as I am concerned, Bill Gates is a greater threat than Adolf Hitler.

Most people are sleep-walking and in five years' time, they will probably still not understand why their lives have changed so dramatically and so much for the worse. The least intelligent and least informed will simply blame the covid fraud – or whatever other fake crisis the globalists, the climate change freaks and the Agenda 21 supporters think up. The collaborators will never know that the pandemic was predicted, in some detail, by many of the main players. By then the one world government will be controlling every aspect of our lives – including our access to our own money and our access to food.

The proponents of the global government condemn all opposition as being worried by threats to their social status, as being racists, as being authoritarian. The monstering, the demonising is done relentlessly and the collaborators are constantly recruited as foot soldiers in the war. Remember, never forget, policewoman Dick's cruel exhortation for collaborators to shame those with hidden disabilities and health problems, as well as those with free spirits and free minds.

Their aim is plainly visible; it is to dehumanise humans, to allow robots to take over the world, to deprive us all of our hearts and souls and of our freedom and democracy. The aim of the fourth industrial revolution is to control who we are as well as what we do and what we think. This is the Great Reset. All babies will be programmed. Robots will take over virtually all jobs. The world population will be reduced by 95%. The UN's stated aim is for the industrialised nations to collapse. 'No one,' says the UN, 'will enter the New Age unless he will take a Luciferian initiation. They want to scare us, divide us and take away all our power.

They want to destroy small businesses and the middle classes and all ambition and all aspirations. They want to confiscate all private property and cause economic chaos so that they can reset the world. They want to install unelected regional governors – just as the EU planned to do – and to ban all manifestations of nationalism. So, for example, nation flags will be outlawed.

In England, the latest figures show that the overall mortality rate in June was lower than average. Fewer people are dying than is usual but the Government is still behaving as though we are living through a plague.

The figures make curious reading.

The number of people dying of heart disease, lung cancer, stroke and bowel cancer are far, far below normal for the month of June.

The only rise is, of course, the number of people dying of covid-19 – a new entrant into the top ten.

But the odd thing is that while the number of people dying of covid-19 is 53 per 100,000, the number of people dying from flu, pneumonia and chronic lower respiratory disease were much lower than usual. Indeed, the number dying of flu and pneumonia was 19.1 per 100,000 lower than is usual for June. The number dying of chronic lower respiratory disease was 16.7 per 100,000 lower than is usual for June. And the number of elderly folk allegedly dying of dementia was 18.5 per 100,000 lower than usual. The dementia figure is relevant first because no one actually dies of dementia and second because the vast majority of dementia patients are over 80 years old and so were the sort of people alleged to have died of covid-19.

Now the really strange thing is, that if you add those three figures together you get 54.3 per 100,000 – which, by one of those odd little coincidences which seem commonplace these days, just happens to be almost the same as the number dying of covid-19.

So there we are.

Those of a suspicious nature might suspect that no one actually died of covid-19 but that the people who would have usually died of flu, pneumonia, dementia or chronic respiratory disease, were bunged down as covid-19 deaths just to keep us all scared witless and to provide an excuse to shut down the whole country – closing down much of the health service, shutting schools, closing factories and shops, restaurants and pubs, bowling alleys, cinemas, theatres and service industries of all kinds.

Naturally, however, you and I are not of a suspicious nature. We would like this video to remain alive and well on the YouTube platform and so we avoid drawing conclusions.

And so we believe that these figures are merely coincidences. Just little oddities; quirks of fate.

The result of closing the country has been disastrous, of course.

So, for example, nearly a third of women with primary breast cancer had their treatment, scans or appointments postponed because of the hysteria. Moreover, a new study showed that patients who had experienced delays were 20% more likely to be depressed and anxious than women whose treatment went ahead as it should have.

Two things about that occur to me.

First, that anyone should be surprised that women with cancer, who were denied essential treatment, were more likely to be depressed. Personally, I can't understand why 100% of the women weren't depressed and anxious.

Second, I am startled by the fact that although the UK health service could not provide essential medical services for women with breast cancer it could, nevertheless, manage to conduct a survey of the women who had been abandoned. I can imagine the conversation. 'Hello, is that Mrs Hancock? It is? Good. You have, as you know, recently been diagnosed as having breast cancer. How do you feel about the fact that your treatment has been delayed indefinitely?'

That's something not even Nero thought of when he set Rome ablaze. He should have sent out a few slaves to conduct a survey of the citizens as their city burnt to cinders.

Meanwhile, the energetic mathematicians at Imperial College, in London, the Bill Gates backed college which shut down the country for the flu, the modelling equivalent of the Three Stooges, have found that the lockdown could lead to an extra 1.4 million deaths from tuberculosis. The imperial College folk reckon that the lockdowns have set back the fight against tuberculosis by at least five to eight years.

And the British Department for Health and Social Care has concluded that the lockdown triggered by Imperial College's scaremongering will have a greater impact on our health and lives than covid-19. I seem to remember mentioning that back in March.

If I had any tears left I would weep.

But there is more to come from Imperial College.

I honestly find this difficult to believe but they are apparently claiming that if we hadn't gone into lockdown then 1.6 more million people would have died.

Yes.

Ferguson and the rest of the gang at Imperial are claiming we should be grateful to them.

They don't seem to have read the reports concluding that their forecasts were about as rubbishy as it is possible to get. We would have all been much better off if the dog had eaten Ferguson's homework. Some are trying to make up their minds whether it was the hysterical nonsense from Imperial College which led to panic or the panic from Imperial College which led to hysteria. I have no such dilemma.

I think Ferguson and imperial College were chosen by the politicians because the politicians knew they'd cock up the forecast. It is, after all, what they've done regularly for years.

I think I've had enough of this lot at Imperial College. They should be given useful work to do. There must be public lavatories somewhere which need cleaning.

Or maybe that would be too tricky for them.

And a document rereleased from the British Government's official advisors at SAGE – surely the most unsuitable acronym in history – confirms what I have been saying for months: that their advice to the Government was to use the media to increase a sense of personal threat and to increase a sense of responsibility to others.

May I remind you that we pay the fat salaries of these bastards.

But instead of looking after us, calming our fears and making us less stressed, they have been deliberately doing everything they could to terrify us and ramp up the scare stories.

Distrust the government, avoid mass media and fight the lies.

Meanwhile, the leaders of the four nations in the UK have been doing everything possible to create confusion and extra anxiety.

I plucked up the courage to take a look at the BBC website the other day and found the official rules on how and when people are allowed to meet one another.

In England six people from multiple households, or up to 30 people from two households can meet together outdoors. They must not get closer than more than three feet three inches. In Scotland up to 15 people from up to five households can meet as long as they all keep six feet six inches apart. In Wales any number of people from two households can meet as long as they are six feet six inches apart. And in Northern Ireland up to 30 people can meet outdoors but must keep three feet three inches apart.

The rules are equally confusing for indoor meetings. In England, two households can meet together, in Scotland eight people from three households can meet, in Wales two households can form one extended household (whatever that means – it sounds like Welsh wife swapping to me) and in Northern Ireland, ten people from four households can meet. There is no advice on what happens to citizens who live on a border between two countries.

The one conclusion from all this bollocks is that there is no science to any of this. Idiot civil servants and politicians have clearly just made it all up.

I bet they couldn't stop laughing to themselves as they wrote this garbage.

Meanwhile, there is increasing evidence that fewer and fewer deaths are being marked down to covid-19 and that more and more people are immune. The testing is a nonsense, as unreliable as Tony Blair, but as the positives turn up with predictable regularity so governments use the results as an excuse for more and tougher new laws.

And all the time the media simply support the fakery, the hoax, the fraud.

The natural inclination of the media is to question, attack and sneer at those in power. Some newspapers will support one point of view and some another view. That's democracy.

But this time the mainstream media has been united in support of the coronavirus hoax. The threat to the public has been massively exaggerated, and official policies have been reported without question. Even in wartime there are always some mainstream journalists who question what is happening. But not much this time. The surveillance methods have all been applauded. Stories have been manipulated and all those protesting about the over-kill have been denounced as morons or worse.

The media have allowed themselves to be used as part of the psychological operations organised by governments. Major internet platforms such as Google, Facebook, Twitter and YouTube have censored critical remarks – even when justified by the facts. I have lost count of the number of videos I have had removed. Not one of those banned videos contained anything untrue or inaccurate. Doctors have been ordered not to speak out. One doctor I know was struck off the medical register in the UK for questioning the official line. The lies have all been coming from politicians and advisors and have been spread with enthusiasm by media organisations such as the BBC in the UK. In my experience, even Wikipedia seems to have become part of the geopolitical damning of individuals.

Back in 2010, the American Rockefeller Foundation described a lockstep scenario in which a pandemic could be used to control a population. The lockstep scenario written a decade ago has been acted out in precise detail. Contact tracking has been introduced despite the fact that over 500 scientists have warned against unprecedented surveillance.

There is evidence that some of those producing fake information – and the guilty include some well-known establishment universities and journals have links to security services.

There is no longer any doubt that health policy is being used to achieve geopolitical goals.

We are at war with our own governments, with many of our universities and with much of our media.

In the long-term, we need to sweep clean the stables and create a new political and administrative system. We need new leaders, new media and new management. Our politicians and public servants have done worse than fail us – they have betrayed us.

August 26th 2020

London Rally August 29th

The coronavirus scare was always a hoax. And today, it's clear to anyone who looks at the facts that the coronavirus was never any more of a threat than the flu. It would make as much sense to sit it somewhere between measles and falling downstairs as to brand it a dangerous plague.

Everything that governments are promoting is wrong headed and indefensible. Their lies, deceit and manipulations are reprehensible. I have repeatedly offered to debate vaccination with Government officials but the silence has been deafening. They won't debate the issues because they know they will lose. Pro-vax conspirators are the biggest threat to health today.

But there are things we can do.

If your local Vlad the Impaler wants to test you point out that the tests are less than 50% accurate and produce more false positives than real positives. Governments keep testing, of course, because the inevitable positive results give them an excuse for more lockdowns. Tony Blair, Britain's most infamous war criminal, supports more testing so you know it's a dangerous, bad idea with an evil purpose. Personally, I prefer my home testing system which is perfectly safe, doesn't collect your DNA and guarantees a rather splendid 50% success rate. Pick a favourite coin. Decide if tails or heads are positive. Toss the coin. Catch it. And there's your answer.

If anyone asks you to wear a mask remind them that masks have already killed children in China. Three boos for Commander Dick head of London's metropolitan police for telling the collaborators to shame those who aren't wearing masks. Presumably, she also intended the collaborators should shame the frail and the sick. I'm told she's lurking behind one of the Trafalgar Squares lions, salivating with excitement as she waits to arrest the magnificently irrepressible Piers Corbyn for the 347th time. If he spends anymore time in police stations they'll charge him rent.

Use the word collaborators to describe the mask wearing, social distancing, sanitising zombies. It's a great psy-op word and it will scare the Government's psychological warfare specialists because it demonises those who wear the masks and effectively defines them as part of the enemy. This is, after all, a war we're fighting. A war for the survival of humanity. And as the French Resistance realised, the collaborators are part of the enemy.

Remember the FDA in the US has banned 149 hand sanitisers because they are very dangerous. If someone asks you to use their sanitiser ask them to check it isn't one of the dangerous ones. They should check their sanitisers against the FDA list at least twice a day. That should keep them busy.

If shops won't take cash – then take your business elsewhere. Once they've got rid of cash they will own us and control us. If you find somewhere which only takes plastic collect a huge pile of shopping and then leave it on the counter. Remember that when they have abolished cash they will be able to switch off your access to your own money at the flick of a switch. Our last remaining vestige of freedom will disappear.

And if your local Vlad the Impaler wants to vaccinate you, demand that he or she gives you a written guarantee that the vaccine is safe and effective – long term. Let them see you write down the date, the batch number and the name of the person giving the vaccination. Tell them you will sue if you have any side effects. Remind them that governments around the world have already paid out billions in compensation for vaccine damage. Point out that Gates, who has boasted of bringing us the final solution, has demanded that the drug companies have legal immunity but that doctors can still be sued. If their legal defence companies go bust, individual doctors will have to pay out themselves. Point out that tens of thousands of doctors and nurses will probably go bankrupt.

This goes for the flu vaccine too which I also fear will genetically modify you. Incidentally, I don't know a single doctor who ever has a flu vaccine.

They want most of us dead, of course.

In England, they are now putting automatic Do Not Resuscitate notices on the over 60s and on all the mentally and physically disabled whatever their age. In Scotland it's rumoured to be the over 45s who are left to die. So watch out for that. All part of the Agenda 21 programme, approved by Prince Charles, to cut the world population. The mask wearing collaborators are soon going to realise how bad things are. In October, unemployment rates are going to hit 25% to 30%. And, tragically, around the world death rates are going to soar as millions die of diseases which should have been treated when hospitals were shut – all for a disease rapidly turning out to be a threat to the over 80s with two or three serious health problems but probably less dangerous than chickenpox for children.

I have spoken in Trafalgar Square on many occasions and I'm sorry I can't be there today.

The last time I spoke there was at a huge anti-hunting rally.

Shortly afterwards hunting in the UK was banned.

So let's hope that today's rally is equally successful.

I genuinely fear that our civilisation is currently under real threat – both as a result of the plans of the United Nations and the World Economic Forum and through the evil work of unelected billionaires who seem to believe they have the right to impose their dangerous views on the rest of us. They've had a lot of support, of course, from organisations such as the BBC and *The Guardian* – and other media groups which have done financial deals with the Bill and Melinda Gates Foundation.

Make no mistake – if we are forced to accept vaccines which result in genetic modification of the human body then the changes will be permanent and multi-generational.

Distrust the Government, avoid mass media – and fight the lies.

Those of you who watch my rapidly disappearing YouTube videos know that I always end by saying 'Please remember, although you may feel like it at times, you are not on your own. More and more people are waking up'. Well, today you can see the proof. We definitely are not alone. Together we will win this war. Thanks for watching an old man in a chair.

August 28ᵗʰ 2020

How the Coronavirus Hoax Has Permanently Destroyed Health Care

Even before the coronavirus fraud closed down many hospital departments, sent waiting lists soaring – even for essential, potentially life-saving surgery – and left millions in constant, unnecessary pain, health care services were in decline.

Indeed, back in January, before most of us had heard of covid-19, I had started to prepare notes for a book explaining why health care today is worse than it was half a century ago, and why, despite all the advances in technology, the health care available in the future will not be as good as it was 50 years ago.

The book got pushed aside as the coronavirus hoax took over our lives and I began researching, writing and recording the Old Man in a Chair series of videos – all of which are available, by the way, as transcripts on my website – vernoncoleman.com.

Today, it is clear that health care is deteriorating by the day and, having been writing about doctors, hospitals and medical treatments for many decades I am now convinced that the majority of patients today are receiving worse treatment than was available in the 1950s. The coronavirus hoax has made things considerably worse and has destroyed what was left of professional health care.

There are some exceptions, of course. The very few patients who have had successful transplant surgery could argue, accurately, that back in the 1950s they would have died. And there are one or two new drugs available that are life-saving.

But those are exceptions. I'm talking about the quality of medical care available for 99% of patients, 99% of the time.

Doubters will, of course, claim that life expectation today is much greater than it was and that, therefore, medical care must have improved.

This is a fallacious argument.

If you look at the figures it is clear that life expectation rose over a century ago when the number of babies and infants dying fell considerably. A little over a century ago, it was commonplace for a woman to have half a dozen babies but for only two of them to survive. It was these infant deaths which lowered life expectation figures. If lots of babies die before they are one-year-old then the average life expectation is brought down dramatically. If one person dies at birth, and another dies at 100, their average life expectancy will be 50 years. But if most babies survive then the average life expectation rises equally dramatically. Back in Victorian times, and even earlier, humans who survived infancy and childhood commonly lived into their 70s, 80s and beyond.

The absence of relatively clean drinking water, and proper sewage systems, meant that serious infections were big killers in the 19th century. And it was infectious diseases such as cholera which meant that infant mortality figures were appallingly high. The death rates fell notably when fairly clean, uncontaminated drinking water supplies were introduced and proper facilities built for dealing with sewage. If you look at the figures it was not vaccinations which helped reduce the number of deaths from infectious diseases – the death rates were largely falling long before vaccinations were introduced – but better living conditions.

In the early part of the 20th century, millions of people lived in damp, cramped conditions and had very little decent food to eat. Drug companies, and their supporters, like to claim that their products are responsible for improved life expectation but the figures prove that to be a falsehood. Drugs have changed our lives in many ways but, with the exception of antibiotics such as penicillin, first introduced just in time for the Second World War, they have not had a major impact and it is not difficult to argue that many of the preparations put on the market have done considerably more harm than good. It is, for example, difficult to claim that benzodiazepine tranquillisers have done anything to improve the quality of human life. Prescription drugs such as benzodiazepines and some painkillers are the causes of the biggest dependency problem in the world.

Even the good drugs, the antibiotics, are now often not as useful as they once were. Overprescribing and the wholesale, routine use of antibiotics on farms have meant that antibiotics which once saved lives are now often useless.

I qualified as a doctor almost exactly 50 years ago and after a year working in hospitals, went straight to work as a general practitioner. I practised much in the way that doctors were practising half a century before that. If patients wanted a consultation they just turned up at the surgery during opening hours. I did a morning surgery and an evening surgery. I gave patients injections and took blood samples. I happily inserted catheters and syringed ears. Patients didn't have to make another appointment to see a care assistant with little training. If you couldn't get to the surgery you telephoned, or sent a message, and the doctor visited. If you needed help outside surgery hours you got in touch and the doctor would visit. Medical care was provided 24 hours a day and 365 days a year. Accident and emergency departments, called casualty departments then, were used largely for victims of road accidents, fights and fires. Why would anyone trek all the way to a hospital when they could have a doctor in their home within minutes? Patients who were elderly or frail or housebound or disabled were often visited routinely once every couple of weeks. District nurses drove themselves round their local community to dress wounds and check on patients discharged from hospital. It now sounds like something out of a history book but I can't be the only one who can remember how things were and why they were better 50 years ago than they are now. It wasn't perfect by any means but it was a damned sight better than things are today.

Today, you're about as likely to get a home visit from a doctor as you are to win the lottery. And your chances of having a doctor visit you at home at night or at the weekend or on a bank holiday are nil – unless you live in a big city and have an arrangement with a private doctor who does house calls. Having a GP always available at the end of a telephone was reassuring; it was good to know that professional help was always available. If a patient had to go into hospital they knew they had someone they could trust if they didn't understand what was happening to them – they could speak to their GP or he would visit them in hospital to help explain things.

Everything has been going wrong for decades – but the slide downhill has accelerated recently. Medical care was never better than it was when people wore hats. Decency disappeared when bare heads became the norm. I'm obviously not saying one caused the other for that would be a simplistic example of post hoc ergo propter hoc, but it's an easy way to define a change. When medicine became more science than humanity the quality of care started to diminish significantly.

Fifty years ago, doctors always strove to keep patients alive. Today, 'Do Not Resuscitate' notices are placed on patients' beds as often as temperature charts. It has got so bad that I have heard reports that DNR notices are put on the notes of any patient over the age of 60 or even 45. Those youngsters who cheer this should be aware that in 10 years' time, the age allowed could be reduced to 40 then, in no time at all, to 30. Remember the film Logan's Run in which 30 was the cut off end of life age.

The ethics committee at Great Ormond Street Hospital, once the standard for quality in the care of sick children, was reportedly criticised by a High Court judge for deciding that a nine-year-old girl should be 'managed' rather than 'treated' and for making this decision without talking to the parents. Lawyers representing the hospital had allegedly asked that Great Ormond Street Hospital not be named. I bet they did.

Today, elderly patients in hospitals are routinely left to die, unfed, unwashed and without fluids. In the UK, it's a government approved programme for the 'care' of the elderly.

The coronavirus hoax gave hospitals the opportunity to shut down whole departments, many of which are still closed, and gave doctors in general practice the excuse to virtually shut down their surgeries. There was never any logical reason for this. GPs claimed that it would be better and safer to conduct all examinations by video rather than in person. It was even seriously suggested that young GPs found their work so onerous that they could not be expected to work more than one day a week – even though they were working 9 until 5 with an hour off for lunch. Patients who had serious symptoms were told that they could not be seen in person by a doctor or even a nurse – because of the coronavirus.

The truth is that video consultations are pretty useless and very dangerous. You can't examine a patient by video. You can't listen to their chest or check their heart or blood pressure. You can't examine lesions properly. You can't palpate an abdomen. You can't look down throats or into ears. You can't even use your sense of smell – useful in the care of diabetics.

Hospital infections, too often untreatable, are now too common to be remarked upon. Fifty years ago a ward sister or a matron would have forty fits if a patient on their ward or in their hospital contracted an infection or developed a pressure sore or any other sign of bad nursing. Hospitals employed almoners whose job it was to make sure that patients didn't have to worry about anything. If an elderly patient was admitted to hospital as an emergency, the almoner would make sure someone went round to feed her cat. If a patient was worried about her bills being paid while she was in hospital, then the almoner would deal with it. If you don't remember those days you probably think I'm joking but I promise you I am not. People working in health care used to understand the meaning of the word 'compassion'. Today, health care staff would probably laugh or sneer if you told them of such realities.

Even in small things, hospitals have gone backwards.

So, for example, many hospitals no longer allow flowers on the ward. The real reason? They make a little more work for the staff. But for several thousand years it has been known that having flowers on a ward cheers up the patients and improves their recovery.

Similarly, when I was young, it was commonplace for someone to come onto a women's ward every day and do the hair and make-up of the patients. That doesn't happen anymore.

When I was a young doctor, all patients requiring hospital treatment were subjected to a full medical examination. They also had a full history taken. Woe betide any young doctor if a patient was seen by a consultant without there being a full medical history in their file.

How can it be an improvement to know virtually nothing about the patients you are looking after? Back in the 1960s, we derided doctors who thought of patients as being 'the liver in the end bed' or 'the kidney problem in the bed third on the left'. But that is what health care has become once again.

Everywhere you look there are problems. Hospitals and general practices are managed by people who don't understand the first thing about medicine. In Europe, the EU has stopped doctors working more than a basic working week and so in hospitals there are frequently no doctors at all available at weekends or at night.

In the UK, the NHS has always been a money wasting machine. The amount now spent on the NHS is so great that if that money were simply handed out to the public, everyone in Britain would be able to buy themselves top level private health care. How can that be? It's simply because there are more administrators than hospital beds in the health service, and vast amounts of money is wasted on pointless bureaucracy. Like all large, bureaucratic organisations, the last people to be fired are the bureaucrats themselves. They just keep hiring and building their empires.

The NHS is regarded worldwide as the pinnacle of socialised medicine. Many around the world look upon it with envy. But that is only because they look at it from a distance: as observers rather than as consumers. The NHS has been a disaster in every possible sense. Most people who work for it say they wouldn't want to be treated in their hospital. The outstanding legal claims in the NHS had reached £85 billion before the coronavirus fiasco hit and left patients untreated and uncared for. Untold thousands of people will be entitled to sue and demand huge damages as a result of the coronavirus hoax – now better referred to as a fraud.

Overall satisfaction with the NHS is low and falling annually. People complain of long waits, staff shortages, lack of money and money being wasted. It is a deadly tale of indifference, incompetence, greed, selfishness and weariness. The incidence of doctor induced disease (iatrogenesis) soars every year.

It has long been recognised, incidentally, that waiting lists of all kinds were and are deliberately created by doctors to enhance their private incomes.

This is a weakness of the system which allows some consultants to work in the NHS and at the same time to have private practices. Their NHS income is the bread, butter and jam and the private income is the piece of cake. Consultants deliberately keep their waiting lists long because they know that this is the great selling point for private care. I once worked at a hospital where, during a consultant's annual holiday, a registrar and I worked hard and got rid of the waiting list completely. It wasn't particularly difficult. Naively we thought that the consultant would be pleased when he returned from his holidays. He was furious. 'Why the devil should people come and see me privately if they can be operated on tomorrow in the health service?' he demanded. He was the norm and not the exception.

Life expectation now is actually falling for women, waiting lists are growing and waiting times are soaring, the amount of illness is rising constantly and the number of patients made ill by doctors has made iatrogenesis an epidemic – up there with cancer and circulatory disease as one of the three major killers in our world. One in six people in hospital is there because they have been made ill by doctors. In half a century, the quality of medicine offered has slumped.

And there have been virtually no breakthroughs in the last 50 years. There are plenty of new drugs – but most of them are merely variations on long established themes. Health care is now controlled by lobbyists working for big drug companies and lies and myths rule our lives in a thousand different ways. The future, we are assured, is vaccination. Vaccination for this, vaccination for that, vaccines in syringes and vaccines in foods. The coronavirus has given drug companies the opportunity to introduce potentially deadly DNA and RNA vaccines. Screening programmes are known to often do more harm than good but they are immensely profitable and so they are popular with businesses and doctors. Medical education is controlled by drug companies and so when doctors are looking for a treatment they think first of pills. Lifestyle changes rarely even figure in their calculations. Laws which control the hours doctors can work mean that even quite large hospitals often have no doctors available at weekends or at night.

Long stay hospitals have been closed with the result that patients who need long-term care spend their days wandering the streets. Celebrities now promote health products and eating habits without having any knowledge or understanding of the harm they are doing. New regulations mean that small hospitals have closed with the result that patients have to travel for hours to visit a hospital.

Charities have become commercially linked with drug companies and use their lobbying skills to influence public policy in favour of their partners. Food companies promote bad eating habits because they are more profitable than good eating habits.

In the UK it can, and does, take weeks or even months for X-rays and scans to be read and for blood results to be recorded, distributed and interpreted. It is for this reason, more than any other, that Britain has the worst cancer survival rates in Europe.

All things considered the modern history of medicine is a deadly tale of indifference, incompetence, greed and selfishness. All of this importance because it was long ago established that when a doctor is sympathetic and compassionate his or her patients will get better quicker – it's a human version of the placebo response which can add a quarter to a half to the effectiveness of a treatment. That has pretty much been lost.

In the UK, the only response to the chaos from the politicians and the collaborating public has been to demand yet more money for the health service, which actually has far too much money but just wastes most of it on unnecessary layers of administration and throws away billions because administrators pay far too much for just about everything from pens and loo rolls to drugs, and to demand that NHS leaflets and so on all be translated into more languages.

When I published the prices the NHS pays for office equipment, washing powder and so on – and proved that the NHS was paying more for stuff bought by the ton than I would pay if I bought the stuff at a supermarket – the NHS responded not by dealing with the waste but by demanding to know where I had obtained the computer print-out containing the NHS prices. They were only interested in covering up the waste – not doing anything about it.

Complex financial schemes, private finance initiatives and absurd bonus schemes for executives have cost the NHS billions. It is hardly surprising that services are deteriorating and that some services, such as dentistry, are likely to be abandoned completely.

The future, I fear, is bleak.

Thanks to the coronavirus hoax, health care is set to deteriorate even faster than before and the relationship between patients and health care professionals is doomed to collapse still further.

Alternative branches of medicine will doubtless blossom and bloom. But for most people the future will involve telemedicine, preventive care and self-care. We all have to learn to look after ourselves and our loved ones.

Doctors haven't yet grasped this, but computer programmes will take over from medical practitioners. Back in 1984, a friend and I wrote the first home doctor programme for computers and ever since then computer programmes have been improving. They are now being fitted into robot physicians and surgeons. In ten years' time, there will be very few jobs for human doctors. Students thinking of entering medical school might like to look for another profession. A career in plumbing might offer better prospects. I am being very serious.This has not happened by accident. It is all part of the United Nations global plan for the future – Agenda 21. We are now living in the future they designed for us.

And unless we speak up, soon and loudly, the future will simply get bleaker and bleaker.

I don't suppose I should admit this but this is my second attempt to make this video.

I had to abandon the first attempt when I suddenly found myself sitting here with tears pouring down my cheeks and quite unable to continue. It saddens me enormously to see my former profession overwhelmed by self-interest and apparently quite without any sense of humanity or vocation. I pray that hope triumphs over current experience.

August 30th 2020

A Conspiracy of Silence

Greek playwrights used to introduce their work with a prologue giving some background details and miscellaneous information. So I am going to begin this video with a short prologue, or introduction. I'm a writer of books by trade, so I suppose this is also in way of a preface or a foreword.

Time is running out for this channel and I fear for us all unless we take action quickly and with as much, if not more determination as our oppressors.

YouTube has been taking down my videos with increasing enthusiasm. I have long since given up wondering why. This morning, I received a rather severe message from the head prefect telling me that they don't allow content that disputes the efficacy of the WHO or local authorities' recommended guidance on social distancing and self-isolation that may lead people to act against that guidance. YouTube sent me a very long list of their rules and, surprisingly, I really don't see how some of the removed videos could possibly be in breach of these guidelines – although there may, I suppose, be a local authority somewhere in the world which doesn't approve of colourful shirts. YouTube said I could appeal but in their Kafkaesque world the appeals button doesn't work so I can't.

The oppression and suppression of the truth is rapidly becoming more blatant. In London, the police fined the organiser of a peaceful demonstration against our loss of freedom but are reported to have given permission for a pro-establishment campaign group, Extinction Rebellion, which ought to be called Exhibition Rebellion, to support the global warming myth behind Agenda 21. The rank and file perhaps don't realise it but I believe they are supporting the fight to destroy mankind, desecrate our planet and put us in thrall to the devil worshippers – a phrase I use not as a term of colourful abuse but as an accurate description.

When the law appears to take sides, you know you're in trouble.

We are living, leaderless, in the early days of a totalitarian world government and it seems to me that YouTube is simply looking for an excuse to terminate channels which provide information or opinions which might inconvenience corrupt politicians, greedy drug companies or psychopaths supporting the global reset and planning to enslave the world population.

This is clearly the beginning of the end for this channel and, unless we up our game, the end for all of us. In an early video entitled, 'Why has YouTube taken down my video?' I explained my views on the freedom of speech.

I'll be putting more practical advice and leaflets to print out on my website.

To make sure I don't miss any more of their threatening messages, I have put YouTube into the special category labelled SPAM which is, I gather, where pompous, totalitarian messages are most safely and appropriately stored. YouTube's prefects won't understand this unless they've seen the original Hitchcock version of The Lady Vanishes but I'm English and a member of the MCC and it is not in my nature to be bullied and told what to do by anyone – especially not by ignorant, humourless, jackbooted carpet knights, gangrels, muggles and scrofulous, oleaginous larrikins. The war 'aint over while the old man has breath.

And so, now to the main feature which, incidentally, does not violate any of the official commandments in the YouTube black prayer book. If they take this one down then we know that this isn't business – it's personal.

They say that the miraculous covid-19 vaccine isn't quite ready yet, though there are those who believe it is ready and sitting in a warehouse waiting until enough people are sufficiently scared to take two knees and beg for it. They say they're still fiddling around with it. You can imagine them at work can't you – add a bit more pepper, some arsenic, a touch of cyanide, I think it needs a splash more mercury to give it that really lethal quality.

So, since the drug company profits aren't going to boom for a while, they want us all to have a flu vaccination this year. They've probably got a few billion doses of something that needs using up.

In the UK, Hancock is like a bad villain in a pantomime.

Oh yes you will.

Oh no we won't, we reply.

Politicians everywhere have for years now been blasting those of us who question the value and safety of vaccination as dangerous idiots who must be ignored, suppressed and silenced in every way possible. The enthusiasm for vaccination is widespread. The EU has apparently been planning a vaccination passport for all EU citizens since 2018. Naturally, the media has obliged with numerous articles following the official line. The media is in thrall to the medical conspiracy which thinks that vaccines are the answer to every disease. As so often happens, journalists ignore the facts and prefer to stick with the myths. And yet the odd thing is that despite the endless propaganda, and the remorseless demonization of those daring to tell the truth, a very large and ever growing proportion of the population distrusts vaccination. A 2018 report by the Royal Society of Public Health in the UK, showed that one in four individuals believes it is possible to be administered too many vaccines. Personally, I suspect that what this shows is that three out of four individuals shouldn't be allowed to get out of bed by themselves.

So, why don't people trust vaccination or the people who promote it? First, they realise that everyone involved in pushing vaccines is making money out of them. Every year, GPs make an absolute fortune out of vaccinating patients. They don't even do the work themselves. A nurse, care assistant or passing cleaner actually does the syringe and needle stuff. The doctor just spends the money.

Second, people are aware that the politicians, advisors and doctors who are promoting vaccination with such enthusiasm won't defend their position. I am prepared to put my reputation on the line and to debate the value of vaccination in general, and the proposed vaccines for covid-19 and the flu in particular, with any senior government figure or senior government medical advisor. In the UK, Boris Johnson and Matt Hancock both claim to know that vaccination is good for us. So, why won't they debate the issue with me or any other doctor who has doubts? I can only think of one explanation – they know they will lose the debate. I would love to debate the issue of vaccination with Bill Gates, who seems to regard himself as an expert on the subject, but we all know there is no chance of that happening. And that's odd because Mr Gates seems to love doing interviews – especially with organisations such as *The Guardian* and the BBC with which he has financial links.

In the past, I used to debate the issue in public with vaccine supporters. But they always lost the debates and so these days they won't take the risk.

If vaccine supporters really believe that vaccines are safe and effective, they should be willing to debate instead of trying to silence the doubters by simply saying, 'we are right and you are wrong so that's that – you're a nutter'.

One of the many, many oddities of the internet is that you can find all sorts of rubbish online but you can't find those debates in which doctors debated with me and struggled, and failed, to defend vaccines and vaccination. Those have all disappeared.

The bottom line is that patients are right to be worried about vaccines. The evidence available suggests that vaccines are neither reliably safe nor effective. There is a solid argument that although profitable for drug companies and doctors, they do more harm than good. The worldwide vaccine market is worth around $60 billion a year and rising fast. The refusal of those in power to debate the science is one of the reasons why people don't trust what they are told.

The scientific evidence proves vaccination is neither safe nor effective. Deceitful, dishonest drug companies haven't done much to improve trust.

Politicians and journalists like to talk a great deal about conspiracy theories but it doesn't occur to them that there is a massive conspiracy of silence about vaccination.

The drug company spin doctors have convinced civil servants and journalists that vaccination is wonderful and essential and that anyone who dares to question vaccination programmes must be a dangerous lunatic and must be suppressed.

But if I am such a lunatic why won't the politicians and experts debate with me? If I am so wrong surely they could destroy me in a public debate?

To be honest I'd have to be stone drunk or fast asleep to lose a debate about vaccination.

I've included scores of facts about vaccines in previous videos but what about the fact that a company called GlaxoSmithKline, GSK, is one of the top earning vaccine companies in the world.

One of its vaccines was Pandemrix, the H1N1 swine flu vaccine. Governments spent fortunes buying the stuff because Neil Ferguson, whose name is now pretty familiar to most of us, had predicted that the swine flu could lead to 65,000 deaths in the UK alone. In the end, the swine flu killed 457 people and had a death rate of just 0.026 per cent of those infected.

And the vaccine?

Well, in Sweden and Finland there were reports of narcolepsy occurring among children who had the H1N1 swine flu vaccine. It is reported that not all the safety problems were made public. I have seen a report that by December 2009, for each one million doses of the vaccine given about 76 cases of serious adverse events were reported though this was not made public. A paper published in the *British*

Medical Journal in 2018 reported that GSK had commented that 'further research is needed to confirm what role Pandemrix may have played in the development of narcolepsy among those involved.'

The writer of the BMJ article commented, 'Now, eight years after the outbreak, new information is emerging from one of the lawsuits that, months before the narcolepsy cases were reported, the manufacturer and public health officials were aware of other serious adverse events logged in relation to Pandemrix. '

In Ireland, the Government kept inviting people to get vaccinated even when it was clear that the pandemic was on the wane and it was nowhere near the catastrophe portrayed by Ferguson, governments, industry and the media.

One member of the Irish parliament, called the adverse effects after Pandemrix a 'completely avoidable catastrophe'. She told the then Prime Minister. 'The Health Service Executive decided to purchase Pandemrix and continued to distribute it even after they knew it was dangerous and untested.'

In Canada, a five-year-old girl died five days after an H1N1 flu shot and her parents sued GSK for $4.2 million. The parents' lawyer alleged that the drug was brought out quickly and without proper testing as the federal government exerted intense pressure on Canadians to get immunised.

In previous videos, I listed some of the massive fines that GSK has had to pay. They make stuff that does a lot of harm and they then cover up the problems.

In 2014, GSK was fined $490 million dollars by China after a Chinese court found it guilty of bribery. The BBC said that GSK had said it had learned its lessons and the BBC added that one of those lessons was 'clearly that foreign companies need to keep a close eye on China's fast changing political and regulatory weather if they are to prosper'. Not that they shouldn't bribe people, you notice, but that they should be careful.

In 2010, GSK paid out $1.14 billion because of claims over a drug called Paxil. And they settled lawsuits over a drug called Avandia for $500 million. In 2011, GSK paid $250 million to settle 5,500 death and injury claims and set aside $6.4 billion for future lawsuits and settlements in respect of the drug Avandia. In 2012, GSK pleaded guilty to federal criminal offences including misbranding of two antidepressants and failure to report safety data about a drug for diabetes to the FDA in America. The company admitted to illegally promoting Paxil for the treatment of depression in children and agreed to pay a fine of $3 billion. That was the largest health care fraud settlement in US history. GSK also reached a related civil settlement with the US Justice Department. The $3 billion fine also included the civil penalties for improper marketing of half a dozen other drugs.

I don't know whether you missed that word, by the way.

Fraud.

'Wrongful or criminal deception intended to result in financial or personal gain.'

Always worth knowing precisely what's meant by the words we use, isn't it?

The British Government alone paid out £60 million to patients who had been damaged by GSK's Pandemrix vaccine and who knew they could claim and how to claim. Naturally, GSK had demanded that the Government indemnify it against claims for damages. Bill Gates has, of course, demanded that everyone involved in the planned covid-19 vaccine will be indemnified. You can't sue them if their vaccine turns out to be deadly. I bet car companies would like that deal.

So, would you want to trust your life, or your children's lives, to GSK? Well, you if you have a vaccine then you may well be doing so because GSK is still making vaccines.

And guess what.

The UK's Chief Scientific Adviser at the moment is someone called Sir Patrick Vallance. He is, I suspect, a key figure in dealing with the coronavirus in the UK and the plans for a vaccine. Vallance worked for GSK between 2006 and 2018. By the time he left GSK, he was a member of the board and the corporate executive team.

And they have the gall to call me a conspiracy theorist?

I could, by the way, produce similar horror stories for just about all the big drug companies. And if I were making this up I'd be facing libel actions that would make your eyes water. Well, they'd make my eyes water.

I got waylaid.

I started by talking about the flu vaccine.

In the UK, the Government is pushing hard to get millions of people vaccinated against the flu this autumn. They will, of course, insist that it is perfectly safe and perfectly effective. It'll probably make hair grow on bald patches, increase your breast size if that's what you want and turn you into a super-being capable of running a three minute mile.

Trust Hancock and Johnson – vaccine salesmen and hucksters to the inept and rather stupid.

Boris Johnson, allegedly the British Prime Minister, claims that anyone who questions the value and safety of vaccination is nuts.

But I do still have a few worries. Millions are worried about the covid-19 vaccine but could it be that the heavily promoted flu vaccine is the one we should be really concerned about?

Here are a few general questions for Boris Johnson to think about.

First, did you know that people who have the flu vaccination may be more susceptible to other respiratory viruses? It's a well-known phenomenon called virus interference. How many people who have the flu vaccine this winter will die as a result of this well documented problem? I could let your government see some research papers if they could find someone able to read them and understand them.

Second, will the new flu vaccine be an RNA or DNA vaccine by any chance? There are, as I am sure you will know, very real potential problems with such vaccines. I know you don't know what the risk will be, but are you aware, Mr Johnson, of the reservations expressed by the World Health Organisation which has said 'many aspects of the immune response generated by DNA vaccines are not understood'? Since your government abides by everything the WHO says, you will naturally be concerned by this.

Third, as I am sure you know, there has always been a link between vaccination and cancer. Are you aware that an FDA researcher has found hundreds of cancer genes in MMR vaccines for example? The FDA has found that cellular matter used in the manufacture of vaccines is often contaminated with serious disease causing viruses. The problem is that the health problems don't occur until years or decades after vaccination. Since no long-term trials are done on vaccination, don't you think it might be a good idea to insist that drug companies start them? The results should be available in 20 or 30 years' time.

Fourth, how much testing will be done on this year's flu vaccine? Or is the vaccine being rushed through like the covid-19 vaccine?

Fifth, how effective will this year's flu vaccine be? Previous vaccines have been pretty useless – providing protection in only just half of adults. And why push vaccines for older patients when vaccines tend to work even less well for the over 65s?

Sixth, it is reported that it was Bill Gates, a software person, who stopped President Trump's planned vaccine safety commission. It is alleged that Gates said, 'No, that's a dead end. That would be a bad thing. Don't do that.' And so the commission didn't happen. Was that true? And if so, why was it a bad thing to have a commission into vaccines?

Seventh, the nasal vaccine proposed for children will be a live flu vaccine. With the live attenuated virus in it. How safe will it be this year – especially when many doctors argue that lockdowns, masks and social distancing mean that immune systems may have been weakened? It's worth remembering that in 2016, the Center for Disease Control and Prevention in the US pulled a nasal flu vaccine because it was only 3% effective. The CDC stated that no protective benefit could be measured and that the vaccine had not been statistically effective for three years running. Did you know that Mr Johnson? Mr Hancock? One vaccine with live flu viruses in it contained 80 million live viruses per dose – attenuated and genetically modified, of course. The side effects with the nasal vaccine are potentially horrific – and include neurological and behavioural problems. I could fill a video with the side effects of this stuff alone. Incidentally, because viruses mutate there is no guarantee that the viruses used won't revert to an infectious version. I wouldn't take a nasal flu vaccine if you gave me a million pounds to have it.

So those are my preliminary questions, Mr Johnson. I know you think I am a nut for asking them but I would appreciate some answers. I hope those who view this video will pass these questions on to their political representatives, asking for answers. And send the questions to radio, TV and newspaper commentators who claim vaccines are always safe and wonderful. The transcript – with these questions – will be on my website. Please, it's important that these questions are asked.

When we've got answers to those, I have another couple of hundred questions I'd like to ask.

Oh, and scientists still don't know if having the flu vaccine makes people more likely to develop covid-19 – or at least to test positive for it. Some research might be a good idea. Come to think of it, maybe that's why there is such enthusiasm about giving the flu vaccine to as many people as possible this autumn.

I think the evidence shows pretty clearly that out of the two of us it's Boris who is the nut, since he supports an indefensible piece of nonsense. We have all the science on our side. The pro-vaxxers have greed, lies, fraud and propaganda on their side. And by any decent definition, Boris is also a conspiracy theorist since he is supporting a pretty untenable conspiracy. It isn't difficult to see why they won't support their point of view by debating the issue. Keep pushing them. Send tweets to Boris and Matt Hancock demanding that they debate vaccination with someone qualified.

Finally, are we supposed to be reassured by the fact that there is a Vaccine Impact Modelling Consortium at Imperial College, London which is apparently funded by a whole bunch of organisations including drug companies, the British Government and, of course, the Bill and Melinda Gates Foundation?

Personally, I find it difficult to have enthusiasm for such an organisation – not least because the acting director is someone called Neil Ferguson.

Now where have I heard that name before?

Wasn't he one of the Three Stooges? Or was he the circus clown who always ended up with the custard pie in his face?

Or was it the bloke whose absurd predictions and lockdown policies seem to me to be likely to be responsible in the end for more global deaths than Hitler?

Meanwhile, the next time a doctor wants to vaccinate you or a relative ask him or her this simple question, 'Will you guarantee that the vaccination is safe and effective and will you take responsibility if things go wrong?'

Ask for the assurance in writing.

I will be very surprised if you get it.

We all very much need to reach and educate more people. Mainstream media continue to lie and mislead and we need to counter that. As far as I know the mass market media didn't even bother to report the fact that in the USA the number of covid-19 deaths had been officially reduced by 94% to just over 9,000. Unbelievably, the NHS in the UK is using vast chunks of taxpayers' money to pay social media celebrities to promote government lies and testing nonsenses.

Please continue to help by sharing existing videos and by printing out material from the website transcripts. This channel isn't monetised and nor is the website, www.vernoncoleman.com. We have no ads and no sponsors and these videos and the website actually cost us money so this isn't about us getting rich – this is a public service channel and we need your help.

Oh, and one other thing. Those of us who question governments, are being silenced in every conceivable way. YouTube videos are being censored and banned almost as soon as I put them up. If the videos disappear completely, something which I fear will happen soon, please go to my website www.vernoncoleman.com

There is one method of silencing which they haven't tried yet. If I suddenly disappear then I'll come back and haunt the bastards for eternity.

It may sometimes seem as though you are alone. But you're not. More and more people are waking up. And together we will win this war. Thanks for watching an old man in a chair.

September 2ⁿᵈ 2020

My Last Video for YouTube

The day before I recorded my first video on the coronavirus hoax, that was March 18th, my Wikipedia entry was comprehensive, respectable and even respectful. They mentioned the TV and radio series I had made, the fact that I had written columns for five national newspapers, the fact that I'd succeeded in changing Government policy on benzodiazepine drugs and so on and so forth. There were a couple of dozen generous quotes from newspaper reviews.

I'd had a Wikipedia entry pretty well since their site started, though I had frequently asked them to take it down, because I think their way of working is absurd. Anyone, with any agenda, can edit a Wikipedia entry except the individual concerned. In my experience, facts about living individuals are never checked properly.

The day after I recorded that video, my Wikipedia entry was changed dramatically. I don't know what it looks like now because I never use Wikipedia any more but all the interesting stuff had been removed and replaced with some very dubious stuff including the allegation that I had been banned by an organisation called the Advertising Standards Authority (ASA). Now I don't know if it still exists but the ASA was a private organisation, funded, I think, largely by big advertisers, which can't ban anyone from anything – though it does I think like to pretend it can. I remember the ASA had itself been reported to the Office of Fair Trading and had about as much power to ban anything as your local window cleaner.

One of the main complaints in the new Wikipedia was that I had been disciplined by the ASA for a claim about a food causing cancer. I remember this well. One of my books, *Food for Thought*, contained a section proving the link between meat and cancer. A representative of the meat trade made a complaint to the ASA and they wrote to me. In reply, I sent them details of 26 scientific papers, from reputable journals, which proved my claim. The ASA wrote back to say that they did not look at scientific references. They then proceeded to find for the complainant and announced that they were banning me from whatever they thought they could ban me from. This was so laughable that I ignored it. I also ignored it when the Press Complaints Commission did exactly the same thing. There's a summary of the evidence I tried to submit to both organisations on my website – headed Meat causes Cancer – the proof.

Wikipedia editors, searching for ways to demonise me, dug these decades' old judgements from page 738 of a search engine and stuck them, and similar nonsenses, and put them on my Wikipedia page. I have written about these absurdities several times and I believe that Wikipedia knows these claims are absurd. But to them they served a purpose because what Wikipedia was doing was demonising or monstering me, in an attempt to persuade users of the Wikipedia site, that I was untrustworthy. This is by no means the first time this has happened to me. Indeed, it has happened scores of times over the years and is, I fear, the price anyone has to pay if they want to oppose dishonesty, corruption and deceit.

Wikipedia was using a well-known technique called 'controlled opposition' or 'opposition research' or 'organised opposition'. It's a military trick which has for years been used widely in politics when members of one party want to demonise the opposition. You simply go through an individual's life history looking for events which can be criticised. The Wikipedia editors know that the individual concerned cannot correct anything on a site which bears their name.

The bottom line, of course, is that if you can't trust one Wikipedia site then you can't trust any of them. I no longer use Wikipedia as a reference source. I am not, by the way, the first person to realise that Wikipedia is suspect. There have been a number of accusations that intelligence officers are editing Wikipedia sites.

It isn't just Wikipedia doing the monstering, of course. The *Bangkok Post*, a publication which I didn't even know existed, published an article about me (without bothering to get in touch of course) which tried to demonise me by claiming that my arguments about AIDS were wrong. In the last century, I had produced evidence proving that AIDS was not going to kill us all – though the establishment line was that it was – and the *Bangkok Post* journalist tried to rubbish my argument by claiming that the rate of HIV diagnoses in the US in 2018 was 24%. This is, perhaps, one of the most absurd claims I have seen anywhere. According to the CDC in the US, a total of 1.2 million people in the US have HIV. Since the population of America is currently over 300 million that means that the rate is not 24% among heterosexuals as claimed by the *Bangkok Post* but about a third of one per cent. Personally, I think that if the *Bangkok Post* had any self-respect they would withdraw the article and send the writer back to school. But I doubt if they will do either. He also claims you can buy my books from my website, as though this were a bad thing, but you can't, I'm afraid.

I am not, of course, the only person whose reputation has been wounded in this war. The BBC has been outrageous. A rally was held in Trafalgar Square on 29th August and well-qualified scientists including Professor Dolores Cahill, Dr Kevin Corbett and Dr Mohammad Adil and the magnificent and seemingly tireless astrophysicist Piers Corbyn spoke to tens of thousands. At 17.17 on Saturday afternoon someone called Marianna Spring, described as a specialist disinformation and social media reporter, wrote what I regard as one of the most disgracefully biased news reports I have ever seen. She claimed, on the BBC website, in an article headed 'Conspiracy theories touted in Trafalgar Square', that some protestors had held placards featuring false claims though I'm not sure that making a judgement about the accuracy or not of a claim is within her capabilities or her remit. Worst of all, however, she wrote that 'various pseudo-scientists who have spread disinformation online about coronavirus were also scheduled to speak at the London demonstration.' I think that was one of the most libellous pieces of writing I have ever seen. I hope that the scientists who were present all sue the BBC and demand massive damages. And I beg everyone watching or reading this to make a formal complaint to the BBC. Just go to their website and then to the complaints section. The BBC must be taught a lesson. They and the rest of the media are a weak point in this war – when the Government stops giving them money they're all going to need our support. I could give many, many more examples of deceit, misreporting and plain dishonesty.

When Piers Corbyn appeared on an ITV morning show, he was attacked by three presenters and a weather girl who holds a world record for folding pancakes. One of them was someone called Dr Hilary Jones who was described in a journal called *Pharmacy Business* as a non-executive director of MedTate which is described as a nutraceutical company – whatever that is – which makes and sells pharmaceutical products. I don't think ITV remembered to mention Dr Jones's commercial relationship. He's always struck me as one of those TV people whose main quality is nice hair. Piers Corbyn did brilliantly but although he is a scientist he is not a medical doctor. What a pity ITV didn't invite a physician to discuss the covid-19 vaccine and so on with Dr Jones and Mr Morgan and the rest of the station's staff.

This is my last video for YouTube. I refuse to collaborate with the collaborators. I refuse to suppress or distort what I know to be true simply to satisfy a platform which has no value, respectability or honour as far as I am concerned. When a government suppresses the truth then the end result is inevitably oppression and tyranny. It is the job of journalists to question everything politicians say. YouTube's policy appears to be to suppress all questioning and to deny scientific truths in the interest of protecting the lies and the myths. No one at YouTube has ever claimed to have found any specific inaccuracy or factual error in any of the videos they have removed and banned.

I am a writer by profession but I have a medical degree and some experience as a practising doctor, and I do not take kindly to being told that I must suppress truths and clinical evidence to satisfy some unnamed censors who seem to me to be working with or for Bill Gates and whose aim seems to me to be to destroy freedom and democracy by censoring and banning scientific truths and suppressing the freedom of expression which is a basic human right.

I can honestly say that I believe that all the information in all my videos is completely accurate. I have always used a script for these videos for two reasons: to make sure that I provide absolutely accurate facts and so that we have a transcript which we can put onto the website. Since YouTube has taken down nearly twenty videos to date, this has proved useful.

This video does not breach any of their guidelines. If they take this one down they will, as far as I am concerned, have proved themselves to be spiteful, vindictive and small-minded. We shall see.

I could keep this channel alive if I were prepared to lie but why on earth would I do that? I resigned as a GP on a matter of principle, I resigned from my last newspaper column on a matter of principle. I'm not going to sell my soul to a platform which disrespects the truth. I shall now add YouTube to the list of organisations which I boycott – I strongly suggest that you do too. There are, I believe, plenty of more honourable alternatives.

I see no point in recording more videos for YouTube. They are taking them down, for absolutely no good reason that I can see, within hours of my putting them up. My videos take much time and effort to research, write and check and it is frustrating and disappointing to see them being banned for what I think are political reasons. It is modern day book burning. YouTube is no longer a reputable site; its commercially inspired intolerance is unacceptable. I described my views on freedom in an early video entitled Coronavirus: Why did

YouTube ban my video? – which they took down and then put back up – perhaps because even they felt embarrassed.

I am sad about this and I suspect that the opposition, the fans of Bill Gates, the 21st century would-be slave owners, will regard this as a victory for them. They would be mistaken to think that. I've been fighting lies and injustices for well over half a century and I'm not going away. I'm regrouping; looking for more favourable ground to continue the fight.

For the time being, I'm moving over to my own website – where nothing is ever censored. At the moment, we don't have the facility to put up videos but we will continue to put up new articles every Wednesday and Sunday and at other times too. And we're going to put up more leaflets that can be printed out and distributed.

My wife who has always been in charge of research, editing and production, and reigning me in when I seem about to get carried away, will choose the appropriate platform. We are both driven by the need to help those who cannot help themselves – especially children, the old, the disabled and the mentally ill. But our new video site will be somewhere which we can control. It might take a while because I am never again going to be in a position where anyone can censor or ban what I've recorded.

Finally, since no one in the Government has accepted my challenge to debate the covid-19 vaccine live on television, and through simple cowardice they're clearly not likely to now, I have another challenge. I am prepared to bet Dr Whitty or Dr Fauci £100,000 that they cannot provide independent clinical evidence proving beyond doubt that the covid-19 vaccine and the newly promoted flu vaccine will be 100% effective and 100% safe not just now but in the long term. If they have the courage to take on the bet, I will share my winnings with groups and websites campaigning for the truth. If they won't take on the bet, we will know that they believe that any new covid-19 vaccine will not be 100% effective or 100% safe in the short and long-term. Let's put a finish date of 31st December 2020 for the bet.

Thank you again for watching the videos. Thank you for sharing them on brandnewtube and bitchute and wherever else. Please share this one too. Thank you for all your support. I'm sorry I cannot reply to messages – but we get many thousands a week and I worked out the other day that if I replied to them all, I would need 48 hour days and there would be no time for anything else. Please forgive me.

Distrust the Government, avoid mass media and fight the lies.

Please remember that although you may at times feel that you are alone – you are not. More and more people are waking up to the truth and we will win this war.

And so, au revoir from the old man in a chair.

I'll be back. But not on YouTube.

September 3rd 2020

Ending YouTube

It saddened us both enormously to end the series of videos which we started last March. In six months the channel had grown from nothing to 168,000 subscribers. But apart from taking down individual videos at a rapid rate, YouTube had also threatened to take down the whole channel if I recorded anything else which breached their bizarre and unscientific WHO rules.

I had four other scripts almost finished, and every one of them contained material about the prevention, diagnosis and treatment of covid-19. All of them would have been removed by YouTube within a day or so at most. I looked through the scripts closely and tried to rewrite them so that they would not break the platform's rules. But I couldn't.

I then realised that it is now impossible to write and record anything about covid-19 (and expect it to stay 'live' on YouTube) without suppressing the truth and avoiding the scientific evidence.

I could have recorded another video but it would have been deleted very quickly and YouTube would have taken down the remaining 80 or so videos which are, I believe, still of value since they contain a mass of valuable material which, among other things, describe the way the hoax has unfolded.

Of course, they may still choose to remove those 80 videos – though that would seem to me to be nothing more than an act of spite.

As I explained in the video – I'll be back. But not on YouTube. I haven't given up. I hope the subscribers who watched the videos on YouTube will join me wherever I end up. Meanwhile, if you haven't watched all the videos there are around 80 of them still there…for the moment.

We are putting together a book containing the scripts of all the videos broadcast in May, June, July and August – together with a foreword and an afterword unpublished elsewhere. It will, I hope, be a valuable guide to how the hoax has unfolded. We'll put a note on this website when it's available.

September 3rd 2020

Afterword

So, what happens if we don't win this war?

Well, in short, it's the end of the human race as we know it. Vaccination will become mandatory and we will all be genetically modified. Heaven knows what effect 5G radiation will have on our bodies. Cash will disappear from circulation and our money will be controlled by banks which will have the legal right to withdraw our access to it. Health care will be rudimentary and the elderly, disabled and mentally ill will all be allowed to die. There will be absolutely no freedom of the press. Very few people will have jobs. We will all be totally dependent on the State. We will be awarded points according to our social value, and those who rebel will be ostracised and denied access to food. Private property will be confiscated and we will be moved into the smart cities promoted by the United Nations.

Anyone who has studied Agenda 21 and the plans defined by the World Economic Forum knows what we are facing.

You will by now be aware that I believe we are fighting the most important war of our lives.

We are constantly researching and investigating and I will try to write more about the future, and what else we can do to protect ourselves, in a future book.

Vernon Coleman, Bilbury, September 2020

Dear Reader

If you found this book useful I would be enormously grateful if you would post a review on Amazon or your preferred online site. It would help a great deal more than I can tell. I have now started work on a book exploring the background to this massive hoax (or fraud). Details of the book will, in due course, be published on my website www.vernoncoleman.com and, I hope, on my author page on Amazon.

Thank you,

Vernon Coleman

P.S. When you finished reading this book might I suggest that you add to it your own thoughts on the greatest and most evil hoax of all time – and then put the book and your notes into a time capsule. I genuinely fear that our civilisation is currently under real threat. If we are forced to accept vaccines which result in genetic modification of the human body then the changes will be permanent and multi-generational. Future generations may like to know how life was, and the details of the war we fought for survival.

About the Author

Biography and reference articles

Vernon Coleman was educated at Queen Mary's Grammar School in Walsall, Staffs. He then spent a year as a Community Service Volunteer in Liverpool where he was the first of Alec Dickson's 'catalysts'. (Ref 1 below). He studied medicine at Birmingham Medical School and qualified as a doctor in 1970. He has worked both in hospitals and as a GP. He resigned from the health service on a matter of principle. (Ref 2 below).

Vernon Coleman has organised many campaigns concerning iatrogenesis, drug addiction and the abuse of animals and has given evidence to committees at the House of Commons and the House of Lords. For example, he gave evidence to the *House of Lords Select Committee on Animals in Scientific Procedures* (2001-2) on Tuesday 12.2.02

Dr Coleman's campaigns have often proved successful. For example, after a 15 year campaign (which started in 1973) he eventually persuaded the British Government to introduce stricter controls governing the prescribing of benzodiazepine tranquillisers. ('Dr Vernon Coleman's articles, to which I refer with approval, raised concern about these important matters,' said the Parliamentary Secretary for Health in the House of Commons in 1988.) (Ref 3 below).

Dr Coleman has worked as a columnist for numerous national newspapers including *The Sun, The Daily Star, The Sunday Express, Sunday Correspondent* and *The People*. He once wrote three columns at the same time for national papers (he wrote them under three different names, Dr Duncan Scott in *The Sunday People*, Dr James in *The Sun* and Dr Vernon Coleman in the *Daily Star*). At the same time he was also writing weekly columns for the *Evening Times* in Glasgow and for the *Sunday Scot*. His syndicated columns have appeared in over 50 regional newspapers in the United Kingdom and his columns and articles have appeared in newspapers and magazines around the world. Dr Coleman resigned from *The People* in 2003 when the editor refused to print a column criticising the Government's decision to start the Iraq War. (Ref 6 below)

He has contributed articles and stories to hundreds of other publications including *The Sunday Times, Observer, Guardian, Daily Telegraph,*

Sunday Telegraph, Daily Express, Daily Mail, Mail on Sunday, Daily Mirror, Sunday Mirror, Punch, Woman, Woman's Own, The Lady, Spectator and *British Medical Journal.* He was the founding editor of the *British Clinical Journal.* For many years he wrote a monthly newsletter called *Dr Vernon Coleman's Health Letter.* He has worked with the Open University in the UK and has lectured doctors and nurses on a variety of medical matters.

Vernon Coleman has presented numerous programmes on television and radio and was the original breakfast television doctor on TV AM. He was television's first agony uncle (on BBC1's *The Afternoon Show*) and presented three TV series based on his bestselling book *Bodypower.* In the 1980s, he helped write the algorithms for the first computerised health programmes – which sold around the world to those far-sighted individuals who had bought the world's first home computers. (Ref 4 below). His books have been published in the UK *by Arrow, Pan, Penguin, Corgi, Mandarin, Star, Piatkus, RKP, Thames and Hudson, Sidgwick and Jackson, Macmillan* and many other leading publishing houses and translated into 25 languages. English language versions sell in the USA, Australia, Canada and South Africa as well as the UK. Several of his books have appeared on both the *Sunday Times* and *Bookseller* bestseller lists.

Altogether, he has written over 100 books which have, together, sold over two million copies in the UK alone. His self-published novel, *Mrs Caldicot's Cabbage War* has been turned into an award winning film (starring Pauline Collins, John Alderton and Peter Capaldi) and the book is, like many of his other novels, available in an audio version.

Vernon Coleman has co-written five books with his wife, Donna Antoinette Coleman and has, in addition, written numerous articles (and books) under a vast variety of pennames (many of which he has now forgotten). Donna Antoinette Coleman is a talented oil painter who specialises in landscapes. Her books include, *My Quirky Cotswold Garden.* She is a Fellow of the Royal Society of Arts. Vernon and Antoinette Coleman have been married for more than 20 years.

Vernon Coleman has received numerous awards and was for some time a Professor of Holistic Medical Sciences at the Open International University based in Sri Lanka.

Reference Articles referring to Vernon Coleman
Ref 1
'Volunteer for Kirkby' – *The Guardian,* 14.5.1965

(Article re VC's work in Kirkby, Liverpool as a Community Service Volunteer in 1964-5)
Ref 2
'Bumbledom forced me to leave the NHS' – *Pulse*, 28.11.1981
(Vernon Coleman resigns as a GP after refusing to disclose confidential information on sick note forms)
Ref 3
'I'm Addicted To The Star' – *The Star, 10.3.1988*
Ref 4
'Medicine Becomes Computerised: Plug In Your Doctor.' – *The Times*, 29.3.1983
Ref 5
'Computer aided decision making in medicine' – *British Medical Journal*, 8.9.1984 and 27.10.1984
Ref 6
'Conscientious Objectors' – *Financial Times magazine*, 9.8.2003

Major interviews with Vernon Coleman include
'Doctor with the Common Touch.' – *Birmingham Post*, 9.10.1984
'Sacred Cows Beware: Vernon Coleman publishing again.' – *The Scotsman*, 6.12.1984
'Our Doctor Coleman Is Mustard' – *The Sun,* 29.6.1988
'Reading the mind between the lines.' – *BMA News Review,* November 1991
Doctors' Firsts – *BMA News Review,* 21.2.1996
'The big league of self-publishing.' – *Daily Telegraph,* 17.8.1996
'Doctoring the books' – *Independent,* 16.3.1999
'Sick Practices' – *Ode Magazine,* July/August 2003
'You have been warned, Mr Blair.' – *Spectator,* 6.3.2004 and 20.3.2004
'Food for thought with a real live Maverick.' – *Western Daily Press,* 5.9.2006
'The doctor will see you now' – *Independent,* 14.5.2008

There is a more comprehensive list of reference articles on www.vernoncoleman.com

Vernon Coleman: What the papers say

'Vernon Coleman writes brilliant books.' – *The Good Book Guide*
'No thinking person can ignore him.' – *The Ecologist*
'The calmest voice of reason.' – *The Observer*
'A godsend.' – *Daily Telegraph*
'Superstar.' – *Independent on Sunday*
'Brilliant!' – *The People*
'Compulsive reading.' – *The Guardian*
'His message is important.' – *The Economist*
'He's the Lone Ranger, Robin Hood and the Equalizer rolled into one.'
– *Glasgow Evening Times*
'The man is a national treasure.' – *What Doctors Don't Tell You*
'His advice is optimistic and enthusiastic.' – *British Medical Journal*
'Revered guru of medicine.' – *Nursing Times*
'Gentle, kind and caring' – *Western Daily Press*
'His trademark is that he doesn't mince words. Far funnier than the
usual tone of soupy piety you get from his colleagues.' – *The Guardian*
'Dr Coleman is one of our most enlightened, trenchant and sensitive
dispensers of medical advice.' – *The Observer*
'I would much rather spend an evening in his company than be trapped
for five minutes in a radio commentary box with Mr Geoffrey
Boycott.' – Peter Tinniswood, *Punch*
'Hard hitting...inimitably forthright.' – *Hull Daily Mail*
'Refreshingly forthright.' – *Liverpool Daily Post*
'Outspoken and alert.' – *Sunday Express*
'Dr Coleman made me think again.' – *BBC World Service*
'Marvellously succinct, refreshingly sensible.' – *The Spectator*
'Probably one of the most brilliant men alive today.' – *Irish Times*
'King of the media docs.' – *The Independent*
'Britain's leading medical author.' – *The Star*
'Britain's leading health care campaigner.' – *The Sun*
'Perhaps the best known health writer for the general public in the
world today.' – *The Therapist*
'The patient's champion.' – *Birmingham Post*
'A persuasive writer whose arguments, based on research and
experience, are sound.' – *Nursing Standard*
'The doctor who dares to speak his mind.' – *Oxford Mail*
'He writes lucidly and wittily.' – *Good Housekeeping*

Books by Vernon Coleman include

Medical

The Medicine Men
Paper Doctors
Everything You Want To Know About Ageing
The Home Pharmacy
Aspirin or Ambulance
Face Values
Stress and Your Stomach
A Guide to Child Health
Guilt
The Good Medicine Guide
An A to Z of Women's Problems
Bodypower
Bodysense
Taking Care of Your Skin
Life without Tranquillisers
High Blood Pressure
Diabetes
Arthritis
Eczema and Dermatitis
The Story of Medicine
Natural Pain Control
Mindpower
Addicts and Addictions
Dr Vernon Coleman's Guide to Alternative Medicine
Stress Management Techniques
Overcoming Stress
The Health Scandal
The 20 Minute Health Check
Sex for Everyone
Mind over Body
Eat Green Lose Weight
Why Doctors Do More Harm Than Good
The Drugs Myth
Complete Guide to Sex
How to Conquer Backache

How to Conquer Pain
Betrayal of Trust
Know Your Drugs
Food for Thought
The Traditional Home Doctor
Relief from IBS
The Parent's Handbook
Men in Bras, Panties and Dresses
Power over Cancer
How to Conquer Arthritis
How to Stop Your Doctor Killing You
Superbody
Stomach Problems – Relief at Last
How to Overcome Guilt
How to Live Longer
Coleman's Laws
Millions of Alzheimer Patients Have Been Misdiagnosed
Climbing Trees at 112
Is Your Health Written in the Stars?
The Kick-Ass A–Z for over 60s
Briefs Encounter
The Benzos Story
Dementia Myth

Psychology/Sociology

Stress Control
How to Overcome Toxic Stress
Know Yourself (1988)
Stress and Relaxation
People Watching
Spiritpower
Toxic Stress
I Hope Your Penis Shrivels Up
Oral Sex: Bad Taste and Hard To Swallow
Other People's Problems
The 100 Sexiest, Craziest, Most Outrageous Agony Column Questions
(and Answers) Of All Time
How to Relax and Overcome Stress
Too Sexy To Print

Psychiatry
Are You Living With a Psychopath?

Politics and General

England Our England
Rogue Nation
Confronting the Global Bully
Saving England
Why Everything Is Going To Get Worse Before It Gets Better
The Truth They Won't Tell You...About The EU
Living In a Fascist Country
How to Protect & Preserve Your Freedom, Identity & Privacy
Oil Apocalypse
Gordon is a Moron
The OFPIS File
What Happens Next?
Bloodless Revolution
2020
Stuffed
The Shocking History of the EU
Coming Apocalypse
Covid-19: The Greatest Hoax in History

Diaries

Diary of a Disgruntled Man
Just another Bloody Year
Bugger off and Leave Me Alone
Return of the Disgruntled Man
Life on the Edge
The Game's Afoot
Tickety Tonk

Animals

Why Animal Experiments Must Stop
Fighting For Animals
Alice and Other Friends
Animal Rights – Human Wrongs

Animal Experiments – Simple Truths

General Non Fiction

How to Publish Your Own Book
How to Make Money While Watching TV
Strange but True
Daily Inspirations
Why Is Public Hair Curly
People Push Bottles Up Peaceniks
Secrets of Paris
Moneypower
101 Things I Have Learned
100 Greatest Englishmen and Englishwomen
Cheese Rolling, Shin Kicking and Ugly Tattoos
One Thing after Another

Novels (General)

Mrs Caldicot's Cabbage War
Mrs Caldicot's Knickerbocker Glory
Mrs Caldicot's Oyster Parade
Mrs Caldicot's Turkish Delight
Deadline
Second Chance
Tunnel
Mr Henry Mulligan
The Truth Kills
Revolt
My Secret Years with Elvis
Balancing the Books
Doctor in Paris
Stories with a Twist in the Tale (short stories)
Dr Bullock's Annals

The Young Country Doctor Series

Bilbury Chronicles
Bilbury Grange
Bilbury Revels

Bilbury Pie (short stories)
Bilbury Country
Bilbury Village
Bilbury Pudding (short stories)
Bilbury Relish
Bilbury Mixture
Bilbury Delights
Bilbury Joys
Bilbury Tales
Bilbury Days
Bilbury Memories

Novels (Sport)

Thomas Winsden's Cricketing Almanack
Diary of a Cricket Lover
The Village Cricket Tour
The Man Who Inherited a Golf Course
Around the Wicket
Too Many Clubs and Not Enough Balls

Cat books

Alice's Diary
Alice's Adventures
We Love Cats
Cats Own Annual
The Secret Lives of Cats
Cat Basket
The Cataholics' Handbook
Cat Fables
Cat Tales
Catoons from Catland

As Edward Vernon

Practice Makes Perfect
Practise What You Preach
Getting Into Practice
Aphrodisiacs – An Owner's Manual

The Complete Guide to Life

Written with Donna Antoinette Coleman

How to Conquer Health Problems between Ages 50 & 120
Health Secrets Doctors Share With Their Families
Animal Miscellany
England's Glory
Wisdom of Animals

Lightning Source UK Ltd.
Milton Keynes UK
UKHW012021250722
406337UK00001B/20